D0858347

Gender and Its Effects on Psychopathology

Gender and Its Effects on Psychopathology

Edited by
Ellen Frank, Ph.D.

American Psychopathological Association

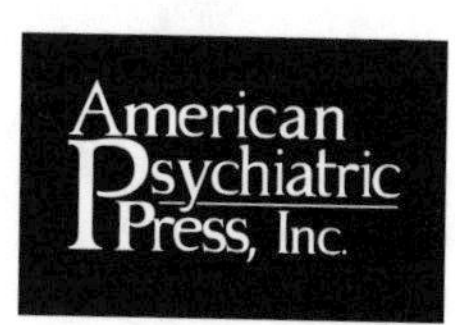

Washington, DC
London, England

Note: The authors have worked to ensure that all information in this book concerning drug dosages, schedules, and routes of administration is accurate as of the time of publication and consistent with standards set by the U.S. Food and Drug Administration and the general medical community. As medical research and practice advance, however, therapeutic standards may change. For this reason and because human and mechanical errors sometimes occur, we recommend that readers follow the advice of a physician who is directly involved in their care or the care of a member of their family.

Books published by the American Psychiatric Press, Inc., represent the views and opinions of the individual authors and do not necessarily represent the policies and opinions of the Press or the American Psychiatric Association.

Manufactured in the United States of America on acid-free paper
03 02 01 00 4 3 2 1
First Edition

American Psychiatric Press, Inc.
1400 K Street, N.W., Washington, DC 20005
www.appi.org

Library of Congress Cataloging-in-Publication Data
Gender and its effects on psychopathology / edited by Ellen Frank.
p. cm. — (American Psychopathological Association series)
Includes bibliographical references and index.
ISBN 0-88048-798-4
1. Mental illness—Sex factors. 2. Sex differences (Psychology). 3. Psychology, Pathological. I. Frank, Ellen, (1944- . II. Series.
[DNLM: 1. Mental Disorders. 2. Sex Factors. WM 140 G325 1999]
RC455.4.S45G465 1999
616.89—dc21
DNLM/DLC 98-33988
for Library of Congress CIP

British Library Cataloguing in Publication Data
A CIP record is available from the British Library.

The ideas for the meeting of
The American Psychopathological Association
on which this volume is based
were developed while the editor was a
John D. and Catherine T. MacArthur Fellow at the
Center for Advanced Study in the Behavioral Sciences,
Palo Alto, California.

Contents

Contributors

Naomi Breslau, Ph.D.
Director of Research for Psychiatry, Departments of Psychiatry and of Biostatistics and Research Epidemiology, Henry Ford Health Systems, Detroit, Michigan; Professor of Psychiatry, Case Western Reserve University School of Medicine, Cleveland, Ohio

Remi Cadoret, M.D.
Professor of Psychiatry Emeritus, Psychiatry Research, University of Iowa, Iowa City, Iowa

Howard D. Chilcoat, Sc.D.
Research Scientist, Department of Psychiatry, Henry Ford Health Systems, Detroit, Michigan

Ulrike Feske, Ph.D.
Assistant Professor of Psychiatry, Western Psychiatric Institute and Clinic, Pittsburgh, Pennsylvania

Ellen Frank, Ph.D.
Professor of Psychiatry and Psychology, Department of Psychiatry, University of Pittsburgh, Western Psychiatric Institute and Clinic, Pittsburgh, Pennsylvania

Catherine Greeno, Ph.D.
Assistant Professor of Social Work and Psychiatry, University of Pittsburgh, Pittsburgh, Pennsylvania

Heinz Häfner, M.D., Ph.D., Dres.h.c.
Professor Emeritus of Psychiatry, University of Heidelberg; and Head of Schizophrenia Research Unit, Central Institute of Mental Health, Mannheim, Germany

Denise Kandel, Ph.D.
Professor of Public Health in Psychiatry, Department of Psychiatry, Columbia University, New York, New York; Chief, Department on the Epidemiology of Substance Abuse, New York State Psychiatric Institute, New York, New York

Ronald C. Kessler, Ph.D.
Professor, Department of Health Care Policy, Harvard Medical School, Boston, Massachusetts

Susan G. Kornstein, M.D.
Associate Professor, Medical College of Virginia, Richmond, Virginia

Mary Jeanne Kreek, M.D.
Professor and Head, Laboratory of the Biology of Addictive Diseases, The Rockefeller University; Senior Physician, The Rockefeller University Hospital, New York, New York; Principal Investigator and Scientific Director, NIH–NIDA Center, New York, New York

Steven O. Moldin, Ph.D.
Chief, Genetics Research Branch, National Institute of Mental Health, National Institutes of Health, Bethesda, Maryland

Barbara Parry, M.D.
Professor of Psychiatry, University of California at San Diego Medical Center, La Jolla, California

Edward L. Peterson, Ph.D.
Biostatician, Department of Biostatistics and Research Epidemiology, Henry Ford Health Systems, Detroit, Michigan

Kristin Riggins-Caspers, Ph.D.
Postdoctoral Fellow in Psychiatric Genetics, Department of Psychiatry, University of Iowa, Iowa City, Iowa

Sarah Rosenfield, Ph.D.
Associate Professor of Sociology, Rutgers University, New Brunswick, New Jersey

Lonni R. Schultz, Ph.D.
Biostatician, Department of Biostatistics and Research Epidemiology, Henry Ford Health Systems, Detroit, Michigan

M. Katherine Shear, M.D.
Professor of Psychiatry, Western Psychiatric Institute and Clinic, Pittsburgh, Pennsylvania

Andrew E. Skodol, M.D.
Professor of Clinical Psychiatry, Columbia University College of Physicians and Surgeons, New York, New York; Director, Department of Personality Studies, New York State Psychiatric Institute, New York, New York

Mark A. Stewart, M.D.[†]
Ida Beam Professor of Child Psychiatry, Department of Psychiatry, University of Iowa, Iowa City, Iowa

Michael E. Thase, M.D.
Professor of Psychiatry and Chief, Division of Adult Academic Psychiatry, University of Pittsburgh School of Medicine, Western Psychiatric Institute and Clinic, Pittsburgh, Pennsylvania

Edward P. Troughton, B.A.
Senior Research Assistant, Department of Psychiatry, University of Oklahoma, Tulsa, Oklahoma

William R. Yates, M.D.
Professor and Chair, Department of Psychiatry, University of Iowa, Iowa City, Iowa

Kimberly A. Yonkers, M.D.
Associate Professor, Department of Psychiatry, Yale University School of Medicine, New Haven, Connecticut

---

[†]Deceased.

Elizabeth Young, M.D.
Professor of Psychiatry, Department of Psychiatry and Mental Health Research Institute, University of Michigan at Ann Arbor

Introduction

Ellen Frank, Ph.D.

One might well ask why the psychopathologist should study gender differences. The answer I would offer is that gender influences the ways in which our brains develop—the neuroendocrine "soup," as Jerome Kagan is fond of calling it, in which our brains and virtually all of our life experiences reside. In other words, gender influences all of the things we believe might be related to susceptibility to psychiatric disorders, the timing of their onset, their course, and their responsivity to treatment.

From the very beginnings of embryonic development, gender has profound influences. In females, estrogen receptors in the brain are involved in neuronal growth and neuroplasticity. In males, androgen receptors are related to stimulation of brain activity and to aggressivity. Thus, endocrine receptors in both the male and the female brain affect cognition, mood, and behavior. We should also note that disorders of the endocrine system are frequently associated with psychological symptoms and that the expression of these symptoms is different in men and women.

At the opposite end of the continuum from this organismic one, we note that in every society, from the most primitive to the most elaborated, gender determines social role—or at least what is perceived as appropriate social role—probably in rough concert with hormonally driven predispositions to behave in particular ways. Having had my own daughters before Gloria Steinem published the first issue of *Ms.* magazine, I still chuckle when I think of how surprised those feminists who came late to motherhood were when confronted by the enormous force of their urge to care for their offspring.

Finally, gender and gender role appear to be key determinants of the kinds of psychosocial experiences we have, particularly the kinds of experiences that many psychopathologists regard as related to psychiatric symptoms and syndromes. Men are rarely raped. Except for a tiny fraction of cultures in the late 20th century, women have rarely been exposed to combat. More normative life experiences are also frequently gendered—from having primary responsibility for the care of children or elderly relatives to taking out the garbage or repairing the roof.

It should not surprise us, then, that men and women have highly replicable differences in risk for many forms of psychopathology—replicable both across time and across cultures. What is more surprising is that they have equivalent risks for other forms of psychopathology and that they appear often to have similar responses to both somatic and psychosocial treatments. Yet on the rare occasions when investigators have looked at what predicts good versus poor response to treatment for men and women separately, they found that different variables correlate with good response in men and women. With prediction of treatment response being one of the most elusive goals in psychiatric research, what further rationale do we need for examining gender differences?

As the various chapters in this volume illustrate, gender is often key to a clear understanding of the initial risk for a disorder, the course of illness once it begins, and the response to treatment. This volume is arranged in four sections. The first addresses possible etiological mechanisms for gender differences, both biological and psychosocial. The second section is devoted to mood and anxiety disorders and includes chapters that address the differential epidemiology of these disorders, possible etiologies for these differences, and treatment response. The third section focuses on schizophrenia and contains both a general overview and a chapter that specifically addresses gender differences in first onset. In the fourth and final section we turn to substance abuse and dependence, examining gender differences in epidemiology, gene–environment interaction, and treatment response. Each of these chapters makes clear that gender is a critical player in psychopathology research and challenges us to never again ignore its possible influence as we examine our own data or try to understand the data of other investigators.

SECTION *I*

Etiological Mechanisms

CHAPTER 1

Hormonal Basis of Mood Disorders in Women

Barbara L. Parry, M.D.

Compared with men, women have a greater lifetime risk for depression. They predominate with respect to unipolar depression (Weissman and Klerman 1977), the depressive subtype of bipolar illness (Angst 1978), and cyclic forms of affective illness such as rapid-cycling manic-depressive illness and seasonal affective disorder (Dunner et al. 1977; Rosenthal et al. 1984). In addition, events associated with the reproductive cycle are capable of inducing affective changes in predisposed individuals. Examples include depression associated with oral contraceptives (Parry and Rush 1979), with the luteal phase of the menstrual cycle (Dalton 1964), with the postpartum period (Brockington and Kumar 1982), and with menopause (Angst 1978; Winokur 1973). The fluctuation of gonadal steroids during specific phases of the reproductive cycle may bear some relationship to women's particular vulnerability to affective changes. The reproductive hormones could exert their effects on mood directly or indirectly through their influence on neurotransmitter, neuroendocrine, or circadian systems (Wehr 1984), all of which have been implicated in the pathogenesis of affective illness.

In this chapter I review the types of depression that women are prone to develop and the specific clinical phenomenology of reproductive-related depressions. Implications for better understanding the hormonal basis of mood disorders in women are also assessed.

Rapid-Cycling Affective Illness

Several clinical models can be used to examine the role of reproductive hormones on affective illness in women. Because most patients with rapid-cycling bipolar illness are women, reviewing the factors that predispose women to the development of rapid cycles in mood may shed light on how reproductive hormones may influence the course of affective illness.

Rapid-cycling manic-depressive illness, defined as four or more affective episodes per year (Dunner et al. 1977), occurs predominantly in women. Kraepelin (1921), in describing patients with regular daily fluctuations of periodic excitement, noted that "in contrast to other forms, in which there was a preponderance of men, two-thirds of these patients were women, in whom the periodicity of sexual life obviously favors this kind of development" (p. 131). Dunner et al. (1977) at the Lithium Clinic of New York State Psychiatric Institute found that in a sample of bipolar patients, 70% of the rapid cyclers and 46% of the non–rapid cyclers were women. In Koukopoulos et al.'s (1980) sample of rapid cyclers, 70% were women. In contrast, in the non–rapid cyclers, women accounted for 47% of the sample. Cowdry et al. (1983) reported that women composed 83% of rapid-cycling bipolar patients and 53% of non–rapid cyclers. A review by Wehr et al. (1988) indicated that 92% of patients with rapid-cycling and 64% of those with non–rapid-cycling affective disorder were women.

Women's Risk Factors for Rapid-Cycling Affective Illness

In addition to being a woman, two other factors appear to be associated with the rapid-cycling form of bipolar illness: 1) treatment with tricyclic and other antidepressants and 2) hypothyroidism. Compared with men, women show an increased incidence of both drug-induced rapid cycling and hypothyroidism (Wehr et al. 1988).

Drug-induced rapid cycling. Among patients whose rapid cycles of mania and depression have been induced by tricyclic antidepressants, women predominate. Wehr and Goodwin (1979) found that of five female bipolar patients in whom rapid cycles developed, all but one had been maintained on antidepressant drugs. Rapid cycles did not develop in either of two male bipolar patients who were maintained on tricyclics. Wehr and Goodwin speculated that the female reproductive neuroendocrine axis, a generator of physiological rapid cycles, may have been instrumental in the expression of drug-induced cycling. Reproductive hormonal disturbances and treatments may have been predisposing factors in their patients' illnesses; all but one (four of five) of the women in their sample had irregular menses, amenorrhea, a history of estrogen or progesterone treatment, or an onset of the illness in the postpartum period.

In a longitudinal study by Koukopoulos et al. (1980), 70% of the patients who developed rapid cycling in response to treatment with tricyclics were women. As summarized by this author, female gender, middle age, and menopause, along with antidepressant drugs, contributed to the establishment of rapid cyclicity. Of the patients in his longitudinal study whose course of illness changed to rapid cycling, 87% were women, and in one-third (25 of 77) of these women, the change in course coincided with menopause. Koukopoulos also noted that the patients with depression and hypomania (i.e., bipolar II disorder) were those most prone to rapid cycling. In this regard, Angst (1978) had previously noted a predominance of women among bipolar II patients. Retrospective data of Squillace et al. (1984) are consistent with those of Angst.

Wehr and Goodwin (1987) concluded that women have a higher risk of drug-induced mania and drug-induced rapid cycling than do men. In contrast, Kupfer et al. (1988) reported that women with recurrent depression were *not* more likely than men to switch into hypomania, and Coryell et al. (1992) deemphasized the rapid-cycling–inducing effects of antidepressant drugs.

Hypothyroidism-associated rapid cycling. In addition to female gender and treatment with antidepressant drugs, thyroid impairment may be associated with rapid cycling (Cowdry et al. 1983; Wehr et al. 1988), and women are more prone to thyroid disease than are men (Ingbar and Woeber 1981). Studies that document gender differences in lithium-induced hypothyroidism (see below) indicate that almost all lithium-treated patients who develop hypothyroidism are female. In studies by Villeneuve et al. (1974), Transbol et al. (1978), and Cho et al. (1979), 90%–100% of bipolar patients with lithium-induced hypothyroidism were women. In a review by Fyro et al. (1973) of 22 reported cases of hypothyroidism that developed during lithium treatment, all but one were in women.

As shown by Cowdry et al. (1983), abnormalities of the thyroid axis, some of which may become apparent only during treatment with $LiCO_3$, are associated with rapid cycling. Cho et al. (1979), examining an affective disorder clinic population, found that post–lithium thyroid medication use was significantly higher among rapid-cycling women (32.2%) than among non–rapid-cycling women (2.1%). Furthermore, thyroid dysfunction was primarily limited to women. Of those patients taking thyroid medication in addition to lithium, 92% were women. Seventy-one percent of women with hypothyroidism had rapid cycling.

In a study by Cowdry et al. (1983), overt hypothyroidism was found in 12 (51%) of 24 rapid-cycling patients and in none of the non–rapid-cycling patients. Elevated thyroid-stimulating hormone (TSH) levels were present (and higher) in 92% of the rapid-cycling group compared with 32% of the non–rapid-cycling group. In this sample, women represented 83% of the rapid-cycling group and 53% of the non–rapid cyclers. In a study by Wehr et al. (1988), 47% of women with rapid-cycling and 39% of women with non–rapid-cycling bipolar illness developed thyroid disease. Of those patients with thyroid disease, the thyroid disease emerged after the onset of affective illness in 90% of the patients, and in the majority of cases it emerged during lithium treatment.

Transbol et al. (1978) evaluated the prevalence of hypothyroidism in lithium-treated manic-depressive outpatients and found elevated TSH levels in 20 (23%) of patients, all of whom were females and all but one of whom were over 40 years of age. None of the men had elevated TSH levels. Rapid-cycling and non–rapid-cycling subgroups were not reported separately in this study.

The relationship of thyroid function to mood state is also illustrated in individual case reports. For one woman, normalization of thyroid function induced mania (Josephson and MacKenzie 1979). Herz (1964) reported on a woman who developed periodic 1- to 2-week depressions that occurred every 1–2 months after she underwent thyroidectomy. In addition, there are reports of induction of rapid cycles of mood in the postpartum period (Herzog and Deter 1974; Protheroe 1969).

Reproductive status may affect the presentation of thyroid disease. It is common for goiter to appear during puberty, pregnancy, and menopause (Ingbar and Woeber 1981). Women are particularly prone to develop hypothyroidism during the postpartum period (Amino et al. 1982). Postpartum hypothyroidism may represent an autoimmune phenomenon, given that the extent of postpartum hypothyroidism correlates with traces of microsomal antibodies early in pregnancy (Jansson et al. 1984). Women with isolated gonadotropin deficiency have blunted basal TSH and blunted TSH responses to thyroid-releasing hormone (TRH) (Spitz et al. 1983). Administration of estrogen restores the TSH response to the level seen in control subjects, and cessation of estrogen treatment reduces the amount of releasable TSH. In hypogonadal men, the TSH response to TRH is similar to that in control men but increases with estrogen treatment. Oral contraceptives increase the TSH response to TRH (Ramey et al. 1975). Thus, estrogens seem to be required to maintain, and may enhance, the normal TSH response to TRH in women.

In summary, cyclic affective disorder in the form of rapid-cycling bipolar illness is more prevalent in women than in men. Treatment with antidepressant drugs often precipitates rapid mood cycling, particularly in women with bipolar II disorder. Thyroid impairment, more prevalent in women, also is associated with the rapid-cycling form of the disorder. Very little information is available on the course of rapid-cycling bipolar illness in men.

Psychopharmacological Treatment of Rapid-Cycling Affective Illness

Thyroid. Thyroid hormone has been used to treat both cyclic and noncyclic forms of affective disorders. Hypermetabolic thyroid treatment was first used by Gjessing in the 1930s to treat periodic catatonia and rapid-cycling affective disorder (see Gjessing 1976). Stancer and Persad (1982) reported treatment of intractable rapid-cycling manic-depressive illness with levothyroxine. Five of the seven women who developed rapid-cycling bipolar disorder during either the postpartum or the involutional period responded to hypermetabolic doses of thyroid hormone. Thyroid hormone had differential effects in males and females; the treatment was unsuccessful in two men and one adolescent girl.

In an uncontrolled and controversial study, women with rapid mood cycling linked to the menstrual cycle were reported to have a high incidence of thyroid disease, and treatment with a thyroid supplement was found to improve their cyclic mood symptoms (Brayshaw and Brayshaw 1986).

Prange et al. (1969) reported that triiodothyronine (T_3) enhanced the antidepressant effect of imipramine in women but not in men. Men responded to initial doses of imipramine more quickly than did women. However, women whose imipramine regimens were supplemented with thyroid hormone responded as rapidly as men treated with imipramine alone. Goodwin et al. (1982) subsequently demonstrated that among tricyclic nonresponders, men benefited as often as women from the addition of T_3.

The mechanisms for thyroid enhancement of responses to antidepressants may be as Whybrow and Prange (1981) suggest, relating to the capacity of thyroid hormone to alter the ratio of α- to β-adrenergic receptors and their sensitivity to noradrenergic neurotransmitters. Depressed women appear to be uniquely responsive to thyroid hormone. Women also are uniquely vulnerable to thyroid impairment.

Estrogen. Women are sensitive to other hormonal treatments in addition to thyroid hormone; estrogen has also been used as a treatment in refractory depression. Klaiber et al. (1979) used 5–25 mg of oral conjugated estrogen in cyclic doses to treat depressive symptoms in pre- and postmenopausal women. With estrogen, compared with placebo, there was a significant drop in Hamilton Rating Scale for Depression (HAMD; Hamilton 1960) scores that correlated with a reduction in previously elevated monoamine oxidase (MAO) levels. Prange (1972) administered 25 mg and 50 mg of estradiol to depressed patients already treated with imipramine, with inconsistent results. Whereas the higher estrogen dose was toxic, the lower dose was associated with a reduction in HAMD scores and improved sleep. In another study, estrogen was also reported to improve the sleep of menopausal women (Thomson and Oswald 1977).

The mechanism by which estrogen exerts its possible antidepressant effect is unknown, but work by Kendall et al. (1981) showed that estrogen is needed for reduction of serotonin receptor binding during imipramine treatment. Ovariectomy blocked the effect of imipramine on serotonin receptors, and estrogen treatment reinstituted it.

Estrogen may also induce rapid cycling or at least predispose women to tricyclic-induced rapid cycling, as reported by Oppenheim (1984). Interestingly, we observed one male rapid-cycling patient who had low testosterone secondary to mumps orchitis. Progesterone, on the other hand, may suppress rapid cycles of mood (Hatotani and Nomara 1983).

Thus, reproductive hormones may alter the course of affective illness via their interaction with thyroid hormone and antidepressant drugs.

Seasonal Affective Disorder

Like rapid-cycling affective disorder, seasonal affective disorder is a cyclic mood disorder that occurs predominantly (80%) in women. Thus, it also may serve as a model to understand the contribution of reproductive hormones to affective illness in women.

Patients with seasonal affective disorder who have recurrent winter depressions have symptoms of major affective disorder with characteristic "atypical" features (such as hyperphagia, hypersomnia, and lethargy), which begin to develop each year in association with shortening of the day length. A majority of these patients respond to high-intensity (2,500 lux) light treatments, which artificially extend the daily photoperiod (Rosenthal et al. 1984). Initially, bright light was thought to exert its antidepressant effect by suppressing melatonin, a hormone that is centrally involved in seasonal reproductive cycles in animals. This hypothesis has since been brought into question, and a multitude of other hypotheses have been proposed (Rosenthal et al. 1985; Wehr et al. 1986).

A large proportion (70%) of women with seasonal affective disorder also have mood changes in association with the menstrual cycle (Rosenthal et al. 1984). Some women with seasonal affective disorder report improvement in their premenstrual symptoms with light therapy. We identified a woman with a family history of bipolar illness who developed severe premenstrual depression with suicidal ideation only during the fall and winter and experienced relief from premenstrual symptoms during the spring and summer (Parry et al. 1987). We found that light was an effective treatment for this patient with seasonal premenstrual syndrome and that its therapeutic effect could be blocked by the simultaneous administration of melatonin. Light also increased this patient's TSH. Propranolol and atenolol, beta-blockers that inhibit the synthesis of melatonin, had a therapeutic effect similar to that of light. Light therapy may also benefit women with nonseasonal premenstrual syndrome (Parry et al. 1989, 1993).

In a study of 12 patients with seasonal affective disorder who experienced summer depression and winter hypomania, Wehr et al. (1987a) reported that 8 of the patients were women and suggested that temperature may influence clinical state in these patients.

It appears that certain women with a genetic vulnerability for mood disorders may be at risk for developing other cyclic affective disorders such as seasonal premenstrual disorders.

Relevance of Rapid Cycling and Seasonal Affective Disorder to Postpartum and Premenstrual Affective Illness

Rapid-cycling bipolar illness and seasonal affective disorder are examples of cyclic forms of mood disorders that occur predominantly in women. The interaction of reproductive hormones, particularly with thyroid hormones in rapid-cycling affective disorder and with melatonin in seasonal affective disorder, may provide clues about the pathogenesis of reproductive-related depressions. The increased incidence of hypothyroidism occurring postpartum (Amino et al. 1982) or in winter may in part account for rapid-cycling mood disorders and depression, respectively, that occurs at these times. Another cyclic mood disorder that can be viewed as a form of rapid cycling is recurrent premenstrual depression, in which thyroid and melatonin (Parry et al. 1990, 1991) disturbances have also been implicated. Melatonin may play a role in the pathogenesis of seasonal premenstrual syndrome (Parry et al. 1987) and of nonseasonal forms of the disorder as well (Parry et al. 1990). Studies have demonstrated that, compared with control subjects, patients with premenstrual depression have circadian disturbances of melatonin secretion and may respond to light treatment (Parry et al. 1989, 1990, 1993). Similar studies of melatonin in postpartum mood disturbances are currently under way.

Postpartum Mood Disorders

A woman's relative risk for developing a major psychiatric illness or psychosis requiring hospitalization is highest during the postpartum period and lowest during pregnancy (Kendell et al. 1987). This finding, as Paffenbarger (reported in Brockington and Kumar 1982, p. 30) has noted, "leads us to ask whether the low attack rate during pregnancy is the result of some protective physiologic, psychological, or social process and whether the sudden increase following delivery is due to release of that defense." First episodes of manic-depressive illness in women often have their onset in the postpartum period (Garvey et al. 1983; Reich and Winokur 1970). Reich and Winokur (1970) observed that not only is there an increased risk for female manic-depressive patients to develop mania or depression in the postpartum period, but having a postpartum affective episode appears to predispose a woman to subsequent postpartum affective episodes (an increased risk of 50%). Furthermore, whereas a woman's initial risk for a postpartum psychosis is 1 in 500 (Kendell et al. 1987), once a woman has had a postpartum psychosis, her risk for psychosis following a subsequent pregnancy is 1 in 3 (Kendell et al. 1987). Thus, in postpartum depression and psychosis, a previous episode predisposes a woman to the development of future episodes with subsequent pregnancies.

Premenstrual Depression

Affective changes associated with the menstrual cycle provide another clinical model for studying the relationship of gonadal hormones to affective illness. Historically referred to as premenstrual syndrome (PMS), this condition has been more rigorously defined as late luteal phase dysphoric disorder (LLPDD) in Appendix A (Proposed Diagnostic Categories Needing Further Study) of DSM-III-R (American Psychiatric Association 1987) and as premenstrual dysphoric disorder (PMDD) in DSM-IV (American Psychiatric Association 1994) under mood disorders. Because of its familiarity, the term *PMS* is used here. In PMS, the mood and behavioral changes are recurrent and predictable and thus can be studied both prospectively and longitudinally.

Similar to winter in seasonal affective disorder and the postpartum period in affective illness, the late luteal phase of the menstrual cycle is a vulnerable time for the development of depressive mood changes. Studies indicate that PMS may be related to major depressive disorders

(Halbreich and Endicott 1985). In support of this hypothesis, patients with PMS and affective disorders, in contrast to patients with anxiety disorders (Roy-Byrne et al. 1986), respond to sleep deprivation: total and late-night partial sleep deprivation temporarily alleviates symptoms in a majority of patients with major affective disorders (Sack et al. 1988a). We found that 80% of patients with premenstrual depression responded to a night of total sleep deprivation and that late-night partial sleep deprivation (in the second half of the night) was more effective than early-night partial sleep deprivation (in the first half of the night) (Parry and Wehr 1987). In a follow-up study, PMS subjects responded equally well to early- and late-night partial sleep deprivations, but only after a night of recovery sleep (Parry et al. 1995). Sleep deprivation lowers prolactin (Parker et al. 1973; Sassin et al. 1973) and increases TSH (Rossman et al. 1981; Sack et al. 1988b), although in at least one study (Kasper et al. 1988) these hormonal changes did not correlate with clinical response. That total or partial sleep deprivation might be an effective intervention in patients with PMS would be consistent with current theories that implicate prolactin and thyroid disturbances (Brayshaw and Brayshaw 1986; Carroll and Steiner 1978) in the pathogenesis of PMS. Sleep reduction may also serve as a final common pathway in the genesis of mania in postpartum psychiatric illness (Wehr et al. 1987b). Thus, the interaction of sleep with a sensitive circadian phase of thyroid or prolactin secretion may be a common predisposing factor for the development of affective illness, premenstrual depression, and possibly postpartum mood disorders.

Sleep and Light Therapies for Cyclic Mood Disorders

Nonpharmacological experimental treatments based on chronobiological models include sleep deprivation and light therapy. One night of total sleep deprivation during the symptomatic premenstrual phase of the menstrual cycle was found to alleviate PMS symptoms (Parry and Wehr 1987). Follow-up studies suggested that 1 night of only *partial* sleep deprivation (sleep 9:00 P.M.–1:00 A.M. or 3:00 A.M.–7:00 A.M.) also might be beneficial (Parry et al. 1995). Light therapy involves sitting in front of a light box 2 hours a day for 1 week. Whereas early studies (Parry et al.

1989) suggested superior efficacy for evening (7:00–9:00 P.M.) bright light (>2,500 lux, or five times brighter than room light), subsequent trials (Parry et al. 1993) have shown equal efficacy for bright evening, bright morning (6:30–8:30 A.M.), and dim (10 lux) red evening light administered in the premenstrual phase to PMS patients.

Although these treatments may show promise, further trials are needed before they can be recommended for general clinical usage. These findings are interesting in view of recent evidence suggesting a seasonal variation in PMS, with approximately 70% of PMS sufferers experiencing fewer symptoms during the summer, when the photoperiod is longer.

Interrelationships Among Reproductive-Related Depressions

A depressive episode occurring in association with the reproductive cycle may predispose a woman to future depression. A previous history of psychiatric illness or of affective changes during pregnancy may predispose a woman to oral contraceptive–induced depressions (Parry and Rush 1979). Postpartum depression may predict menopausal depressions (Protheroe 1969). Severe premenstrual depression may predispose a woman to postpartum depression (Brockington and Kumar 1982); in addition, premenstrual depression, like affective illness, may have its onset or be exacerbated after a postpartum depression. Alternatively, a major depressive episode? major depressive disorder may be exacerbated or precipitated during the premenstrual period (Halbreich and Endicott 1985). There are anecdotal reports of bipolar patients whose premenstrual and seasonal mood cycles persisted or became more prominent after lithium treatment. Price and Dimarzio (1986) reported that patients with rapid-cycling disorders are more likely to have more severe forms of PMS, although Wehr et al. (1988) found no convincing relationship between manic-depressive cycles and menstrual cycles in their patients with rapid-cycling disorders.

Thus, the cyclicity of affective disorders in the form of rapid-cycling bipolar illness or seasonal affective disorder may be compounded by periodic affective changes occurring in association with the premenstruum, with pregnancy and the postpartum period, and with altered reproductive hormonal milieus induced by oral contraceptives or gonadal hormone treatments.

Mechanisms of Reproductive-Related Depressions

Bearing in mind the kindling model of depression (Post et al. 1984), one wonders whether such periodic reproductive-related depressions may sensitize women to future affective episodes (Zis and Goodwin 1979). Most longitudinal studies to date have not specifically focused on gender-related differences in the course of the illness. Gender differences in depression begin to appear after the onset of puberty in adolescence (Kandel and Davies 1982; Weissman and Klerman 1977). There is a marked increase in major depression in females beginning at approximately 16 years of age. In contrast, males exhibit a gradual increase in depression across all ages, with considerably lower absolute rates in comparison with females. Furthermore, the onset of major depression is earlier (i.e., 12–13 years of age) in both male and female offspring of depressed probands than in offspring of healthy probands (Weissman et al. 1987), and the rates of affective disorders appear to be increasing over time (Gershon et al. 1987; Hagnell et al. 1982; Weissman et al. 1984, 1987).

How cyclic depressions related to reproductive events may affect other forms of cyclic mood disorders is unknown, but a relationship does seem to exist. Research in animals may provide models for and possibly shed light on the mechanisms involved. For example, the predisposition of women with thyroid impairment to cyclic forms of depression has a parallel in an animal model: Richter et al. (1959) found that partial thyroidectomy produced abnormal cycles of motor activity in female but not male rodents. As occurs in humans with rapid-cycling mood disorders, treatment with thyroid extract abolished the abnormal behavioral cycles, which returned after cessation of treatment. Richter and colleagues hypothesized that the abnormal periodic cycles of activity were produced by the effect of thyroid deficiency on homeostatic mechanisms controlling luteotropin (prolactin) release (possibly related to the effect of TRH on prolactin). He used daily subcutaneous injections of prolactin to induce similar cycles. Such cycles were also produced by inducing pseudopregnancy. This condition stimulates pituitary secretion of prolactin, which acts on the ovary to produce persistent corpora lutea and to secrete progesterone. Ovariectomy abolished running-wheel activity; estrogen administration increased it. Longer abnormal activity cycles were produced by giving the rats anhydrohydroxy progesterone. As occurs in affective illness, the abnormal activity cycles become shorter with time. Also of relevance here is our own clinical work demonstrating higher baseline prolactin levels (Parry et al. 1994) and increased prolactin response to TRH in women with rapid cycling in mood related to the menstrual cycle (i.e., PMS) (Parry et al. 1991).

Reproductive hormones modulate hormonal and neurotransmitter mechanisms and the regulation of biological rhythms, each of which has been the focus of hypotheses about the pathophysiology of affective disorders. Estrogen and progesterone can alter the biosynthesis, release, uptake, degradation, and receptor density of norepinephrine, dopamine, serotonin, and acetylcholine (McEwen and Parsons 1982). In addition, the gonadal steroids modulate other hormonal mechanisms (thyroid, cortisol, prolactin, and opiates) that also affect neurotransmitter systems.

Gonadal hormones affect circadian systems, which also have been implicated in the pathophysiology of affective disorders. Estrogen shortens the duration of the approximate 24-hour circadian activity in ovariectomized hamsters and rats (Albers et al. 1981; Morin et al. 1977). In intact hamsters, the onset of activity occurs earlier on days of the estrous cycle when endogenous titers of estradiol are high. In intact rats, progesterone delays the onset of activity by antagonizing the effect of estrogen (Axelson et al. 1981). Clinically, progesterone is associated with an exacerbation of depressive symptoms (Sherwin 1991). Estrogen, in addition to shortening the free-running period (i.e., the duration of the approximate 24-hour cycle of rest and activity without a structured light–dark cycle under constant conditions) and altering the phase relationship of the activity rhythm to the light–dark cycle, increases the total amount of activity and *decreases the variability* of day-to-day onsets of activity.

These findings parallel those of Wever (1984), who reported that the mean free-running period of the sleep–wake cycle is significantly shorter in women than in men by an average of 28 minutes. The wake episode is shorter (by 1 hour, 49 minutes) and the sleep episode longer (by 1 hour, 21 minutes) in women compared with men. Thus, the fraction of sleep (i.e., the part of sleep over the diurnal sleep–wake cycle) is longer for women than for men. The circadian temperature rhythm is similar in both genders. According to Wirz-Justice et al. (1984), women sleep longer than men at all times of the year. Under free-running conditions (i.e., in temporal isolation when the subject is free of external time cues), women, unlike men, tend to become internally desynchronized, particularly in the summer, the period in which the sleep–wake cycle becomes shorter.

Estrogen also serves to enhance coupling between different circadian pacemaker components (Albers et al. 1981). Ovariectomized female rodents develop rhythm desynchronies; estrogen replacement restores the normal coupling relationship between these disparate rhythms. This factor may be involved in some of the therapeutic effects of estrogen.

Summary

Thus, the decline in ovarian hormones common to the premenstrual, postpartum, and menopausal periods, and these hormones' inherent cyclicity, may destabilize or sensitize neurotransmitter, neuroendocrine, and biological clock mechanisms and thereby set the stage for the development of cyclic affective disorders.

Although the cyclicity of the endocrine milieu may increase the vulnerability to episodic depressions in women, it may protect against the development of many chronic illnesses that are more characteristic in men. Investigation of hormonal contributions to affective illness in women and examination of the way in which the course of these illnesses is affected by reproductive events of the life cycle may increase our understanding of affective illness and potentially provide alternative treatment strategies.

References

Albers EH, Gerall AA, Axelson JF: Effect of reproductive state on circadian periodicity in the rat. Physiol Behav 26:21–25, 1981

American Psychiatric Association: Diagnostic and Statistical Manual of Mental Disorders, 3rd Edition, Revised. Washington, DC, American Psychiatric Association, 1987

American Psychiatric Association: Diagnostic and Statistical Manual of Mental Disorders, 4th Edition. Washington, DC, American Psychiatric Association, 1994

Amino N, More H, Iwatani Y, et al: High prevalence of transient postpartum thyrotoxicosis and hypothyroidism. N Engl J Med 306:849–852, 1982

Angst J: The course of affective disorders, II: typology of bipolar manic-depressive illness. Arch Psychiatr Nervenkr 226:65–73, 1978

Axelson JF, Gerall AA, Albers E: Effect of progesterone on the estrous activity cycle of the rat. Physiol Behav 26:631–635, 1981

Brayshaw ND, Brayshaw DD: Thyroid hypofunction in premenstrual syndrome. N Engl J Med 315:1486–1487, 1986

Brockington IF, Kumar R: Motherhood and Mental Illness. London, Academic Press, 1982

Carroll BJ, Steiner M: The psychobiology of premenstrual dysphoria: the role of prolactin. Psychoneuroendocrinology 3:171–180, 1978

Cho JT, Bone S, Dunner DL, et al: The effects of lithium treatment on thyroid function in patients with primary affective disorder. Am J Psychiatry 136: 115–116, 1979

Coryell W, Endicott J, Keller M: Rapidly cycling affective disorder: demographics, diagnosis, family history, and course. Arch Gen Psychiatry 49:126–131, 1992

Cowdry RW, Wehr TA, Zis AP, et al: Thyroid abnormalities associated with rapid cycling bipolar illness. Arch Gen Psychiatry 40:414–420, 1983

Dalton K: The Premenstrual Syndrome. London, Heineman Medical, 1964

Dunner DL, Patrick V, Fieve R: Rapid cycling manic depressive patients. Compr Psychiatry 18:561–566, 1977

Fyro B, Peterson U, Sedvail G: Time course for the effect of lithium on thyroid function in men and women. Acta Psychiatr Scand 49:230–236, 1973

Garvey MJ, Tuason VB, Lumry AE, et al: Occurrence of depression in the postpartum state. J Affect Disord 5:97–101, 1983

Gershon ES, Hamovit JH, Guroff JJ, et al: Birth-cohort changes in manic and depressive disorders in relatives of bipolar and schizoaffective patients. Arch Gen Psychiatry 44:314–319, 1987

Gjessing RR: Contribution, in Somatology of Periodic Catatonia. Edited by Gjessing LR, Jenner FA. Oxford, Pergamon, 1976, pp 370–380

Goodwin FK, Prange AJ, Post RM, et al: Potentiation of antidepressant effects by l-triiodothyronine in tricyclic nonresponders. Am J Psychiatry 139:34–38, 1982

Hagnell O, Lanke J, Rorsman B, et al: Are we entering an age of melancholy? Depressive illness in a prospective epidemiological study over 25 years: the Lundby Study, Sweden. Psychol Med 12:279–289, 1982

Halbreich U, Endicott J: Relationship of dysphoric premenstrual changes to depressive disorders. Acta Psychiatr Scand 71:331–338, 1985

Hamilton M: A rating scale for depression. J Neurol Neurosurg Psychiatry 23: 56–62, 1960

Hatotani N, Nomara J: Neurobiology of Periodic Psychoses. New York, Igaku-Shoin Toyko, 1983

Herz M: On rhythmic phenomena in thyroidectomized patients. Acta Psychiatr Scand 40 (suppl 180):449–456, 1964

Herzog A, Deter T: Postpartum psychoses. Diseases of the Nervous System 35: 556–559, 1974

Ingbar SH, Woeber KA: The thyroid gland, in Textbook of Endocrinology. Edited by Williams RH. Philadelphia, PA, WB Saunders, 1981, pp 95–232

Jansson R, Bernander S, Karlesson A, et al: Autoimmune thyroid depression in the postpartum period. J Clin Endocrinol Metab 58:681–687, 1984

Josephson AM, MacKenzie TB: Appearance of manic psychosis following rapid normalization of thyroid status. Am J Psychiatry 136:846–847, 1979

Kandel DB, Davies M: Epidemiology of depressive mood in adolescents. Arch Gen Psychiatry 39:1205–1212, 1982

Kasper S, Sack DA, Wehr TA, et al: Nocturnal TSH and prolactin secretion during sleep deprivation and prediction of antidepressant response in patients with major depression. Biol Psychiatry 24:631–641, 1988

Kendall DA, Stancel AM, Einna SJ: Imipramine: effect of ovarian steroids on modification in serotonin receptor binding. Science 211:1183–1185, 1981

Kendell RE, Chalmers JC, Platz C: Epidemiology of puerperal psychoses. Br J Psychiatry 150:662–673, 1987

Klaiber EL, Broverman DM, Vogel W, et al: Estrogen therapy for severe persistent depressions in women. Arch Gen Psychiatry 36:550–554, 1979

Koukopoulos A, Reginaldi P, Laddomada GF, et al: Course of the manic depressive cycle and changes caused by treatments. Pharmacopsychiatry 13:156–167, 1980

Kraepelin E: Manic Depressive Insanity and Paranoia. Edinburgh, Scotland, E & S Livingstone, 1921

Kupfer DJ, Carpenter LL, Frank E: Possible role of antidepressants in precipitating mania and hypomania in recurrent depression. Am J Psychiatry 145: 804–808, 1988

McEwen BS, Parsons B: General steroid action on the brain: neurochemistry and neuropharmacology. Annu Rev Pharmacol Toxicol 22:555–598, 1982

Morin LP, Fitzgerald KM, Zucker I: Estradiol shortens the period of hamster circadian rhythms. Science 196:305–307, 1977

Oppenheim G: A case of rapid mood cycling with estrogen: implications for therapy. J Clin Psychiatry 45:34–35, 1984

Parker DC, Rossman LG, Vanderloom EF: Sleep related, nyctohemeral and briefly episodic variation on human plasma prolactin concentrations. J Clin Endocrinol Metab 36:1119–1124, 1973

Parry BL, Rush AJ: Oral contraceptives and depressive symptomatology: biologic mechanisms. Compr Psychiatry 20:347–358, 1979

Parry BL, Wehr TA: Therapeutic effect of sleep deprivation in patients with premenstrual syndrome. Am J Psychiatry 144:808–810, 1987

Parry BL, Rosenthal NE, Tamarkin L, et al: Treatment of a patient with seasonal premenstrual syndrome. Am J Psychiatry 144:762–766, 1987

Parry BL, Berga SL, Mostofi N, et al: Morning vs. evening bright light treatment of late luteal phase dysphoric disorder. Am J Psychiatry 146:1215–1217, 1989

Parry BL, Berga SL, Kripke DF, et al: Altered waveform of plasma nocturnal melatonin secretion in premenstrual depression. Arch Gen Psychiatry 47: 1139–1146, 1990

Parry BL, Gerner RH, Wilkins JN, et al: CSF and endocrine studies of premenstrual syndrome. Neuropsychopharmacology 5:127–137, 1991

Parry BL, Mahan AM, Mostofi N, et al: Light therapy of late luteal phase dysphoric disorder: an extended study. Am J Psychiatry 150:1417–1419, 1993

Parry BL, Hauger R, Lin E, et al: Neuroendocrine effects of light therapy in late luteal phase dysphoric disorder. Biol Psychiatry 36:356–364, 1994

Parry BL, Cover H, Mostofi N, et al: Early versus late partial sleep deprivation in patients with premenstrual dysphoric disorder and normal comparison subjects. Am J Psychiatry 152:404–412, 1995

Post RM, Rubinow DR, Ballenger JC: Conditioning, sensitization and kindling: Implications for the course of affective illness, in Neurobiology of Mood Disorders. Edited by Post RM, Ballenger JC. Baltimore, MD, Williams & Wilkins, 1984, pp 432–466

Prange AJ: Estrogen may well affect response to antidepressant. JAMA 219: 143–144, 1972

Prange AJ, Wilson IC, Rabon AM, et al: Enhancement of imipramine antidepressant activity by thyroid hormone. Am J Psychiatry 126:457–469, 1969

Price WA, Dimarzio L: Premenstrual tension syndrome in rapid-cycling bipolar affective disorder. J Clin Psychiatry 47:415–417, 1986

Protheroe C: Purperal psychoses: a long-term study. Br J Psychiatry 115:9–30, 1969

Ramey JN, Burrow GN, Polackwich RJ, et al: The effect of oral contraceptive steroids on the response of thyroid stimulating hormone to thyrotropin releasing hormone. J Clin Endocrinol Metab 40:712–714, 1975

Reich T, Winokur G: Postpartum psychoses in patients with manic depressive disorder. J Nerv Ment Dis 151:60–68, 1970

Richter CP, Jones GS, Biswanger L: Periodic phenomena and the thyroid. Arch Neurol Psychiatry 81:117–139, 1959

Rosenthal NE, Jacobsen FM, Sack DA, et al: Atenolol in seasonal affective disorder: a test of the melatonin hypothesis. Am J Psychiatry 45:52–56, 1975

Rosenthal NE, Sack DA, Gillin JC, et al: Seasonal affective disorder: a description of the syndrome and preliminary findings with light therapy. Arch Gen Psychiatry 41:72–80, 1984

Rosenthal NE, Sack DA, James SP, et al: Seasonal affective disorder and phototherapy. Ann N Y Acad Sci 453:260–269, 1985

Rossman LG, Parker DC, Pekary AE, et al: Effect of an imposed 21-hour sleep wake cycle upon the rhythmicity of human plasma thyrotropin, in Human Pituitary Hormones: Circadian and Episodic Variations. Edited by van Cauter E, Capinochi G. Boston, MA, Martinus Ninjhoff, 1981, pp 96–117

Roy-Byrne PP, Uhde TW, Post RM: Effects of one night's sleep deprivation on mood and behavior in panic disorder: patients with panic disorder compared with depressed patients and normal controls. Arch Gen Psychiatry 43:895–899, 1986

Sack DA, Duncan W, Rosenthal NE, et al: The timing and duration of sleep in partial sleep deprivation therapy of depression. Acta Psychiatr Scand 77:219–224, 1988a

Sack DA, James SP, Rosenthal NE, et al: Deficient nocturnal surge of TSH secretion during sleep and sleep deprivation in rapid cycling bipolar illness. Psychiatry Res 23:179–191, 1988b

Sassin JF, Frantz AG, Kapen S, et al: The nocturnal rise of human prolactin is dependent on sleep. J Clin Endocrinol Metab 37:436–440, 1973

Sherwin BB: The impact of different doses of estrogen and progestin on mood and sexual behavior in postmenopausal women. J Clin Endocrinol Metab 72:336–343, 1991

Spitz IM, Zylber-Haran A, Trestian S: The thyrotropin (TSH) profile in isolated gonadotropin deficiency: a model to evaluate the effect of sex steroids on TSH secretion. J Clin Endocrinol Metab 57:425–430, 1983

Squillace K, Post RM, Savard R, et al: Life charting of recurrent affective illness, in Neurobiology of Mood Disorders. Edited by Post RM, Ballenger JC. Baltimore, MD, Williams & Wilkins, 1984, pp 38–59

Stancer HC, Persad E: Treatment of intractable rapid cycling manic depressive disorder with levothyroxine. Arch Gen Psychiatry 39:311–312, 1982

Thomson J, Oswald I: Effect of oestrogen on the sleep, mood, and anxiety of menopausal women. BMJ 2(6098):1317–1319, 1977

Transbol I, Christiansen C, Baastrup PC: Endocrine effects of lithium, I: hypothyroidism, its prevalence in long-term treated patients. Acta Endocrinol (Copenh) 87:759–767, 1978

Villeneuve A, Gautier J, Jus A, et al: The effect of lithium on thyroid in man. Int J Clin Pharmacol 9:75–80, 1974

Wehr TA: Biological rhythms and manic depressive illness, in Neurobiology of Mood Disorders. Edited by Post RM, Ballenger JC. Baltimore, MD, Williams & Wilkins, 1984, pp 190–206

Wehr TA, Goodwin FK: Rapid cycling in manic depressives induced by tricyclic antidepressants. Arch Gen Psychiatry 36:555–559, 1979

Wehr TA, Goodwin FK: Can antidepressants cause mania and worsen the cause of affective illness? Am J Psychiatry 144:1403–1411, 1987

Wehr TA, Sack DA, Jacobsen FM, et al: Phototherapy of seasonal affective disorder: time of day and suppression of melatonin are not critical for antidepressant effects. Arch Gen Psychiatry 43:870–875, 1986

Wehr TA, Sack DA, Rosenthal NE: Seasonal affective disorder with summer depression and winter hypomania. Am J Psychiatry 144:1602–1603, 1987a

Wehr TA, Sack DA, Rosenthal NE: Sleep reduction as a final common pathway in the genesis of mania. Am J Psychiatry 144:201–204, 1987b

Wehr TA, Sack DA, Rosenthal NE: Rapid cycling affective disorder: contributing factors and treatment responses of 51 patients. Am J Psychiatry 145: 179–184, 1988

Weissman MM, Klerman GL: Sex differences and the epidemiology of depression. Arch Gen Psychiatry 34:98–111, 1977

Weissman MM, Leaf PJ, Holzer CE III, et al: The epidemiology of depression: an update on sex differences in rates. J Affect Disord 7:179–188, 1984

Weissman MM, Gammon D, John K, et al: Children of depressed parents: increased psychopathology and early onset of major depression. Arch Gen Psychiatry 44:847–853, 1987

Wever RA: Properties of human sleep–wake cycles: parameters of internally synchronized free running rhythms. Sleep 7:27–51, 1984

Whybrow PC, Prange AJ: A hypothesis of thyroid-catecholamine receptor interaction. Arch Gen Psychiatry 38:106–113, 1981

Winokur G: Depression in the menopause. Am J Psychiatry 130:92–93, 1973

Wirz-Justice A, Wever RA, Aschoff J: Seasonality in freerunning rhythms in man. Naturwissenschaften 71:316–319, 1984

Zis AP, Goodwin FK: Major affective disorder as a recurrent illness: a critical review. Arch Gen Psychiatry 36:835–839, 1979

CHAPTER 2

Gender and Dimensions of the Self

Implications for Internalizing and Externalizing Behavior

Sarah Rosenfield, Ph.D.

Differences by gender are among the most consistent patterns in the epidemiology of mental illness. Gender differences encompass two of the major types of psychopathology. The first is internalizing disorders, including anxiety and depression, which are more prevalent in females than in males. The second is externalizing disorders, including antisocial behavior and substance abuse, in which males predominate. Internalizing and externalizing disorders both originate in childhood or early adolescence. On the social side, these findings suggest that socialization processes and dimensions of the self may have a central role in the formation of these disorders. Toward this end, in this chapter I search for socialized aspects of the self that differentiate the genders, that arise (or are accentuated) in adolescence, and that have implications for both antisocial behavior and depressive disorders. Given these clues, I suggest that sociocultural conceptions of masculinity and femininity—which are activated and applied most strongly in adolescence—differentially shape dimensions of the self that, in turn, contribute to the development of externalizing and internalizing disorders. Guided by this perspective, I examine evidence for the relationships among socialized conceptions of gender, dimensions of the self, and psychopathology. Finally, I review some of the literature and present findings from ongoing research.

Socialization

There are several perspectives on socialization that apply to the social acquisition of gender. Many of these—such as social learning theory and classic cognitive developmental theory—have been criticized for tending to conceptualize children as passive recipients of messages from the adult world. In this chapter I draw on symbolic interactionist perspectives. This approach holds that our ability to take ourselves as an object is a central foundation for the development of the self (Mead 1934). Using shared meanings in symbols, we imagine the responses of others to our own words and gestures. Through this act of imagination, we can assume others' perspectives toward ourselves as well as toward the world. By taking the role of the other and identifying with that position, we incorporate the outlooks of others. This process begins in childhood, with forms of play. As children pretend and play games, they infer who they are from the perspectives of all the other parts and roles. As they develop, they interpret and internalize the attitudes toward themselves of larger and larger numbers of persons and groups, culminating in a "generalized other" within the self that represents the perspective of the larger (dominant) culture.

In this process, we are both active agents—the "I" in Meadian terms—and the recipients of culture—the "me" for Mead. Individuals use the attitudes of others as tools to construct their own viewpoints. Socialization throughout life is characterized by choice and active construction within limits.

Even considering the element of choice, the process of taking the role of the other tends to reproduce the existing social structure (Thoits 1996). Desiring positive reflected appraisals, people tend to modify their thoughts, feelings, and behaviors to mirror their image of others' expectations about them. Such expectations are largely shaped by social categories. Because gender constitutes a fundamental social category, conceptions of masculinity and femininity are a central part of the attitudes and expectations we internalize and re-create in taking the role of the other.

Conceptions of Masculinity and Femininity

In our culture, conceptions of masculinity and femininity embody social practices that divide work, power, and social relations by gender. Ideals of masculinity have been associated with the public sphere of production and primary economic responsibilities and with the consonant characteristics of assertiveness, competitiveness, independence, and dominance. Ideologies of femininity associate women with the private sphere of domesticity and consumption, carrying primary responsibilities for caretaking and "emotion work" and possessing related characteristics of nurturing, sensitivity, and emotional expressiveness.

This division of public and private spheres has implications for inequality. The skills and rewards of the public sphere—and thus its power—are more transferable, since the value of money remains the same across exchanges. In contrast, the skills and rewards of the private sphere—and thus its power—are nontransferable, focusing on the characteristics of a particular spouse and particular children. Given their greater ties to the public sphere, men hold more generalizable forms of power than do women.

Interpersonal dynamics and the negotiations of dominance between individual males and females are carried out within this context of inequality (Foucault 1978). Such inequalities and demands shape social relationships, including the boundaries drawn between the self and others and the balance of giving and receiving support.

Along with these differences, there appears to be a more fundamental opposition between male and female. The dichotomies made in Western culture between body and mind and between emotion and reason are infused with value. Paralleling the public–private split, masculinity has come to be associated with reason and the mind, and femininity with nature and emotion. Given the cultural premium placed on mind and on reason, that which is associated with males and masculinity has become by definition the norm—what Tavris (1995) calls the "universal male." If the reference point is male, female is defined as other. The differences ascribed to males and females are not mere differences. They are charged with meaning. That which is associated with femininity is weak, needs apology, is wanting too much. This fundamental dichotomy and the standard of the universal male colors the interpretation of everything associated with maleness and femaleness.

The above description outlines some of our dominant conceptions of gender. As Connell (1995) shows, there are multiple masculinities and femininities that contend with these conceptions in some form, if only by rebelling against them. For example, conceptions of masculinity and femininity differ to some degree by social class, a point I do not have room to get into here.

Basic Assumptions and Internalizing and Externalizing Disorders

How do these conceptions of gender affect the formation of the self? It seems evident that the power one holds or will inherit conveys messages about one's value in and control over the world. The nature and valuation of day-to-day labor and the balance of support similarly provide information on mastery and worth. These differences also carry messages about the nature of social relationships—for example, the degree of connection to or separation from others and the importance of one's own interests and desires relative to others'.

I thus argue that our conceptions of masculinity and femininity give rise to certain views about reality. Dimensions like those above constitute some of the assumptions that we use to make sense of the world and that govern our actions and reactions. Using the capacity for judging themselves and others as objects, we derive basic assumptions about ourselves, the world, and relationships from such cultural conceptions and the social practices they embody or reflect. This formulation has similarities with gender schema theories and cognitive theories such as cognitive–experiential self-theory, insofar as these focus on organized ways of seeing and interpreting the world that come from social experiences.

Thus, individuals take an active part in constructing their assumptions about the world. They carry these as hypotheses into each situation to be altered or reinforced, but with a slant toward seeing things as they have done in the past—another of the prisms of gender. Thus, basic assumptions are not completely automatic or unchangeable. Furthermore, assumptions apply and are applied more in some situations than in others, depending on the demands of the situation and the relevance of the assumption. In sum, basic assumptions are formed from an interaction between messages from the outside—taken in through identification with others—and our own internal interpretations.

Focusing on the dimensions described above, individuals' judgments about their own worth and value obviously constitute one of the basic assumptions about the self. Perceptions of personal control form a similarly fundamental assumption about the world. The boundaries we draw between self and others—that is, the degree of individuation from or connection to other people we assume—represent a basic assumption about the relationship of ourselves to others (Chodorow 1978). Finally, the salience we confer on others' versus our own needs, desires, and interests also constitutes a basic relational assumption. Individuals rank the importance of their own interests, feelings, desires, and thoughts relative to others, which varies from the extreme of self-salience on one end, in which the self is given complete primacy, to the extreme of other-salience, in which others are given total priority.

I argue that such basic assumptions are related to psychopathology by blocking some reactions and facilitating others. In the present case, these assumptions facilitate either internalizing or externalizing disorders and protect individuals from the opposing extreme. On the facilitation side, for example, assumptions of mastery, self-salience, and self-containment more easily allow externalizing behavior. Elevating the importance of one's own interests to the exclusion of others' interests and lacking a sense of identification with others allows one to act against them. Others are viewed as obstacles to obtaining what one wants. In addition, assumptions of self-sufficiency and emotional detachment encourage minimization of expression of emotional pain, discomfort with most emotions, and thus the tendency toward actions that push away or anesthetize emotional pain or discomfort. Drugs are one means of blocking or numbing painful feelings, thus suppressing emotions. Such tendencies are reinforced by basing self-esteem on the ascendancy of reason and using abstract rules as the measure of success. On the protective side, acting according to one's own interests and a sense of self-containment—in addition to possessing a positive sense of self and personal control—interferes with the perceptions of helplessness and hopelessness and with the tendencies toward self-attack that characterize internalizing disorders. Extreme assumptions of entitlement make it unimaginable to hurt oneself.

Turning to the other side, a strong identification with others' interests interferes with the possibility for action on one's own behalf, generating feelings of helplessness and tendencies toward self-blame. To the extent that others' interests come first, individuals deny the desires of the self. In contrast, having doubts about one's ability to have an impact on the world interferes with engaging in risky, antisocial actions. Identifying with others' interests as similar and, at the least, equal to one's own interferes with harming another person. Under these conditions, an act against another is experienced as an act against oneself.

In sum, I have argued that we internalize conceptions of masculinity and femininity by taking the attitudes of others toward ourselves. We use these culturally based conceptions and the practices they embody in formulating our basic assumptions about the self, the world, and relationships with others. These, in turn, shape tendencies toward and protections against specific forms of psychopathology. Thus, the specific ways we construct gender have implications for gender differences in the prevalence of externalizing and internalizing disorders.

Gender Differences in Socialization Experiences

In examining evidence for these connections, we would expect to find differences in socialization experiences between males and females that are accentuated in adolescence. Therefore, what are the differences in socialization for boys and girls? Much of the research focuses on the immediate family and whether parents treat sons and daughters differently. There is some evidence for this. For example, sons receive more physical stimulation than daughters and are given more freedom and independence (Best and Williams 1995). Greater instrumental control or supervision over their daughters' activities discourages risk taking and independence, in preparation for a primary emphasis on domesticity. Parents exercise less control over sons, thus encouraging a risk-taking, entrepreneurial spirit that fits into the public sphere of production (Hagan et al. 1987).

One clear difference that emerged from a large meta-analysis was that parents encourage gender stereotypes in play activities and household chores. In relation to emotions, parents showed greater warmth toward and more discouragement of aggression in daughters (Lytton and Romney 1991). These differences are greater in observational studies and experimental studies than in self-reports, which means that parents think they treat sons and daughters more similarly than they actually do.

Teachers also do socialization work. Research finds that males are treated as more important and more competent by teachers in nursery schools, elementary schools, and college classrooms (Geis 1993). Teachers also respond more often to boys' aggression, a reaction that serves to maintain aggressive interchanges, whereas they ignore girls' aggression, a response that tends to terminate such interactions (Fagot and Hagen 1985).

Differential socialization also occurs in play. Insofar as play is direct preparation for adulthood, gender-typed play is the antecedent for gender-typed social and achievement behaviors (Tittle 1986). Playing dolls calls for the practice and development of nurturing skills—as opposed to the demands of sports such as football and basketball, which call for the practice and development of competitive and physical skills. When adults offer playthings to children, their choice of objects strongly depends on the child's gender: dolls go to girls and footballs to boys.

There is reason to believe that differential socialization practices by gender and the basic assumptions derived from them are activated or accentuated in adolescence. The physical changes in girls and boys at adolescence identify them to others as women and men. These changes invoke images of the perfect woman and man (Brown and Gilligan 1992). Adolescents evaluate themselves against the cultural ideals of masculinity and femininity, as mirrored in the reactions of others. Parents also begin to apply more stereotyped ideas of womanhood and manhood to their daughters and sons (Nolen-Hoeksema 1990). Purposive gender-role socialization in general intensifies in adolescence (Gove and Herb 1974; Chodorow 1978). Thus, the differences in socialization by gender appear to achieve their full expression in adolescence, a finding that may underlie the gender differences in the prevalence of internalizing and externalizing disorders that emerge at this point.

Gender Differences in Basic Assumptions

Brown and Gilligan's (1992) work traces the effects of this intensified gender training on girls and shows its consequences for girls' assumptions about themselves and their social relationships. Brown and Gilligan's interviews over time with girls in the first through tenth grades document dramatic changes. The youngest girls, 7- and 8-year-olds, are outspoken about how they think and feel: they face conflict with friends and family directly and negotiate differences of opinion with little hesitation about clashes in feelings or ideas. Girls eventually move to a stance of not speaking openly about their feelings and to not knowing what their thoughts and feelings are. By adolescence, they become dependent on others to define their wishes and ideas. It becomes more important to preserve connections than to hold onto one's own feelings and beliefs.

Other more structured research shows gender differences in basic assumptions about the self, the world, and social relationships. Females exhibit lower mastery and greater learned helplessness than males (Pearlin et al. 1981).

In terms of relational assumptions, females perceive more interpersonal dependency and emotional reliance on others than do males. Females also report a stronger identification with the feelings of others, or empathy. Although no direct measures of self–other salience are available, we have some evidence for differences, in that men have a better memory for information encoded with respect to the self, and women have a better memory for information encoded with reference to others. Research on life events also shows that women are more likely than men to see the well-being of their family members as important sources of concern, and that stressful events that happen to others are more distressing to women than to men.

Evidence that these differences are socially based comes from cross-cultural research. Boys and girls are more similar in aggression and nurturance when both are assigned to care for younger siblings and when both perform housework (Edwards and Whiting 1974; Whiting and Edwards 1973, 1988; Whiting and Whiting 1975). This reminds us that what is at issue here is not the inherent *capacity* for traits or behaviors but rather the differences as they are developed by social practices.

Basic Assumptions and Psychopathology

There is some evidence that these kinds of basic assumptions are related to internalizing and externalizing disorders. Low mastery, low self-esteem, and high interpersonal dependence are each linked to elevations in depressive symptoms. A greater willingness to take risks is associated with delinquency, in acts against both people and property. Males' predominance in antisocial behavior is in part explained by the differences in risk taking and risk aversion between males and females.

Furthermore, there is some evidence that relational assumptions are linked to internalizing and externalizing disorders. In a large-scale study of adolescents, an extremely high degree of identification with others' feelings was associated with depressive symptoms. Conversely, an extremely low degree of identification with others was connected with antisocial behavior (Rosenfield et al. 1994). These differences in emotional identification help explain girls' higher levels of depressive symptomatology and, to a lesser extent, boys' higher levels of antisocial behavior.

A Report From Ongoing Research

The underlying claim here is that changes in socialization by gender at adolescence are reflected in changes in the assumptions girls and boys hold about themselves, the world, and social relations. These changes, in turn, are linked to internalizing and externalizing symptoms and disorders. In a collaborative study with Helene White, our group analyzed data from the Rutgers Health and Human Development Project (Pandina et al. 1984), a prospective longitudinal study that followed adolescents from age 12 to age 18 years. Subjects were recruited through a random-digit-dial telephone survey conducted from 1979 to 1981 in 16 of New Jersey's 21 counties. The resulting sample was evenly divided by age into three groups (ages 12, 15, and 18 years), each divided evenly by gender. Subjects were interviewed every 3 years for four waves. A total of 1,380 subjects were interviewed in the first wave, with a completion rate of 87% across all waves.

Findings from these data illustrate some of the issues discussed here (all findings reviewed below are summarized from Rosenfield 1998). I report here on analyses of the youngest cohort, followed at 12, 15, and 18 years of age. This cohort contained a total of 430 subjects.

We first looked at socialization by gender and at whether differences arise or are accentuated in adolescence. The subjects in this study were asked a number of questions about what adults expect from a boy or girl of their age. For example, subjects were asked how much adults expect independence, self-confidence, and superiority—from "not at all" to "a great deal." They were also asked about how much adults expect competitiveness, understanding others, and being helpful. These questions provide an indication of the "generalized other," in Mead's (1934) terms. Also, that the expectations are from the subjects' own reports captures the active role of each person in interpreting the messages of others.

As an example of what subjects said at different ages, I review our findings on how much young people thought that adults expect independence. At 12 years of age, girls and boys were very similar in how much independence was expected. Both boys and girls thought it was encouraged a fair amount by adults—3.5 on a 4.0 scale. The gender difference was not statistically significant. By age 15 years, however, boys and girls were beginning to have different ideas about how important independence was, and the difference between them had become statistically significant. By age 18, boys thought of independence as a strong expectation for them—scoring on average nearly at the highest level—whereas girls had changed very little from their assessment at age 12. Thus, there was clearly a change in ideas about how much independence was expected for a person like themselves. Beginning at age 15 years, boys and girls differed in the importance they assigned to independence, with girls assigning it less value than boys. We found similar results for perceived expectations about being superior to others and being confident.

These data also contain information on some of the basic assumptions postulated as important. For example, to examine self–other salience, researchers in the Rutgers study used the abasement scale, a scale in the Personality Research Form (Jackson 1974) that measures other-salience to the extreme. This scale asks subjects how closely their own attitudes are described by statements such as "I apologize when someone bumps into me"; "When people try to make me feel important, I feel uncomfortable"; and "Several people have taken advantage of me, but I try to take it like a good sport." We found large changes in abasement between 12 and 15 years of age. At age 18, these questions were not asked. At age 12, there were no gender differences in how other-salient children were. But by the time they reached age 15 years, boys' scores on this kind of relational assumption had plummeted and girls' scores had sharply increased. The differences at age 15 were highly significant. Results on other types of basic assumptions such as identification with others and self-esteem showed similar patterns of change.

Do these changes in basic assumptions from ages 12 to 15 and 18 years correspond to the changes that occur in internalizing and externalizing symptomatology? We used data on depressive symptoms and alcohol use problems as examples of internalizing and externalizing symptoms, respectively. Results with the depression subscale of the Johns Hopkins Symptom Checklist (SCL-90; Derogatis et al. 1974) showed that there were no gender differences in the level of depressive symptoms when boys and girls were 12 years old. But at age 15 this changed, and in a surprising way. The gender difference increased, but only because boys had decreased in their levels of depressive symptoms.

Levels of alcohol problems were measured with the Rutgers Alcohol Problems Index, a 23-item self-administered screening tool for assessing problem drinking. This instrument asks about the frequency of experiencing negative consequences, such as physical effects and interpersonal problems, as a result of drinking or while drinking within the preceding 3 years. We found that boys and girls do not differ in problems related to alcohol when they are 12 or 15 years of age. Between the ages of 15 and 18 years, however, problems become more frequent for boys than for girls.

Thus, in these data, we found that gender differences in internalizing and externalizing symptoms develop in adolescence and that boys and girls do not differ in these symptoms before that time. But do the differences that emerge in adolescence in socialization, basic assumptions, and masculinity and femininity contribute to the changes in these symptoms? Our data indicate that they do. The increase in expectations of independence, self-confidence, and superiority, the large jump in self-esteem, and the decline in extreme levels of other-salience for males help explain why they have fewer depressive symptoms over time. When we controlled for any one of these factors, the gender difference in depressive symptoms was reduced to nonsignificance.

I theorized earlier in this chapter that the attitudes imparted during socialization and the basic assumptions derived from this process are embodied in our conceptions of masculinity and femininity. The data set discussed above included questions from the Personal Attributes Questionnaire (Spence and Helmreich 1978), which asks respondents to indicate how close they feel they are to opposite extremes of gender-linked characteristics. For example, respondents are asked to indicate where they fall on a 5-point scale between contradictory characteristics such as "not at all aggressive" versus "very aggressive." Also included in the same general format are questions asking respondents how independent they think they are, how emotional, how submissive versus dominant, how self-confident, how competitive, and so forth. At 12 years of age, girls and boys both scored fairly high on masculine traits such as independence, competitiveness, and dominance. By age 15, boys' scores on masculinity had risen and girls' scores had declined. On the other hand, although both boys and girls increased in "feminine" characteristics such as nurturance, empathy, and devotion to others as they got older, girls endorsed these characteristics to a much greater degree than did boys.

Examining conceptions of gender as the distal cause, we found that the degree of masculinity contributes to gender differences in depression. Controlling for masculinity reduced these differences to nonsignificance. On the other hand, the changes in gender differences in femininity accounted for the increase in differences in alcohol problems over time. When gender differences in femininity were controlled (as if men and women were equal in "feminine" characteristics), gender differences in alcohol problems were reduced to nonsignificance.

Because we examined factors overlapping in time, the causal direction of these relationships was not clear. To investigate whether these factors are also predictors across time, we analyzed the full sample of 1,380 subjects at the second wave, when they were 15, 18, and 21 years old. We examined the relationship of basic assumptions and masculinity and femininity at the first wave to internalizing and externalizing symptoms at the second wave. Looking at internalizing symptoms, we found that masculinity and high self-esteem similarly protected individuals from depressive symptoms. Femininity—and, in particular, nurturance—reduced the occurrence of alcohol problems. This evidence indicates that the causal direction goes from assumptions to symptoms.

Conclusion

In conclusion, these analyses and the literature reviewed in this chapter indicate that conceptions of gender—and the socialization processes and basic assumptions that are involved in realizing these conceptions—have facilitating and preventive roles in relation to psychological problems. In some ways, the preventive role seems stronger—it is certainly the more surprising of the two. Expectations and assumptions associated with femininity seem both to increase the propensity for depressive symptoms and to decrease the tendency for externalizing behavior. Expectations and assumptions associated with masculinity seem to form a primarily protective barrier against experiencing depressive and anxious symptomatology. Given the continuing debates about which gender's traits and values are "superior," this finding provides additional support for the notion that it is essential to combine the best of both sides. It appears that the traits we define as masculine block depression. Traits we define as feminine protect us against substance abuse. Only the combination appears to reduce the threat of going to either extreme.

References

Best D, Williams J: A cross-cultural viewpoint, in The Psychology of Gender. Edited by Beale A, Sternberg R. New York, Guilford, 1995, pp 215–250

Brown L, Gilligan C: Meeting at the Crossroads. Boston, MA, Harvard University Press, 1992

Chodorow N: The Reproduction of Mothering. Berkeley, CA, University of California Press, 1978

Connell RW: Masculinities. Berkeley, CA, University of California Press, 1995

Derogatis LR, Lipman RS, Rickels K, et al: The Hopkins Symptom Checklist (HSCL): a self-report symptom inventory. Behav Sci 19:1–15, 1974

Edwards CP, Whiting BB: Women and dependency. Politics and Society 4: 343–355, 1974

Fagot BL, Hagen R: Aggression in toddlers: responses to the aggressive acts of boys and girls. Developmental Psychology 22:440–443, 1985

Foucault M: The History of Sexuality. New York, Vintage Books, 1978

Geis F: Self-fulfilling prophesies: a social psychological view of gender, in The Psychology of Gender. Edited by Beale A, Sternberg R. New York, Guilford, 1993, pp 9–54

Gove W, Herb T: Stress and mental illness among the young: a comparison of the sexes. Social Forces 53:256–265, 1974

Hagan J, Simpson J, Gillis AR: Class in the household: a power-control theory of gender and delinquency. American Journal of Sociology 92:788–816, 1987

Jackson DN: Personality Research Form Manual. Goshen, NY, Research Psychologists Press, 1974

Lytton H, Romney DM: Parents' differential socialization of boys and girls: a meta-analysis. Psychol Bull 109:267–296, 1991

Mead GH: Mind, Self, and Society. Chicago, IL, University of Chicago Press, 1934

Nolen-Hoeksema S: Sex Differences in Depression. Stanford, CA, Stanford University Press, 1990

Pandina R, Labouvie E, White H: Potential contributions of the life span developmental approach to the study of adolescent alcohol and drug use: the Rutgers Health and Human Development Project. Journal of Drug Issues 14:253–268, 1984

Pearlin LI, Lieberman MA, Menaghan E, et al: The stress process. J Health Soc Behav 22:337–356, 1981

Rosenfield S: Gender, Race, and Mental Health. San Francisco, CA, Society for the Study of Social Problems, 1998

Rosenfield S, Vertefuille J, McAlpine D: The emergence of sex differences in depression. Paper presented at the Society for the Study of Social Problems, Los Angeles, CA, August 1994

Spence J, Helmreich R: Masculinity and Femininity: The Psychological Dimensions, Correlates, and Antecedents. Austin, TX, University of Texas Press, 1978

Thoits PA: Me's and we's: forms and functions of social identities, in Self and Identity: Fundamental Issues. Edited by Ashmore RD, Jussim L. New York, Oxford University Press, 1996

Tittle CK: Gender research and education. Am Psychol 41:1161–1168, 1986

Whiting BB, Edwards CP: A cross-cultural analysis of sex differences in the behavior of children aged three through eleven. J Soc Psychol 91:171–188, 1973

Whiting BB, Edwards CP: Children of Different Worlds: The Formation of Social Behavior. Cambridge, MA, Harvard University Press, 1988

Whiting BB, Whiting JW: Children of Six Cultures: A Psychocultural Analysis. Cambridge, MA, Harvard University Press, 1975

CHAPTER 3

Gender-Specific Etiologies for Antisocial and Borderline Personality Disorders?

Andrew E. Skodol, M.D.

Are there gender-specific etiologies for antisocial personality disorder (ASPD) and borderline personality disorder (BPD)? It is reasonable to ask this question, given that both personality disorders share problems with impulse control, yet their gender ratios are reversed: approximately 75% of persons with ASPD are male and approximately 75% of persons with BPD are female (American Psychiatric Association 1994).

A search for gender specificity in factors involved in the genesis of ASPD and BPD can at best lead only to relative specificity. There are antisocial women, believed by many to be increasing in number (Mulder et al. 1994), as well as borderline men. ASPD and BPD are themselves not discrete, but rather show substantial comorbidity. Certain risk factors may be common to both disorders; other risk factors may be more specific to one disorder than to the other. There may be different mechanisms or pathways to each disorder for men and for women, or similar contributing factors at different strengths.

In this chapter I review research on biological, psychological, and social factors believed to be etiologically significant in the development of ASPD, BPD, or both. A discussion of the possible etiology of a condition relies on a model for understanding, in general, how that condition might develop. Therefore, I begin with an etiological model for the development of personality disorders, with specific reference to the continuity of traits and behaviors represented by ASPD and BPD. I then discuss selected potential risk factors for ASPD and BPD from a long list of candidate risk factors. I begin with the most fundamental biological factors and proceed through more complex factors, such as behavior and personality traits, concluding with social factors, which, in concert with more basic biological and psychological factors, might help to explain both the pathogenesis of personality psychopathology and the observed differences in gender distribution across types. Because many individual risk factors are involved and virtually all relevant research is limited by one or more design problems, I have focused on recent research reporting substantial findings on representative factors that themselves appear to show gender differences. I conclude the chapter by attempting to synthesize findings and offering suggestions for future research.

An Etiological Model for Personality Disorders

Although attempts to unravel the etiologies of personality disorders are still in the early stages, in order to approach the subject of risk factors or etiological mechanisms, a model for how personality disorders develop is necessary. Both ASPD and BPD have been shown to run in families, although the evidence for the familiality of ASPD is considerably stronger than that of BPD. Familiality of a disorder suggests roles for both inherited vulnerability and family environment, risk factors that often interact. A simple definition of personality might be the product of temperament (i.e., fundamental behavioral predispositions, such as emotionality, activity, and sociability, present at birth) and character (i.e., complex organizing and integrative systems, including cognitive and motivational components, that result from experience). Personality *disorders* may result when particular temperaments or derivative personality traits or attributes interact repeatedly with deleterious experiences to the point that the person's characteristic way of perceiving, thinking about, and relating to him- or herself and the environment (i.e., personality) becomes inflexible and maladaptive, resulting in substantial functional impairment or subjective distress.

Continuity of Personality Traits and Disorders Over Time

Personality traits are assumed to be relatively enduring characteristics of a person, stable over time and consistent across situations. The features of personality disorders usually become recognizable during adolescence or early adult life and in many cases even before that time. The diagnostic criteria for ASPD in DSM-IV (American Psychiatric Association 1994) and its predecessors require evidence of conduct disorder with onset before age 15 years, as well as a pervasive pattern of disregard for and violation of the rights of others into adulthood, thereby specifying continuity from at least midadolescence to early adult life. In fact, longitudinal studies of disruptive behavior problems of childhood have found a thread of continuity that may stretch back as far as early childhood oppositional behavior, attentional problems, hyperactivity, and childhood-onset conduct disorder in a group of persons who have a lifelong pattern of antisocial behavior typifying ASPD (Caspi and Moffitt 1995). Although the BPD diagnosis has no required childhood or adolescent antecedents, both clinical literature and recent longitudinal research suggest that traits or behaviors that are forerunners of BPD (e.g., conduct problems, impulsivity, and mood lability) are recognizable in childhood and adolescence (Bernstein et al. 1996; Rey et al. 1995). Factors associated with or responsible for persistent patterns of maladaptive behaviors indicative of a personality disorders are likely to be involved in their etiologies.

Candidate Risk Factors for Antisocial or Borderline Personality Disorder

The list of potential risk factors for ASPD or BPD is long. It includes the following:

- genes
- childhood temperament or predispositions
- psychophysiological factors, such as autonomic nervous system arousal and reactivity
- neurotransmitters
- brain structure and functioning, including brain size, regional cerebral blood flow (rCBF), and glucose metabolism

- other biological factors, including head injury, birth complications, minor physical anomalies, soft neurological signs, body size, gonadal and adrenal hormones, hypoglycemia, and environmental toxins
- cognitive and other neuropsychological factors, such as conditionability, learning, intelligence, moral reasoning, linguistic functions, and executive functions
- antecedent childhood or adolescent problems or disorders
- personality structure or traits
- family factors, including parental psychopathology and criminality; harsh, erratic, and inconsistent punishment; parental affection and control; inadequate parental supervision; marital conflict and divorce; and child abuse or neglect
- extrafamilial factors, such as peer influences, academic failure, socioeconomic status (SES), and poor living conditions

These are obviously not mutually exclusive categories; most are interrelated factors, and some are simply different levels of conceptualization or analysis of similar processes or phenomena. My review of risk factors in this chapter is necessarily selective and illustrative and focuses on factors for which gender differences may exist.

A few caveats concerning the research reviewed should be mentioned. One or more of these criticisms apply to most if not all of the studies cited. In addition to the previously mentioned problem of comorbidity, there are other definitional problems associated with the target behaviors studied. For example, research pertinent to the ASPD construct may focus on criminality, violent offending, delinquency, or psychopathy as well as on conduct disorder or ASPD. However, these are overlapping but not identical constructs. Even the criteria for conduct disorder and ASPD have undergone changes in recent years that affect their gender distributions and thus, conceivably, their risk factors. Because both ASPD and BPD involve complex behavioral patterns, it is inevitable that time and resources will be expended in studying processes that—although involved in the genesis of some aspect of the disorder—do not necessarily account for the entire clinical picture. Invariably, samples studied are patients as opposed to community populations, in the case of BPD, and are often incarcerated prisoners or other documented offenders, in the case of ASPD or psychopathy. Thus, sampling biases are prevalent. Much of the available research is cross-sectional, retrospective, and correlational as opposed to longitudinal, prospective, and predictive, thus limiting conclusions that can be drawn as to cause and effect. For ideological, economic, and practical reasons, most research is conducted in relative isolation from other research perspectives or traditions. Thus, most biologically oriented research is conducted without consideration of social factors, and vice versa. Although lip service is often paid to the importance of other factors and the potential of such factors to mediate or moderate the factor under examination, opportunities to compare the relative strengths of different types of risk factors in the same research design are rare. Most research on ASPD has been conducted in men, and most research on BPD has been conducted in women. Therefore, relatively less is known about the minority gender in each disorder. Finally, gender differences are sometimes obscured in studies that combine small numbers of the minority gender in samples and report overall findings.

Genes

Twin and adoption studies estimate that criminal behavior is between 30% and 60% heritable (Nigg and Goldsmith 1994). The evidence of heritability is more convincing for petty criminality than for violent offending. There is some suggestion that there is stronger heritability for female criminality than for male criminality, although the data are not unequivocal. It has been suggested that females at genetic risk for ASPD might also be at risk for other symptoms or disorders, such as somatization disorder, histrionic personality disorder, and even BPD (Lilienfeld 1992). These possibilities suggest that Cluster B personality disorders may represent variable expressions of a common diathesis, perhaps influenced by gender. What exactly is inherited is not known. Rutter (1996) has suggested that "the roots of antisocial behavior may lie in a broad behavioral propensity rather than in any predisposition to commit illegal acts as such" (p. 3).

The heritability estimates for criminal behavior leave room for environmental contributions. Most theories of crime include interactions between genetic predispositions and environmental factors. In a study of Iowa adoptees, Cadoret and associates (1995) showed that 1) ASPD in a biological parent predicted increased child conduct disorder, adolescent aggression, and adult antisocial behaviors; and 2) adverse adoptive home environments, including adoptive parents who had marital or legal problems or anxiety, depressive, or substance use disorders independently predicted increased adult antisocial behaviors. Adverse adoptive home environment interacted with biological background of ASPD to result in increased aggressivity and conduct disorder in the presence of, but not in the absence of, a biological background of ASPD. There were no gender differences in these effects.

Studies of juvenile delinquency have generally yielded lower estimates of heritability and higher estimates of environmental effects than have been found in studies of adult criminality (Raine 1993). This finding, in turn, may indicate that only a subset of adolescents are predisposed to delinquency for genetic reasons and that others engage in transient delinquency for other reasons, such as peer pressure. Given that the ASPD diagnosis requires a continuous pattern of antisocial behavior from childhood to adulthood, a focus on continuous as opposed to transient antisociality is necessary in identifying risk factors for ASPD.

Although family history studies of BPD have indicated some elevations in the rates of BPD in the relatives of BPD probands, all of the existing studies are in some way flawed. Only two family studies have been conducted that directly interviewed relatives (Reich 1989); both found modest rates of BPD. The only published twin study of BPD, conducted by Torgersen (1984), reported no evidence of genetic transmission of BPD in a small subgroup of BPD twins.

The study of behavioral dimensions thought to underlie BPD or ASPD in family and twin designs is also informative. Elevated rates of impulsive and affective behaviors have been found via family informants in the relatives of BPD probands (Silverman et al. 1991). Neuroticism (Loehlin 1992), negative emotionality (Tellegen et al. 1988), and novelty or stimulus seeking (Heath et al. 1994; Koopmans et al. 1995) (see section titled "Personality Traits," later in this chapter) have each been shown to have substantial heritability. Twin and adoption studies of MMPI psychopathic deviate (Pd) scale scores have shown heritabilities of about 50% (Gottesman and Goldsmith 1994).

Childhood Temperament

As mentioned earlier, *temperament* refers to a person's constitutional behavioral style, evident as early as the first few months of life. Several models of temperament have been proposed, beginning with the nine categories of behavior described originally by Thomas and Chess (Thomas et al. 1963). "Difficult temperament"—consisting of low approach, high intensity, negative mood, distractibility, nonpersistence, high activity, and aggression—has been hypothesized to be a source of gender differences in psychiatric disorders, its presence particularly predisposing an individual to externalizing disorders.

A recent study of early childhood temperament by Schwartz et al. (1996) tested the degree of temporal stability of temperamental inhibition and disinhibition from ages 21–31 months (early childhood) into adolescence. Adolescents of both genders who had been classified as inhibited at 21 months of age had significantly lower externalizing scores on the Achenbach Youth Self-Report (Achenbach 1991) than those classified as uninhibited. Girls scored lower than boys, and inhibited girls had the lowest externalizing scores. The results were similar for both the delinquent behavior and the aggressive behavior problem scales. Uninhibited boys and girls also scored higher on the attentional problems scale. Overall, being uninhibited as a toddler quadrupled a girl's probability of scoring in the clinical range on the externalizing dimension as an adolescent.

There is some evidence that boys and girls begin in infancy with similar temperaments but diverge in middle childhood, with boys becoming more difficult in temperament than girls and remaining so (Bezirganian and Cohen 1992). Temperamental differences by themselves are unlikely to result in psychopathology in the absence of an interaction with socialization experiences (i.e., parenting). Thus, the concept of "fit" between a child's temperament and his or her caregivers' parenting styles has developed. Unfortunately, for the most part, few strong links have been demonstrated between infant temperament and later childhood or adolescent disorder, despite the intuitive appeal of such a theory.

Autonomic Arousal: Heart Rate

Resting heart rate is an indicator of autonomic nervous system arousal. Low resting heart rate has been related to fearlessness (Raine 1993); high heart rate in infants and young children is associated with anxiety and fearful, inhibited temperament (Kagan 1989). Young, noninstitutionalized, nonpsychopathic antisocial individuals have been shown to have low resting heart rates. Lack of fear, especially in childhood, would help to explain poor socialization, since reduced fear of punishment would reduce the effectiveness of conditioning. Autonomic underarousal may lead to stimulus-seeking behavior, passive coping, withdrawal in the face of threat, and insensitivity to socializing punishments.

To my knowledge, resting heart rate or other indicators of autonomic nervous system reactivity have not been studied in patients with BPD; however, there is some suggestion that such rates in patients with BPD either may not be as low as those in antisocial patients or may show different responses to stress. In a study by Cloninger's group of the seven-factor model of temperament and character (Svrakic et al. 1993), patients with BPD had significantly increased harm avoidance, rather than decreased, as had been originally predicted. In our own studies (Skodol et al. 1995), we found increased odds of anxiety disorders in BPD patients, most of whom were female. In general, males have lower resting heart rates than females (Burns 1995). Since low resting heart rate is one of the best-replicated biological findings in delinquency to date and also seems to be associated with milder antisocial behavior, it may tie into the genetic finding that heritability of criminal behavior is especially strong for petty criminality.

Serotonin

Reduced cerebrospinal fluid serotonin levels have been found in violent offenders and in patients with ASPD, with BPD (Raine 1993), with impulsive–aggressive behavior (Coccaro et al. 1989), with conduct disorder (Stoff et al. 1987), with attention-deficit/hyperactivity disorder (ADHD) (Halperin et al. 1994; Kruesi et al. 1990), and with suicide attempts, particularly attempts with high lethality (Malone et al. 1996). Serotonin is linked to central nervous system behavioral inhibition, which is obviously deficient in impulsive patients. There is some indication that women have greater serotonergic responsivity than do men (McBride et al. 1990). Patients with ASPD or with BPD may also have enhanced noradrenergic activity, which contributes to extraversion, sensation seeking, irritable aggression, other-directed aggression, and affective instability.

Hypofrontality

Brain studies show reduced frontal activity in violent offenders and in children with ADHD (Raine 1993). Prefrontal dysfunction has been associated with generalized loss of inhibition; increases in risk taking, rule breaking, emotional and aggressive outbursts, and argumentative behavior; impulsivity and poor judgment; reduced concentration and reasoning ability; and decreased problem-solving skills and verbal communication ability. All of these behaviors would seem to characterize the antisocial individual, and most would describe the patient with BPD. Women appear to have enhanced frontal activity compared with men, as measured by tests of resting and task-related rCBF (Gur and Gur 1990) and glucose metabolism (Baxter et al. 1987). Dysfunction of frontal regions of the brain could disrupt serotonin activity because efferents from those regions go to nuclei where the cells of origin of the serotonin system are located.

Gonadal Hormones

Gonadal steroids have early *organizing* effects on the brain influencing masculinization and defemininization and later *activating* effects, which mobilize existing neural systems to influence behavior (Collaer and Hines 1995). Excess prenatal androgens, such as in congenital adrenal hyperplasia, are associated with increased aggression and rough and tumble play. Individual differences in androgens have been related to traits of aggression, assertiveness, and impulsiveness. Specifically, a lower threshold for stimuli to instigate aggressive behavior and increased gratification from motor pathways for aggressive behavior have been proposed to result from the impact of androgens on the prenatal organization of brain structures that mediate aggression (Maccoby and Jacklin 1974). Links between testosterone and aggression are strongest for males (Susman et al. 1987) and for behavioral aggression (Archer 1991).

Aggression, active play by children, and assertiveness all have moderate to large male–female gender differences. There are relatively small male:female prepubertal testosterone ratios with overlapping gender distributions and a 10:1 ratio by late adolescence without gender distribution overlap. Therefore, testosterone has been implicated both in the predisposition to aggressive behavior and in the great increase in aggression, at least in males, during the teenage years.

Testosterone has been linked during embryogenesis to delays in the development of the left cerebral hemisphere and fluctuating female hormones to changes in left hemisphere functioning and in verbal fluency. Estrogens may be responsible for increased heart rate, pulse pressure, and cardiac index in women, which in turn might be responsible for increased rCBF and glucose metabolism. At least one study has demonstrated, however, that although males at puberty had a much higher level of testosterone than females, there was little effect of testosterone on a stable extroversion personality trait, because girls' personalities responded much more to each additional unit of testosterone than did the personalities of boys (Udry and Talbert 1988). There still are questions concerning whether normal variations in hormones relate to individual differences within each gender in behaviors that show gender differences.

Cognitive Deficits

Criminals and delinquents show poor conditionability. Their IQs are also 8–10 points lower than those of control subjects (Hirschi and Hingelang 1977; Wilson and Herrnstein 1985). Lower IQ and learning problems may contribute to underdeveloped conscience, preference for highly stimulating activities, school failure, and social information–processing deficits, all of which are associated with delinquency and criminality. Learning disabilities are also common in the histories of patients with BPD, especially males (Andrulonis 1991). Boys have more learning disabilities than girls (American Psychiatric Association 1994). Girls have better verbal communication skills, which might reflect differences in brain structure or organization (e.g., less lateralization) in females. Individuals with psychopathy (especially males) may have impaired left-hemisphere function related to their lower verbal IQs and higher prevalence of left-handedness (Raine 1993). Some of these effects may be under hormonal control.

Childhood Antecedents

Although there has been some debate regarding appropriate criteria for conduct problems in girls, available evidence from epidemiological surveys, independent of clinical referral patterns, strongly identifies a preponderance of boys with childhood disruptive behavior disorders (Zoccolillo 1993). In children 12 years of age or younger, oppositional defiant disorder is twice as common in boys as in girls, ADHD 4–10 times as common, and conduct disorder 3–4 times as common (American Psychiatric Association 1994). Although by adolescence, these gender differences in conduct problems have disappeared, they resurface in the gender-ratio difference in ASPD mentioned above.

These changes in gender ratios suggest different pathways to conduct problems in boys than in girls. For example, in the longitudinal study conducted by Bernstein and associates (1996), childhood immaturity—a variable that measured clumsiness and distractibility, noncompliance, nonpersistence, and low school achievement separate from conduct problems and hyperactivity—predicted adolescent behavior problems indicative of Cluster B personality disorders only in girls. The temporary rise in conduct disorder in adolescent girls also suggests that girls may account for a greater proportion of transient conduct disturbance of adolescence than of life-persistent antisocial behavior leading to ASPD, while a subgroup of boys possess traits and have experiences that account for enduring antisociality.

During preadult development, emotional problems show a gender pattern different from that of behavioral problems. In childhood, the gender ratio for depressive disorders is about 1:1. By adolescence, more girls than boys are affected. All childhood anxiety disorders, including separation anxiety disorder and posttraumatic stress disorder but excluding obsessive-compulsive disorder, are more common among girls than boys. This pattern holds true into adolescence and early adult life (American Psychiatric Association 1994).

It should be noted that continuities between childhood and adolescent behavioral or emotional disorders and personality disorder type, although evident, are not specific. Conduct and attentional problems in childhood have been shown to be associated with the development of other Cluster B personality disorders as well as of personality disorders from Clusters A and C. Childhood mood and anxiety disturbances accompany childhood behavior problems in many cases and may result in adolescent behavior problems such as substance abuse. The evolution of childhood conduct problems and affective disturbance or instability into adolescent BPD would be consistent with Siever and Davis's (1991) proposition that BPD lies at the intersection of two biologically based diatheses, one of impulsivity/aggression and the other of affective dysregulation. At the conceptual level of child or adolescent mental disorder, despite differential gender distributions and some evidence of continuity over time, to argue specificity would stretch existing evidence.

Personality Traits

Personality disorders may represent extremes of normal personality traits. According to this model, a person at the extreme end of the distribution for certain traits might, as a consequence of adverse experiences, develop the maladaptive behaviors of a personality disorder.

Various personality trait systems have been used to theoretically and empirically describe ASPD and BPD. According to the currently popular five-factor model (FFM) of personality (Digman 1990), both ASPD and BPD are high in neuroticism and low in agreeableness (high antagonism), but ASPD is also low in conscientiousness. At the facet or subscale level, several subtle differences may be evident. Neuroticism in persons with ASPD may be expressed as hostility and impulsiveness, whereas in BPD it may be expressed as anxiety, depression, and self-conscious vulnerability (Widiger et al. 1994). According to Cloninger's three-factor model of personality (Cloninger 1987), both ASPD and BPD (as a variant of histrionic personality disorder) were predicted to be high in novelty seeking (a behavioral activation system) and low in harm avoidance (a behavioral inhibition system). However, ASPD was predicted to be low in reward dependence (a behavioral maintenance system), whereas BPD was expected to be high. These theoretical predictions have received modest empirical support (particularly for increased novelty seeking and neuroticism in both disorders) (Goldman et al. 1994; Svrakic et al. 1993). Nonetheless, a consensus prevails that ASPD involves a deficiency in impulse control, whereas BPD involves both deficient impulse control and emotional (affective) dysregulation.

Problems with impulse control can be a function of personality traits reflecting increased impulsivity, decreased constraints on behavior, or both. The personality traits may be heightened activity, novelty seeking, sensation seeking, aggression, risk taking, impulsivity, or other personality constructs related to behavioral activation. Conversely, the personality traits may be inattention, neuropsychological or cognitive dysfunction, harm avoidance, or impaired autonomic responsivity related to behavioral inhibition. Any number of these traits or predispositions are thought to be at least partially under genetic control.

Males account for the majority of extreme low scores on the agreeableness factor (77% male) of the FFM and its facets of altruism (83%), tender-mindedness (80%), straightforwardness (79%), and compliance (65%) (Corbitt and Widiger 1995). These traits of low agreeableness (and its facets) are similar to the traits of deceit and lack of empathy characteristic of individuals with psychopathy. Males also score in the highest range on the extroversion facet of excitement seeking and have very low scores on certain facets of neuroticism, especially vulnerability (69%) and anxiety (64%). These findings are consistent with an antisocial personality characterized by sensation seeking, emotional underreactivity, and interpersonal antagonism and exploitation.

Neuroticism may be the personality trait most relevant to BPD. Neuroticism encompasses many facets of borderline psychopathology, including anxiety, depression, poor psychological defenses, impulsivity, and vulnerability to stress. As such, it captures the major behavioral dimensions—that is, emotional dysregulation and impulsivity—thought to be impaired in BPD patients. There is some empirical evidence for genetic effects on the negative affectivity and vulnerability aspects of neuroticism, but not on the aggressive aspects. These findings are consistent with an etiological process in BPD encompassing a constitutional contribution to stress vulnerability, resultant anxiety and depression, and an adverse family environment that contributes to increased aggression. Evidence of both shared and unshared environmental effects, in addition to genetic effects, on neuroticism also invites consideration of unique environmental etiological agents in BPD, such as physical or emotional abuse (Nigg and Goldsmith 1994).

Women tend to score higher than men on neuroticism and its facets of impulsiveness (78% female), anxiety (71%), self-consciousness (68%), vulnerability (67%), and depression (64%) (Corbitt and Widiger 1995).

A recent meta-analysis of gender differences in personality traits combined results from different inventories according to facets of the FFM (Feingold 1994). The two major gender differences observed—in the personality traits of assertiveness (males scored higher than females) and tender-mindedness (females scored higher than males)—were consistent with the traditional theory that males score higher than females on traits of agency (i.e., instrumental traits) and females score higher than males on traits of communality (i.e., expressive traits). These findings suggest that compared with females, males would be more inclined to the active, physical, aggressive, and antagonistic pursuits characteristic of the individual with ASPD.

In a study by Krueger et al. (1994), male and female adolescents who engaged in delinquent activities had low scores on the Tellegen constraint factor—in particular, the traditionalism and control scales—and high scores on aggression. To a lesser degree, both genders exhibited alienation (a sense of betrayal by friends) and stress reaction (a tendency to become easily upset and irritable) on the Tellegen negative emotionality factor, which is similar to neuroticism. The only gender difference was that girls scored low on achievement, a scale measuring hard work and ambition. There were few overall differences between males and females in personality correlations with delinquency.

Child Abuse

Child maltreatment is a prime example of a "failure in the expectable environment" (Cicchetti and Lynch 1995). Child maltreatment has been associated with a range of negative outcomes, including physical injury (and death); attentional problems, learning disorders, and poor school performance; anxiety and depression; alcohol and substance abuse; self-destructive behaviors and suicide attempts; poor peer relationships; and physical aggression and violence (Browne and Finkelhor 1986; Malinosky-Rummell and Hansen 1993). Many of these problems are associated with ASPD, BPD, or both. Abuse and neglect have been related to the development of externalizing symptoms and disorders, violent offending, and ASPD in males (Luntz and Widom 1994; Widom 1989). Child physical abuse is more related to adult violence than is child sexual abuse, but it has not been shown to be more influential in the development of ASPD. Abuse and neglect have been related to the development of internalizing symptoms, depression, suicide attempts, and alcohol abuse in females (Widom 1998).

Epidemiological studies report that sexual abuse is 10 times more common in females than in males, whereas physical abuse is more equal between the genders (Jason et al. 1982). There are many reports of childhood sexual abuse in patients with BPD. In their studies comparing patients with BPD and with non-BPD personality disorders, Paris and colleagues found that childhood sexual abuse was a risk factor for BPD in both males and females, although the percentage of female patients reporting childhood sexual abuse (as high as 70%) (Paris et al. 1994a) was greater than that of males (50%) (Paris et al. 1994b). Interestingly, in these similarly selected samples of males and females with BPD, female BPD patients reported significantly more physical abuse than did female patients with non-BPD personality disorders, but male BPD patients did not report more physical abuse than did male patients with non-BPD personality disorders. Childhood sexual abuse was not specific to BPD, and not all BPD patients reported abuse. The same was true for abuse and ASPD. These findings suggest the existence of multiple pathways to ASPD and BPD and also underscore the importance of protective factors and resilience.

Abused and neglected children often have antisocial or substance-abusing parents, which further serves to obscure the relative contributions of genetics and environmental experiences to adverse outcomes.

Social Processes

Negative peer influences, academic failure, large family size, unemployment, poor living conditions, and a variety of other adverse social situations are associated with delinquency and criminality. In terms of gender differences, there is some suggestion that compared with girls, boys are more susceptible to peer influence and are more likely to instigate delinquent behavior. As examples of the latter, it has been shown that large family size increases delinquency when there are more male siblings; having more female siblings exerts a protective effect (Jones et al. 1980). Brothers are more likely to spread delinquent behavior to siblings of either gender—a so-called contagion effect. Also, a longitudinal study of the development of delinquency in girls found that early menarche was a risk factor, but only for girls who attended a coed high school, where they could associate with older boys and be negatively influenced (Caspi et al. 1993).

Studies examining very young children (i.e., before age 6 years) for gender differences in aggressive behaviors such as fighting, arguing, and other actions intended to do harm have not found statistically significant differences, a result that casts doubt on theories of constitutional determinants of aggression and raises questions about the effect of early gender-role socialization on aggressive behavior (Tieger 1980). Some investigators have suggested that infant boys and girls are handled differently by caregivers, such that boys receive more gross motor stimulation than girls. Parents seem more concerned about "appropriate" gender-role behavior with boys than with girls and will attempt to get boys to conform to gender-role-appropriate behavior by physically punishing "inappropriate" behavior. Gender-role stereotypes traditionally pervade culture and tend to support male aggressiveness and female passivity. Media portrayals of aggression teach aggressive skills and provide motivation for disinhibition because aggressive acts are often successful. Boys' behavior has been shown to be more susceptible to the influence of media aggression (Eron and Huesmann 1986). The current trend toward more aggressive behavior among women (e.g., higher proportions in prison populations, higher auto insurance rates) may be a sign that Western cultural norms inhibiting women's aggressiveness are changing.

To my knowledge, the effects of peers, siblings, and other social processes in BPD have not been investigated. Lack of adequate epidemiological data renders premature any definitive statements regarding the SES correlates of BPD. Some theories attempting to explain the rise in the incidence of BPD in the past few decades implicate broken homes and underinvolvement of parents with children as well as the decline of stabilizing institutions and of the extended family (Millon and Davis 1995).

Conclusion

The search for gender-specific etiological factors in ASPD and BPD has identified a number of potential risk factors on which males and females differ. Few of the risk factors are highly specific either for one of the genders or for one of the personality disorders. Perhaps this should come as no surprise, since, in general, for any trait on which the genders differ, variability within each gender is greater than that between the genders. In the case of delinquency, at least, it has been shown that basically the same factors that account for delinquency variation within a given gender account for the difference between the genders in the mean rates of delinquency (Rowe et al. 1995). This finding would go against theories that postulate strikingly different etiological pathways for male and female delinquency.

Longitudinal research is beginning to demonstrate continuity of personality traits and behavior patterns over time. Of particular significance for the development of ASPD is a pattern of impulsive and aggressive personality and behavior; for BPD, both impulsive aggression *and* affective instability are involved. Although both of these fundamental behavioral/emotional proclivities are substantially heritable, the environment exerts considerable influence over their development into personality styles and disorder.

It is not clear how infant boys and girls differ on these dimensions. Differences quickly emerge in early childhood, however, as boys show more aggression and externalizing behavior patterns and disorders and girls show more behavioral inhibition and internalizing problems. Some relevant (and possibly genetic) differences have been demonstrated in autonomic and central nervous system functioning: compared with females, males have lower levels of autonomic arousal, less serotonergic responsivity, and reduced frontal activity in the brain. Some of these differences might be influenced by prenatal gonadal hormones. All of them would contribute to poorer socialization, less behavioral inhibition, weaker verbal problem-solving skills, and the like in boys versus girls and thus would potentially contribute to males' greater antisociality. Research on how these factors differ in healthy children versus children with behavioral or emotional precursors of adult personality disorders is now under way. Some of the biological sex differences between boys and girls could help explain why girls are more likely than boys to experience fear, to develop strong consciences, to experience guilt and depression, and, consequently, to show an affective component to an impulse-control disturbance.

Socialization differences between boys and girls cannot be ignored, however. Girls are clearly reinforced for less aggressive behavior patterns than are boys and girls who develop delinquent or antisocial behavior patters have probably been exposed to harsher, more unusual environmental experiences than have delinquent boys. An uninhibited, aggressive temperament in girls may, in fact, increase the chances of their exposure to adverse environments. Thus, until recently at least, a reasonable explanation for the gender differences in ASPD and BPD might be that girls are more biologically and socially influenced toward internalizing problems, such as anxiety or depression, but with increasing "doses" of biological and/or social factors influencing impulsive aggression, they may develop BPD. Extreme exposures could result in ASPD. The reverse process would hold for aggressive boys, who as a result of high genetic loadings for affective dysregulation or exposure to environmental circumstances engendering emotional disequilibrium would develop BPD in addition to or instead of ASPD. To date, however, these theories are mostly speculations.

Future research should continue to investigate the causal pathways for different types of personality psychopathology in prospective, longitudinal studies of at-risk children in which methods and measures from diverse traditions and perspectives are employed simultaneously. Samples of males and females should be examined and compared for risk factors and mechanisms. Because of the complexity of personality disorder behavioral patterns, greater emphasis might be placed on the search for risk factors for the fundamental emotional and behavioral disturbances that constitute personality psychopathology. Understanding gender differences in the rates of psychiatric disorders may increase our knowledge about both etiology and prevention.

References

Achenbach TM: Manual for the Youth Self-Report and 1991 Profile. Burlington, VT, University of Vermont Department of Psychiatry, 1991

American Psychiatric Association: Diagnostic and Statistical Manual of Mental Disorders, 4th Edition. Washington, DC, American Psychiatric Association, 1994

Andrulonis PA: Disruptive behavior disorders in boys and the borderline personality disorder in men. Ann Clin Psychiatry 3:23–26, 1991

Archer J: The influence of testosterone on human aggression. Br J Psychol 82: 1–28, 1991

Baxter LR Jr, Mazziotta JC, Phelps ME, et al: Cerebral glucose metabolic rates in normal human females versus normal males. Psychiatry Res 21:237–245, 1987

Bernstein DP, Cohen P, Skodol AE, et al: Childhood antecedents of adolescent personality disorders. Am J Psychiatry 153:907–913, 1996

Bezirganian S, Cohen P: Sex differences in the interaction between temperament and parenting. J Am Acad Child Adolesc Psychiatry 31:790–801, 1992

Browne A, Finkelhor D: Impact of child sexual abuse: a review of the research. Psychol Bull 99:66–77, 1986

Burns JW: Interactive effects of traits, states, and gender on cardiovascular reactivity during different situations. J Behav Med 18:279–303, 1995

Cadoret RJ, Yates WR, Troughton E, et al: Genetic–environmental interaction in the genesis of aggressivity and conduct disorders. Arch Gen Psychiatry 52: 916–924, 1995

Caspi A, Moffitt TE: The continuity of maladaptive behavior: from description to understanding in the study of antisocial behavior, in Developmental Psychopathology, Vol 2: Risk, Disorder, and Adaptation. Edited by Cicchetti D, Cohen DJ. New York, Wiley, 1995, pp 472–511

Caspi A, Lynam D, Moffitt TE, et al: Unraveling girls' delinquency: biological, dispositional, and contextual contributions to adolescent misbehavior. Dev Psychopathol 29:19–30, 1993

Cicchetti D, Lynch M: Failures in the expectable environment and their impact on individual development: the case of child maltreatment, in Developmental Psychopathology, Vol 1: Theory and Methods. Edited by Cicchetti D, Cohen DJ. New York, Wiley, 1995, pp 32–71

Cloninger CR: A systematic method for clinical description and classification personality variants: a proposal. Arch Gen Psychiatry 44:573–588, 1987

Cocarro EF, Siever LJ, Klar H, et al: Serotonergic studies of personality disorder: correlates with behavioral aggression and impulsivity. Arch Gen Psychiatry 46:587–599, 1989

Collaer ML, Hines M: Human behavioral sex differences: a role for gonadal hormones during early development? Psychol Bull 118:55–107, 1995

Corbitt EM, Widiger TA: Sex differences among the personality disorders: an exploration of the data. Clinical Psychology: Science and Practice 2:225–238, 1995

Digman JM: Personality structure: emergence of the five-factor model. Annu Rev Psychol 50:116–123, 1990

Eron LD, Huesmann LR: The role of television in the development of prosocial and antisocial behavior, in Development of Antisocial and Prosocial Behavior: Research, Theories, and Issues. Edited by Olweus D, Block J, Radke-Yarrow M. New York, Academic Press, 1986, pp 285–314

Feingold A: Gender differences in personality: a meta-analysis. Psychol Bull 116:429–456, 1994

Goldman RG, Skodol AE, McGrath PJ, et al: Relationship between the Tridimensional Personality Questionnaire and DSM-III-R personality traits. Am J Psychiatry 151:274–276, 1994

Gottesman II, Goldsmith HH: Developmental psychopathology of antisocial behavior: inserting genes into its ontogenesis and epigenesis, in Threats to Optimal Development: Integrating Biological, Psychological and Social Risk Factors. Edited by Nelson CA. Hillsdale, NJ, Lawrence Erlbaum, 1994, pp 69–104

Gur RE, Gur RC: Gender differences in regional cerebral blood flow. Schizophr Bull 16:247–254, 1990

Halperin JM, Sharma V, Siever LJ, et al: Serotonergic function in aggressive and nonaggressive boys with attention-deficit hyperactivity disorder. Am J Psychiatry 151:243–248, 1994

Heath AC, Cloninger CR, Martin NG: Testing a model for the genetic structure of personality: a comparison of the personality systems of Cloninger and Eysenck. J Pers Soc Psychol 66:762–775, 1994

Hirschi I, Hingelang MJ: Intelligence and delinquency: a revisionist review. American Sociological Review 42:571–587, 1977

Jason J, Williams SL, Burton A, et al: Epidemiologic differences between sexual and physical child abuse. JAMA 247:3344–3348, 1982

Jones MD, Offord DR, Abrams N: Brothers, sisters, and antisocial behavior. Br J Psychiatry 136:139–145, 1980

Kagan J: Temperamental contributions to social behavior. Am Psychol 44:668–674, 1989

Koopmans JR, Boomsma DI, Heath AC, et al: A multivariate genetic analysis of sensation seeking. Behav Genet 25:349–356, 1995

Krueger RF, Schmutte PS, Caspi A, et al: Personality traits are linked to crime among men and women: evidence from a birth cohort. J Abnorm Psychol 103:328–338, 1994

Kruesi MJP, Rapoport JL, Hamburger S, et al: Cerebrospinal fluid monoamine metabolites, aggression, and impulsivity in disruptive behavior disorders of children and adolescents. Arch Gen Psychiatry 47:419–426, 1990

Lilienfeld SO: The association between antisocial personality and somatization disorders: a review and integration of theoretical models. Clin Psychol Rev 12:641–662, 1992

Loehlin JC: Genes and Environment in Personality Development. Newbury Park, CA, Sage, 1992

Luntz BK, Widom CS: Antisocial personality disorder in abused and neglected children grown up. Am J Psychiatry 151:670–674, 1994

Maccoby EE, Jacklin CN: The Psychology of Sex Differences. Stanford, CA, Stanford University Press, 1974

Malinosky-Rummell R, Hansen DJ: Long-term consequences of childhood physical abuse. Psychol Bull 114:68–79, 1993

Malone KM, Corbitt EM, Shuhua LI, et al: Prolactin response to fenfluramine and suicide attempt lethality in major depression. Br J Psychiatry 168:324–329, 1996

McBride PA, Tierney H, DeMeo M, et al: Effects of age and gender on CNS serotonergic responsivity in normal adults. Biol Psychiatry 27:1143–1155, 1990

Millon T, Davis RD: The development of personality disorders, in Developmental Psychopathology, Vol 2: Risk, Disorder, and Adaptation. Edited by Cicchetti D, Cohen DJ. New York, Wiley, 1995, pp 633–676

Mulder RT, Wells JE, Joyce PR, et al: Antisocial women. J Personal Disord 8:279–287, 1994

Nigg JT, Goldsmith HH: Genetics of personality disorders: perspectives from personality and psychopathology research. Psychol Bull 115:346–380, 1994

Paris J, Zweig-Frank H, Guzder J: Psychological risk factors for borderline personality disorder in female patients. Compr Psychiatry 35:301–305, 1994a

Paris J, Zweig-Frank H, Guzder J: Risk factors for borderline personality in male outpatients. J Nerv Ment Dis 182:375–380, 1994b

Raine A: The Psychopathology of Crime: Criminal Behavior as a Clinical Disorder. San Diego, CA, Academic Press, 1993

Reich JH: Familiality of DSM-III dramatic and anxious personality clusters. J Nerv Ment Dis 177:96–100, 1989

Rey JM, Morris-Yates A, Singh M, et al: Continuities between psychiatric disorders in adolescents and personality disorders in young adults. Am J Psychiatry 152:895–900, 1995

Rowe DC, Vazsonyi AT, Flannery DJ: Sex differences in crime: do means and within-sex variation have similar causes? Journal of Research on Crime and Delinquency 32:84–150, 1995

Rutter M: Introduction: concepts of antisocial behavior, of cause and of genetic influences, in Genetics of Criminal and Antisocial Behavior (Ciba Foundation Symposium 194). Edited by Bock GR, Goode JA. Chichester, England, Wiley, 1996, pp 1–20

Schwartz CE, Snidman N, Kagan J: Early childhood temperament as a determinant of externalizing behavior in adolescence. Dev Psychopathol 8:527–537, 1996

Siever LJ, Davis KL: A psychobiological perspective on the personality disorders. Am J Psychiatry 148:1647–1658, 1991

Silverman JM, Pinkham L, Horvath TB, et al: Affective and impulsive personality traits in the relatives of patients with borderline personality disorder. Am J Psychiatry 148:1378–1385, 1991

Skodol AE, Oldham JM, Hyler SE, et al: Patterns of anxiety and personality comorbidity. J Psychiatr Res 29:361–374, 1995

Stoff DM, Pollack L, Vitiello B, et al: Reduction of ^{3}H-impramine binding sites on platelets of conduct disordered children. Neuropsychopharmacology 1:55–62, 1987

Susman EJ, Inoff-Germain G, Nottelmann ED, et al: Hormones, emotional dispositions, and aggressive attributes in young adolescents. Child Dev 58: 1114–1134, 1987

Svrakic DM, Whitehead C, Przybeck TR, et al: Differential diagnosis of personality disorders by the seven-factor model of temperament and character. Arch Gen Psychiatry 50:991–999, 1993

Tellegen A, Lykken DT, Bouchard TJ, et al: Personality similarity in twins reared apart and together. J Pers Soc Psychol 54:1031–1039, 1988

Thomas A, Chess S, Birch HG, et al: Behavioral Individuality in Early Childhood. New York, New York University Press, 1963

Tieger T: On the biological basis of sex differences in aggression. Child Dev 51:943–963, 1980

Torgersen S: Genetic and nosological aspects of schizotypal and borderline personality disorders: a twin study. Arch Gen Psychiatry 41:546–554, 1984

Udry JR, Talbert LM: Sex hormone effects on personality at puberty. J Pers Soc Psychol 54:291–295, 1988

Widiger TA, Trull TJ, Clarkin JF, et al: A description of the DSM-III-R and DSM-IV personality disorders with the five-factor model of personality, in Personality Disorders and the Five-Factor Model of Personality. Edited by Costa PT, Widiger TA. Washington, DC, American Psychological Association, 1994, pp 41–56

Widom CS: The cycle of violence. Science 244:160–165, 1989

Widom CS: Childhood victimization: early adversity and subsequent psychopathology, in Adversity, Stress, and Psychopathology. Edited by Dohrenwend BP. New York, Oxford University Press, 1998, pp 81–95

Wilson JQ, Herrnstein R: Crime and Human Nature. New York, Simon & Schuster, 1985

Zoccolillo M: Gender and the development of conduct disorder. Dev Psychopathol 5:65–78, 1993

SECTION II

Mood and Anxiety Disorders

CHAPTER 4

Gender Differences in Major Depression

Epidemiological Findings

Ronald C. Kessler, Ph.D.

One of the most widely documented findings in psychiatric epidemiology is that women have higher rates of major depression than men. This has been found consistently throughout the world in community epidemiological studies using a variety of diagnostic schemes and interview methods (Bebbington et al. 1981; Bland et al. 1988a, 1988b; Canino et al. 1987; Cheng 1989; Hwu et al. 1989; Lee et al. 1987; Weissman and Myers 1978; Wells et al. 1989; Wittchen et al. 1992; for reviews, see Bebbington 1988; Nolen-Hoeksema 1987; Weissman and Klerman 1977, 1985, 1992; Weissman et al. 1984). The prevalence of depression among women in these studies has typically been between 1.5 and 3 times that among men. In this chapter I review the literature on this relationship between gender and depression and discuss and evaluate plausible explanations.

The report contained in this chapter is based on data from the National Comorbidity Survey (NCS), a collaborative epidemiological study of the prevalences, causes, and consequences of psychiatric morbidity and comorbidity in the United States. The NCS (Ronald C. Kessler, Principal Investigator) is funded by the National Institute of Mental Health (R01 MH46376, R01 MH49098, and RO1 MH52861), with supplemental support from the National Institute on Drug Abuse (through a supplement to MH46376) and the W. T. Grant Foundation (90135190). Preparation of this report was also supported by a Research Scientist Award (K05 MH00507) to Dr. Kessler.

Proposed Explanations for Gender Differences in Depression

Differential Survey Validity Due to Response Bias

Before turning to substantive issues, it is useful to consider the possibility that societal norms and gender-role socialization experiences make it easier for women than it is for men in epidemiological surveys to admit having experienced depression (Phillips and Segal 1969; Young et al. 1990). If this is so, then the higher reported rate of depression among women in such surveys might be due to nothing more than differential reporting bias. However, my reading of the available evidence suggests that this is not a plausible hypothesis, for two reasons. First, a number of methodological studies have been conducted to study this type of response bias in community surveys of nonspecific psychological distress (Clancy and Gove 1972; Gove 1978; Gove and Geerken 1977). These studies used standard psychometric methods to assess potential biasing factors such as social desirability (i.e., the tendency to give responses that will put the respondent in a more favorable light), expressivity (i.e., the tendency to choose exaggerated response categories in characterizing intensity of emotion or severity of impairment), lying, and yeasaying/naysaying (i.e., the tendency to give the same positive or negative response to a long string of parallel questions without seriously considering the content of the questions). No evidence was found in any of these studies that the significantly higher levels of self-reported distress found among women were due to these biasing factors.

Second, a more direct evaluation of the impact of response bias on the gender difference in major depression was carried out by Young et al. (1990). They hypothesized that lower reluctance to admit depression should lead women to be more likely than men to acknowledge ever having had a period lasting 2 weeks or longer of being sad, blue, or depressed but should not affect reports of the less-stigmatizing symptoms that cluster with depressed mood to make up a major depressive episode, such as sleep disturbance, eating disturbance, and lack of energy. Yet the opposite was found by Young and his colleagues in an analysis of a representative sample of nonpatient relatives of depressed probands. The female:male ratio of a 2-week period of depressed mood or anhedonia (1.3) was much smaller than the ratio of less-stigmatizing associated symptoms (1.7). As shown in Table 4–1, we found very similar results in the National Comorbidity Survey (NCS; Kessler et al. 1993). The female:male odds ratio in the NCS increased steadily from 1.26 for endorsement of the major depression diagnostic stem question to 2.50 for endorsement of the stem question plus all eight of the other "A" criteria stipulated in DSM-III-R (American Psychiatric Association 1987). It is implausible that a pattern of this sort would be due to greater reluctance on the part of men to admit depression.

It is important to recognize, however, that this pattern is exactly what one would expect to see with invalidity due to differential forgetting. The notion here is that although men might remember the vague outlines of past depressive episodes as well as women do, they might be more likely than women to minimize in memory the impairment and constellation of symptoms associated with these episodes. Angst and Dobler-Mikola (1984) reported a pattern of this sort in a longitudinal study of young adults. Prospective data in their study showed no gender difference in the period prevalence of depression, despite the fact that retrospective data over the same recall period suggested that women had higher rates of depression than men. Wilhelm and Parker (1994) subsequently found a similar pattern regarding male underreporting in a separate sample and added the important finding that women were more likely than men to overreport depression (i.e., retrospectively to report a previously reported subclinical episode as having met full criteria). These results argue persuasively that the gender difference in reported lifetime depression is at least partially due to a gender difference in accuracy of retrospective reporting.

Nonetheless, as noted by Ernst and Angst (1992), it is unlikely that this differential retrospective reporting bias completely explains the gender difference in reported depression. The most important evidence in this regard comes from studies of current or recent prevalence, in which recall becomes unimportant. Women consistently have higher rates of current depression than men in these studies (e.g., Blazer et al. 1994; Weissman et al. 1991). It is likely, though, that recall bias plays a part in evidence of a gender difference in the course of depression, most of which has been based on retrospective data. Indeed, Ernst and Angst (1992) found that evidence for a higher recurrence risk of major depres-

TABLE 4–1.

Sex ratio of lifetime diagnosis of DSM-III-R major depressive episode (MDE), by varying diagnostic criteria: the National Comorbidity Survey

	Percentage meeting MDE lifetime diagnosis			
Diagnostic criteria	**Male**	**Female**	**Female:Male**	**Total**
Stem	45.70	57.60	1.26	51.70
Stem plus 1 or more symptoms	25.20	35.90	1.43	30.60
Stem plus 2 or more symptoms	20.90	32.00	1.53	26.50
Stem plus 3 or more symptoms	16.60	26.90	1.62	21.80
Stem plus 4 or more symptoms	12.70	21.30	1.68	17.10
Stem plus 5 or more symptoms	8.50	16.60	1.95	12.60
Stem plus 6 or more symptoms	5.70	11.00	1.93	8.40
Stem plus 7 or more symptoms	3.30	6.10	1.85	4.80
Stem plus all 8 symptoms	1.20	3.00	2.50	2.10

Note. DSM-III-R = Diagnostic and Statistical Manual of Mental Disorders, 3rd Edition, Revised (American Psychiatric Association 1987).
Source. Reprinted from Kessler RC, McGonagle KA, Swartz M, et al.: "Sex and Depression in the National Comorbidity Survey, I: Lifetime Prevalence, Chronicity and Recurrence." *Journal of Affective Disorders* 29:88, 1993. Copyright © 1993, Elsevier Science Inc. Used with permission.

sion among women than among men disappeared entirely when adjustments were made for recall bias. Furthermore, in the NCS, in which special procedures were used to stimulate active memory search (Kessler et al., in press), no gender difference in recurrence risk was found (Kessler et al. 1994). The NCS also failed to find evidence of a gender difference in either speed of episode recovery from or chronicity of depression. A recent report from the National Institute of Mental Health (NIMH) Collaborative Program on the Psychobiology of Depression reported prospective data consistent with these results, finding no gender difference in the subsequent course of first episodes of depression (Simpson et al. 1997).

These results regarding absence of a gender difference in course of depression are not definitive. It could be that a higher proportion of depressed men than women consistently refuse to admit their depression to survey interviewers. However, this result is inconsistent with the fact that a higher prevalence of depression in women versus men is found not only in studies that rely on self-report but also in those that use informant reports (Kendler et al. 1997). Another possibility is that men are as likely to be depressed as women but mask their depression so completely that neither they nor those close to them are aware of it. A more plausible scenario is simply that women are more likely to be depressed than men. Assuming that this is in fact the case, we now turn to explanations.

Mood Amplification

One explanation for the gender differences in depression relates to the results shown in Table 4–1. This explanation, proposed by Nolen-Hoeksema (1987), argues that men and women do not differ in the frequency with which they experience brief episodes of sadness but that women are more likely than men to allow these episodes to escalate into full-blown episodes of major depression. The reason, according to Nolen-Hoeksema, is that men tend to respond to depressed mood with distraction methods that blunt the mood, whereas women are more likely to ruminate upon and amplify the mood. Consistent with this hypothesis, empirical studies by Nolen-Hoeksema and her colleagues have shown that ruminative responses to distress exacerbate depressed mood (Nolen-Hoeksema et al. 1994) and that women are more likely than men to adopt these ruminative responses when they become sad (Nolen-Hoeksema et al. 1993).

It is conceivable that the gender difference in rumination explains why the studies reviewed in the previous section found that associated symptoms are more likely to cluster with depressed mood among women than among men. Related possibilities have been proposed by other researchers. These include the observations that women are more introspective than men (Hansell and Mechanic 1986) and have more depressogenic attributional styles than men (Abramson and Andrews 1982). The argument that mood amplification due to some combination of these characteristics can lead to a gender difference in clinical depression may be questioned by claiming that major depression is not an extreme variant of depressed mood but something qualitatively different. However, genetic models estimated with general-population twin data cannot refute the hypothesis that a single latent liability underlies depressed mood, minor depression, and major depression (Kendler et al. 1992). Furthermore, epidemiological studies find no evidence of sharp distinctions between minor and major depression in terms of family history or other predictors, presence of comorbidity, course of illness, or degree of impairment (Kessler et al. 1997; Sherbourn et al. 1994). On the basis of these considerations, it is not implausible that variation in the amplification of normal depressed mood might account for the gender difference in depression.

It is important to appreciate that the mood amplification argument makes predictions more about time than about symptom clustering. Men and women are assumed to be equally likely to become sad initially, but women are thought to be more likely than men to persist in a depressed mood. The limited evidence that is available on this point, yielded from only two studies, offers no support for this argument. One of these studies was carried out by Nolen-Hoeksema et al. (1993) in a small sample of male and female college students; the other was conducted by Almeida and Kessler (1998) in a community sample of married couples. Both studies used daily diaries to assess stress and mood over a period of several weeks. Both studies found that women were significantly more likely than men to report high daily distress. But disaggregation showed that there was no significant gender difference in the probability of continuation of a distress episode into a subsequent day in either study. Instead, the overall higher prevalence of daily distress among women was due to a significantly higher probability of new-onset daily distress among women than among men on days subsequent to distress-free days. This result is inconsistent with the mood amplification hypothesis.

Gender Roles

This last result highlights a problem that has traditionally plagued research on gender differences in depression: theories have often been designed to explain patterns that do not exist. A good example comes from feminist theories designed to explain the higher prevalence of depression in women than in men. These theories have usually argued that there is something about the position of women in contemporary society that is depressogenic (see review in McGrath et al. 1990; Mirowsky and Ross 1989). This argument was originally based on the observation of survey researchers in the early 1970s that the higher levels of nonspecific psychological distress in women versus men in general-population surveys were confined to married people (Gove and Tudor 1973). This observation led to the speculation that there is something about marriage that is bad for the mental health of women, a view that persists even today in the thinking of some gender-role theorists (e.g., R. W. Simon 1995).

A more cautious examination of the data suggests, rather, that marriage is benign for men but not malign for women. Levels of distress among women are not higher in the married than in the unmarried. Indeed, nonspecific psychological distress varies little by marital status among women and, if anything, is somewhat lower among married than among never-married or previously married women. Distress varies powerfully with marital status among men, however, with the levels of distress much lower among married men than among either never-married or previously married men. In terms of gender differences, this pattern manifests in equal levels of nonspecific psychological distress among the young and the never married, lower levels among the married (although distress levels are lower for men than for women, so that a significant gender difference appears), and elevated levels among the widowed or divorced (although the increase is much higher for men than for women, so that the previous gender difference disappears). This kind of pattern raises the possibility that conventional adult gender roles are involved in women's higher rates of depression compared with men—that the typical life situations of women are either more stressful or less fulfilling than those of men, or perhaps that women have less access than do men to the kinds of coping resources that can protect against the onset of depression or ameliorate depression once it begins.

Before speculating further, we must pause to consider precisely what we are trying to explain, a task never undertaken by advocates of the gender-role perspective. The epidemiological evidence shows that the gender difference in depression begins much earlier in life than this theory would predict. As shown in Figure 4–1, retrospective data from the NCS suggest that the gender difference in lifetime risk of major depression begins in the age range of 10–14 years, which implies that the gender difference in depression precedes adult gender-role differentiation and greatly predates marriage.

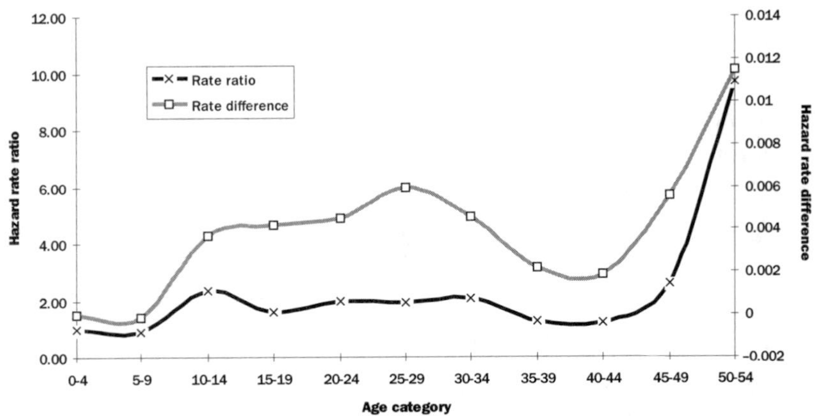

	0-4	5-9	10-14	15-19	20-24	25-29	30-34	35-39	40-44	45-49	50-54
Hazard rate ratio	1.00	0.90	2.33	1.58	2.00	1.92	2.09	1.26	1.24	2.60	9.71
95% lower CI	1.00	0.46	1.35	1.14	1.42	1.35	1.22	0.73	0.72	0.85	0
95% upper CI	1.00	1.76	4.04	2.19	2.82	2.72	3.58	2.17	2.12	7.97	∞

FIGURE 4–1. Major depressive episode hazard rate ratios (female:male) and rate differences (female –male) in the National Comorbidity Survey. CI = confidence interval.
Source. Reproduced from Kessler RC, McGonagle KA, Swartz M, et al.: "Sex and Depression in the National Comorbidity Survey, I: Lifetime Prevalence, Chronicity and Recurrence." *Journal of Affective Disorders* 29:90, 1993. Copyright © 1993, Elsevier Science Inc. Used with permission.

There is also another aspect of the gender-role perspective that does not fit the epidemiological data. The argument holds that women are more depressed than men because their day-to-day life situations are more depressogenic: chronic isolation and lack of fulfillment for homemakers, unremitting and unconditional demands for mothers, and chronic overloads and exposure to the conflicting demands of family and work roles for women who try to maintain careers while still fulfilling household responsibilities. But if such chronic stresses really account for the higher prevalence of depression among women, we would expect female depression to be more chronic. This is not the case. Women are much more likely than men to become depressed (that is, to have a lifetime history of depression), but women with a lifetime history of depression are not more likely than comparable men to have chronic depression (Kessler et al. 1994). Among individuals with a history of depression, there is no gender difference in risk of recurrent depression (Simpson et al. 1997) or in speed of recovery from depressive episodes (McLeod et al. 1992).

Biological Influences

One might speculate that hormones are involved, given that the observed gender difference emerges at about the time of puberty (Angold and Worthman 1993). Angold and colleagues (1998) are currently conducting an important study that investigates this issue by following cohorts of prepubertal boys and girls through puberty with direct measures of sex hormones from blood samples. Preliminary results suggest that the increase in depression among girls relative to boys occurs sharply at midpuberty (Tanner stage III) and that pubertal status is more important than age in predicting the gender difference in depression.

An intriguing finding in earlier work that must be considered when evaluating these findings is that a gender difference in low self-esteem, which often accompanies depression, emerges at different ages, depending on the timing of the transition from primary to secondary school and the beginning of girls' exposure to the pressures associated with dating older boys. Simmons and Blythe (1987) found that the gender difference in low self-esteem emerges in the seventh grade when students are situated in a school system that has a grades-seven-through-nine middle school but does not emerge until the ninth grade when students hail from a system that has a kindergarten-through-eighth-grade primary school and a 4-year high school. Clearly, even if sex hormones are involved, this finding strongly suggests that this differential vulnerability is potentiated by environmental stresses related to gender roles.

It is also possible to search for a biological basis of the gender difference in depression at the genetic level. The twin research of Kendler and associates (1993) has shown clearly that there is a strong genetic basis for major depression among women. Until recently, this work was confined exclusively to female–female twin pairs. Over the past few years, however, male–male pairs and male–female pairs have been added to the Kendler twin data set, and a separate nationally representative sample of both same-sex and opposite-sex twin pairs has been collected (Brim and Featherman, in press). These new studies, results of which have not yet been reported, will soon provide important information on the extent to which genes are involved in the gender difference in depression.

Cohort Effects

One important aspect of the picture that cannot be explained by sex hormones or genes is that the prevalence of depression has increased dramatically over the past few decades, whereas the gender difference in depression has narrowed during this time. Estimates based on retrospective age-at-onset reports obtained in the NCS (Kessler et al. 1994) suggest that the lifetime prevalence of major depression among men in the age range of 20–24 years increased from 3.7% in the early 1960s to 17.8% in the early 1990s (an increase of 14.1%) and among women in the same age range over this time period from 5.7% to 28.1% (an increase of 22.4%). Neither the population distribution of sex hormones nor the gene pool changes this quickly, which means that the influence of changing environmental conditions must be at work in accounting for these dramatic increases.

Before considering what these environmental conditions might be, it is important to recognize that controversy exists about the meaning of the cohort effect. Recall failure and/or reluctance to admit depression might increase with age; if so, this would create the false impression that the prevalence of depression had increased in recent cohorts. Another possibility is that selective mortality or other forms of sample censoring due to depression might increase with age. We do not know if these influences are at work, although there is at least some indirect evidence consistent with the possibility of age-related recall bias (G. E. Simon and VonKorff 1995). In addition, findings from simulations suggest that it would not be difficult to produce cohort effects similar to those found in retrospective surveys by assuming plausible levels of censoring and recall biases (Giuffra and Risch 1994). However, other evidence suggests that the cohort effect might represent a real temporal increase and a narrowing of the gender difference. Data indicating the latter possibility come from several long-term prospective epidemiological surveys (Hagnell et al. 1982; Kessler and McRae 1981; Srole and Fisher 1980) and from time-series data on suicide rates.

One finding within the retrospective cohort data that is unlikely to be bias driven is that the cohort effect is much more pronounced for secondary major depression than for "pure" or primary major depression (Kessler et al. 1996). Specifically, disaggregated analyses of the NCS data suggest that the lifetime prevalence of primary major depression (that is, major depression that occurred in people who had no history of a prior psychiatric disorder) has not changed over the past four decades. The prevalence of major depression subsequent to other disorders, in comparison, increased substantially over this same period. It is unlikely that such a finding is caused by recall bias. Indeed, in light of the fact that comorbid depression is generally more severe than pure depression (Kessler et al. 1996) and the plausible assumption that severe disorders are less likely to go unreported than nonsevere disorders, we might expect the opposite pattern to have occurred if recall error explained the cohort effect. Another finding that we would not expect if recall error were the primary reason for the observed intercohort difference in the survey data is that the concentration of the cohort effect in secondary depression would be attributable to increases in the prevalences of other primary disorders, such as anxiety and drug addiction, and not to increases in the transition probabilities from these primary disorders to secondary depression.

Summary of Epidemiological Studies

We have seen that there is a gender difference in onset risk of major depression that begins in the adolescent years and persists at least through the end of midlife. There appears to be no gender difference in chronicity of, recurrence of, or speed of episode recovery from major depression. It would seem likely from the available evidence that the gender difference in onset risk is genuine rather than attributable to men's relatively greater reluctance to admit depression or relatively poorer memory for past depressive episodes. The lifetime risk of major depression has increased over the past few decades, and the gender difference has increased with it. This cohort effect has been especially pronounced for secondary depression, due largely to an increase in the prevalences of primary anxiety disorders and primary addictive disorders.

Although we have not yet considered plausible etiological mechanisms in any detail, the evidence reviewed thus far seems to be inconsistent with the mood amplification hypothesis to the extent that this hypothesis implies that the depression of women should be more persistent than that of men. The data are also inconsistent with the gender-role hypothesis to the extent that this hypothesis predicts that the gender difference in onset risk should not begin until adulthood and that depression in women should be more chronic than that in men. However, there is an interesting finding suggesting that whereas the onset of the gender difference in low self-esteem, an important correlate of depression, occurs at the beginning of junior high school (typically the seventh grade) in parts of the country that have junior high schools, it is delayed until the beginning of senior high school (ninth grade) in parts of the country that do not have junior high schools (Simmons and Blythe 1987). This finding strongly suggests that environmental experiences, possibly related to the pressures associated with gender-role differentiation, are importantly involved in the gender difference in depression.

Other Possible Causes of Gender Differences in Depression

The Effect of Traumatic Experience

There are a number of directions one could imagine exploring to learn more about the gender difference in depression. My research group has taken one of these paths by looking at differential exposure and vulnerability to environmental experiences that might either trigger or predispose to the onset of depression. We have been especially interested in adverse experiences that are more likely to happen to women than to men and that might have become increasingly prevalent in recent cohorts. One class of experiences of special interest that we have examined in the NCS involves rape and other forms of sexual trauma. We know that these events are much more likely to occur to women than to men, that their frequency has been increasing over time, and that they are powerful predictors of the 2:1 higher prevalence of posttraumatic stress disorder (PTSD) among women than among men in the United States (Kessler et al. 1995). Indeed, our analyses suggest that if we were able to prevent all sexual trauma from occurring, the observed gender difference in PTSD would totally disappear (Kessler et al. 1995).

Might it be that sexual trauma also plays a major part in the higher risk of major depression among women than men? We investigated this question in the NCS. When we controlled for rape and other forms of sexual trauma in a conventional survival analysis in which exposure to these traumas was treated as a series of time-varying predictors of first onset of major depression, the residual gender difference in risk of first onset of depression was halved. It seems that the fact that women are more likely than men to be exposed to sexual trauma does explain a substantial part of the observed gender difference in depression. It is important to clarify what we mean by "explain." There are a great many different types of traumatic life experiences. Some of them, like rape, are more likely to occur to women, and others, such as combat exposure in a war, are more likely to occur to men. If we focus exclusively on the former, it is not difficult to "explain" the higher risk of depression among women than men. This is not a trivial exercise. It is of real interest to know that we can explain fully half the gender difference in depression by taking into consideration both the prevalence of exposure to rape and the impact of rape on depression. But it is a somewhat artificial exercise. It is not terribly surprising to find that a simulation of the expected impact on depression of eradicating all the bad things that happen to women but not those that happen to men produces a greater reduction in the predicted levels of depression among women than men.

The more interesting exercise is to compare the relative importance of the traumatic stresses that typically occur to women with those that typically occur to men. We did this in the NCS by estimating a more complex survival model in which we controlled for sexual trauma, combat exposure in a war, other kinds of assaultive violence such as mugging, and a wide range of other traumatic experiences such as the sudden, unexpected death of a loved one; exposure to a natural disaster, being involved in a life-threatening accident, witnessing the death or serious injury of another person, and discovering a traumatic experience that occurred to a close loved one. We found quite a different result than when we controlled only for sexual trauma (Kendler et al. 1997). While the female:male odds ratio for risk of major depression in the survival model without any controls was approximately 1.9 (i.e., women had a 90% higher odds of depression than men) and the odds ratio in the model controlling only for sexual trauma was approximately 1.45 (i.e., the excess risk among women in the uncontrolled model was halved), the odds ratio in the model that controlled for all of the more than two dozen types of trauma assessed in the NCS yielded a residual female:male odds ratio of 2.0, virtually the same as when there were no controls at all. Furthermore, when we focused on the subsample of respondents who reported never experiencing any of the traumas assessed in the survey, the female:male odds ratio was 1.9. These results strongly suggest that differences in trauma exposure do not explain an important part of the observed gender difference in depression.

The Effect of Prior Psychopathology

Breslau et al. (1995) hypothesized that the gender difference in depression is partly due to a difference in prior anxiety. Breslau supported this claim by showing that the odds ratio of gender predicting major depression substantially attenuates when controls are introduced for the prior existence of anxiety. A similar result was recently reported by Wilhelm et al. (1997). This finding is indirectly consistent with the finding, reported above, that the cohort effect for major depression is largely confined to secondary depression. However, this finding is limited in the same way as the finding regarding sexual trauma in that it focuses on a predictor that is more characteristic of women (i.e., anxiety) and ignores other comparable predictors that are more characteristic of men (e.g., alcohol/drug abuse, conduct disorder, antisocial personality disorder).

In an effort to investigate this issue, we replicated the result of Breslau and colleagues (1995) in the NCS by estimating a series of survival models to predict first onset of major depression. The only predictor used in the first model was gender. As previously reported, the female:male odds ratio in this model was 1.9. The second model introduced a series of controls for prior anxiety disorders (panic, simple phobia, social phobia, agoraphobia, generalized anxiety disorder, and posttraumatic stress disorder). Consistent with Breslau et al. (1995), we found that the introduction of these controls reduced the female:male odds ratio to 1.6. However, we also estimated a third model in which we controlled for prior substance use disorders and conduct disorder rather than prior anxiety disorders. The female:male odds ratio in this third model increased to 2.4. What this means is that the higher risk of depression among women versus men would be even greater than it is were it not for the fact that men are more likely than women to have a history of substance abuse and conduct problems. Finally, we estimated a model in which we controlled simultaneously for prior anxiety disorders, substance use disorders, and conduct disorder. The female:male odds ratio in this fourth model was 1.9—exactly what it was in the model that had no controls. Furthermore, in the subsample of respondents with no history of any of these prior disorders, the female:male odds ratio was 2.2.

These results show clearly, contrary to Breslau et al.'s conclusion, that a history of prior psychiatric disorders does not play an important part in explaining the observed gender difference in onset risk of major depression in the NCS data. However, as reported by Breslau in the current volume, prior anxiety *did* explain the gender difference in depression in her Detroit data even when analyses were carried out in the way we did here (Breslau et al., Chapter 7, this volume). It would be useful to investigate the effects of prior disorders in other data sets in order to determine the generalizability of our results in the NCS.

The Effect of Childhood Experience

We next adjusted for retrospective reports about the child-rearing style experienced by respondents, reasoning that parents are likely to be more overprotective of female than male children and that this might play some part in the subsequent gender difference in depression. Parker's Parental Bonding Instrument (Parker et al. 1979) was used to measure maternal and paternal warmth and overprotectiveness. This had no effect on the female:male odds ratio. We then controlled for size of sibship and birth order, thinking that women who were oldest children or perhaps only children might have had mastery experiences as part of their childhood socialization that placed them at lower risk of depression. No effects of this sort were found either in models that controlled for these factors or in more complex models that studied gender differences in depression onset risk within subsamples defined in terms of the cross-classification of sibship size and birth order. Finally, we constructed subsamples defined in terms of complex multivariate profiles of life histories involving the conjunction of childhood socialization experiences, social class origins, trauma exposure, and subsequent adult roles. The relationship between gender and onset risk of depression was found to be the same in all of these subsamples.

Gender Differences in Current Depression

This is not to say that the gender difference in current depression is the same in all of these subsamples. For example, it has been known for nearly two decades, since the early empirical studies of the relationship between gender roles and mental illness (e.g., Gove 1972; Gove and Tudor 1973), that the gender difference in depressed mood is stronger for married people than for the unmarried. The same is true for current major depression. But contrary to the interpretation of gender-role theorists, this pattern is not due to a greater protective effect of marriage on men than on women. As previously noted, the gender difference in risk of first onset of major depression is the same among married as among never-married or previously married individuals. Instead, there are two other processes at work that lead to a stronger gender difference in depression among married versus unmarried people.

First, our analyses of the NCS data show that depression has different consequences for men and for women, including different effects on educational attainment, teen childbearing, marital timing, marital stability, selection into a violent marriage, and selection into other forms of adversity associated with employment, interpersonal relations, finances, and health. Second, although there is no gender difference in the chronicity or recurrence of major depression, the environmental experiences that are associated with chronicity and recurrence are different for men and women. For example, financial pressures are more depressogenic for men than for women, and family problems are more depressogenic for women than for men. Together, these two processes create variation in the relationship between gender and current depression across sectors of the population defined in terms of roles. It is a mistake to be misled into thinking that these findings afford insight into the causes of the gender differences in depression.

An important example of this confusion can be found in the recent work of Nazroo et al. (1997) on the differential effects of life events on men and women. Nazroo and colleagues argue that the gender difference in risk of past-year episodes of major depression is due in large part to a greater vulnerability in women to the effects of stressful life events and difficulties. However, given that the vast majority (>90% in the NCS) of past-year episodes of major depression in the adult general population are recurrences rather than first episodes, this line of thinking is attempting to explain something that does not exist: a gender difference in recurrence risk of depression.

How is it that Nazroo et al. (1997) were able to find a gender difference in their analysis if no such difference exists? The answer is that by failing to distinguish first episodes from recurrences in the analysis of past-year episode onset, Nazroo et al. confounded three separable processes: 1) the gender difference in risk of first onset in the subsample of respondents who had never been depressed before the past year (a difference that was statistically significant); 2) the gender difference in recurrence risk in the subsample of respondents who were asymptomatic at the beginning of the past-year but who subsequently experienced a recurrence of major depression (a difference that was not significant); and 3) the gender difference in the proportion of respondents who had an elevated risk of episode onset by virtue of having a history of depression (a difference that was significant).

Furthermore, exposure to stressful life experiences is higher among people with a history of depression than among those without such a history. In addition, the impact of stress on the onset of depressive episodes is stronger among people with a history of depression than among those without such a history. Given that women are more likely than men to have a history of depression, these differences in exposure and impact will create the impression that the higher rate of past-year episode onset among women versus men is due to a combination of differential exposure and differential reactivity to stress, when in fact the higher rate is largely due to a higher proportion of women than men having a history of depression and to the fact that such a history is associated with risk of subsequent episode onset.

To illustrate: The female:male odds ratio for past-year episode onset of major depression in the total NCS sample was 2.2. This odds ratio was reduced by controlling for past-year stressful events and difficulties. However, when we disaggregated the data into the subsample of respondents with a history of depression, the odds ratio became 1.0, regardless of whether past-year stress was controlled. By comparison, the odds ratio was 2.6 in the subsample of respondents with no prior history of depression before controlling for stress. This odds ratio decreased to 2.3 after controlling for stress. There was no significant interaction between gender and stress in predicting past-year first onset of major depression.

Our work with the NCS has shown that a number of putative predictors of the gender difference in depression work in exactly the same way. One of the most important of these predictors is personality. There has been considerable discussion of the possibility that personality differences account for the higher prevalence of depression among women than among men. Low self-esteem, interpersonal dependency, pessimistic attributional style, low perceived control, expressiveness, and instrumentality have all been implicated in this way (Abrahams et al. 1978; Abramson and Andrews 1982; Bassoff and Glass 1982; Baucom and Danker-Brown 1984; Klerman and Hirshfeld 1988; Nolen-Hoeksema 1987; Whiteley 1985). However, few of the empirical studies that have documented these effects controlled for prior history of depression, and those that did failed to find powerful effects of personality on the gender difference in depression (Hirshfeld et al. 1983, 1984). When we carried out similar analyses in the NCS, we found that personality differences appeared to explain part of the association between gender and current depression in the total sample when we did not control for a prior history of depression. When we *did* control for history, however, all such significant associations disappeared.

Summary

I have attempted to clarify what it is that we need to explain when considering the gender difference in depression. We must explain why women are more likely than men to have a first onset of depression beginning in adolescence and continuing through the end of midlife. As I have tried to demonstrate, much previous research and theorizing is ill conceived because it labors to explain a gender difference in the chronicity of depression when in fact such a difference does not exist. Nor is there a gender difference in past-year recurrence of depression or in speed of episode recovery from depression. Theories and empirical studies that are designed to explain these nonexistent differences are fatally flawed.

I have also attempted to focus future research by presenting evidence that allows us to discard otherwise plausible hypotheses. Based on the evidence reviewed in this chapter, it seems unlikely that the gender difference in onset risk of major depression is due to a higher rate of dissembling on the part of men compared with women. Nor is it likely that gender differences in mood amplification or in exposure or reactivity to traumatic life experiences or recent major stressors are involved. This means that interventions aimed at these factors are unlikely to result in a decrease in the gender difference in depression. The same can be said for interventions aimed at changing socialization experiences linked to the ways in which parents relate to their sons and daughters. Finally, there is no evidence that a history of prior psychiatric disorder is involved in the gender difference in depression. Instead, sex hormones, genes, subtle socialization experiences, and gender-role-related experiences that create vulnerabilities to depression remain as plausible possibilities.

As noted above, exciting new initiatives are under way to study the effects of hormones on gender differences in depression. Other studies are in progress to examine gender differences in depression among twins in ways that could yield insight into genetic influences. Also under way are several new NIMH initiatives designed to carry out prospective studies of child and adolescent mental health in ways that are apt to shed light on reasons for the emergence of the gender difference in onset risk in adolescence.

It is important that the investigators in these studies clearly focus on what they are trying to explain. This is a very complex problem, and it is easy to become distracted by patterns in the data that are due to differential consequences of depression rather than to differential causes. It is also easy to lose sight of the fact that we need to explain onset risk rather than other aspects of depression. If we can avoid these pitfalls and blind alleys, the new and exciting research currently being conducted may well be able to expand our understanding and facilitate the development of interventions that will help reduce the risk of depression in women and men alike.

Acknowledgments

The National Comorbidity Survey (NCS) is a collaborative epidemiological study of the prevalences, causes, and consequences of psychiatric morbidity and comorbidity in the United States that is supported by the National Institute of Mental Health, the National Institute on Drug Abuse, and the W. T. Grant Foundation. Collaborating NCS sites and investigators are as follows: The Addiction Research Foundation (Robin Room), Duke University Medical Center (Dan Blazer, Marvin Swartz), Harvard Medical School (Richard Frank, Ronald Kessler), Johns Hopkins University (James Anthony, William Eaton, Philip Leaf), the Max Planck Institute of Psychiatry Clinical Institute (Hans-Ulrich Wittchen), the Medical College of Virginia (Kenneth Kendler), the University of Miami (R. Jay Turner), the University of Michigan (Lloyd Johnston, Roderick Little), New York University (Patrick Shrout), the State University of New York at Stony Brook (Evelyn Bromet), and Washington University School of Medicine (Linda Cottler, Andrew Heath).

A complete list of all NCS publications, along with abstracts, study documentation, interview schedules, and the raw NCS public-use data files, can be obtained directly from the NCS home page (http://www.hcp.med.harvard.edu/ncs).

References

Abrahams B, Feldman S, Nash SC: Sex-role self concept and sex-role attitudes: enduring personality characteristics or adaptations to changing life situations? Dev Psychol 14:393–400, 1978

Abramson LY, Andrews DE: Cognitive models of depression: implications for sex differences in vulnerability to depression. International Journal of Mental Health 11:77–94, 1982

Almeida DM, Kessler RC: Everyday stressful events and gender differences in daily distress. J Pers Soc Psychol 75:670–680, 1998

American Psychiatric Association: Diagnostic and Statistical Manual of Mental Disorders, 3rd Edition, Revised. Washington, DC, American Psychiatric Association, 1987

Angold A, Worthman CW: Puberty onset of gender differences in rates of depression: a developmental, epidemiologic and neuroendocrine perspective. J Affect Disord 29:145–158, 1993

Angold A, Costello EJ, Worthman CW: Puberty and depression: the roles of age, pubertal status, and pubertal timing. Psychol Med 28:51–61, 1998

Angst J, Dobler-Mikola A: Do the diagnostic criteria determine the sex ratio in depression? J Affect Disord 7:189–198, 1984

Bassoff ES, Glass GV: The relationship between sex roles and mental health: a meta-analysis of twenty-six studies. The Counseling Psychologist 10:105–112, 1982

Baucom DH, Danker-Brown P: Sex role identity and sex stereotyped tasks in the development of learned helplessness in women. J Pers Soc Psychol 46:422–430, 1984

Bebbington PE: The social epidemiology of clinical depression, in Handbook of Social Psychiatry. Edited by Henderson AS, Burrows GD. Amsterdam, Elsevier, 1988, pp 87–102

Bebbington PE, Hurry J, Tennant C, et al: The epidemiology of mental disorders in Camberwell. Psychol Med 11:561–579, 1981

Bland RC, Newman SC, Orn H: Period prevalence of psychiatric disorders in Edmonton. Acta Psychiatr Scand Suppl 338:33–42, 1988a

Bland RC, Orn H, Newman SC: Lifetime prevalence of psychiatric disorders in Edmonton. Acta Psychiatr Scand Suppl 338:24–32, 1988b

Blazer DG, Kessler RC, McGonagle KA, et al: The prevalence and distribution of major depression in a national community sample: the National Comorbidity Survey. Am J Psychiatry 151:979–986, 1994

Breslau N, Schultz L, Peterson E: Sex differences in depression: a role for preexisting anxiety. Psychiatry Res 58:1–12, 1995

Brim OG, Featherman D: Surveying midlife development in the United States. Aging and Society (in press)

Canino GJ, Bird HR, Shrout PE, et al: The prevalence of specific psychiatric disorders in Puerto Rico. Arch Gen Psychiatry 44:727–735, 1987

Cheng TA: Sex difference in the prevalence of minor psychiatric morbidity: a social epidemiological study in Taiwan. Acta Psychiatr Scand 80:395–407, 1989

Clancy K, Gove W: Sex differences in mental illness: an analysis of response bias in self-reports. American Journal of Clinical Hypnosis 14:205–216, 1972

Ernst C, Angst J: The Zurich Study, XII: sex difference in depression—evidence from longitudinal epidemiological data. Eur Arch Psychiatry Clin Neurosci 241:222–230, 1992

Giuffra LA, Risch N: Diminished recall and the cohort effect of major depression: a simulation study. Psychol Med 24:375–383, 1994

Gove WR: The relationship between sex roles, marital status, and mental illness. Social Forces 51:34–44, 1972

Gove WR: Sex differences in mental illness among adult men and women: an evaluation of four questions raised regarding the evidence on the higher rates of women. Soc Sci Med 12(3B):187–198, 1978

Gove WR, Geerken MR: Response bias in surveys of mental health: an empirical investigation. American Journal of Sociology 82:1289–1317, 1977

Gove WR, Tudor JF: Adult sex roles and mental illness. American Journal of Sociology 78:812–835, 1973

Hagnell O, Lanke J, Rorsman B, et al: Are we entering an age of melancholy? Depressive illness in a prospective epidemiological study over 25 years: the Lundby Study, Sweden. Psychol Med 12:279–289, 1982

Hansell S, Mechanic D: The socialization of introspection and illness behavior, in Illness Behavior: A Multidisciplinary Model. Edited by McHugh S, Vallis TM. New York, Plenum, 1986, pp 253–260

Hirshfeld RMA, Klerman GL, Clayton PJ, et al: Assessing personality: effects of the depressive state on trait measurement. Am J Psychiatry 140:695–699, 1983

Hirshfeld RMA, Klerman GL, Clayton PJ, et al: Personality and gender-related differences in depression. J Affect Disord 7:211–221, 1984

Hwu HG, Yeh EK, Chang LY: Prevalence of psychiatric disorders in Taiwan defined by the Chinese Diagnostic Interview Schedule. Acta Psychiatr Scand 79:136–147, 1989

Kendler KS, Neale MC, Kessler RC, et al: A population-based twin study of major depression in women: the impact of varying definitions of illness. Arch Gen Psychiatry 49:257–266, 1992

Kendler KS, Neale MC, Kessler RC, et al: A longitudinal twin study of 1-year prevalence of major depression in women. Arch Gen Psychiatry 50:843–852, 1993

Kendler KS, Davis CG, Kessler RC: The familial aggregation of common psychiatric and substance abuse disorders in the National Comorbidity Survey: a family history study. Br J Psychiatry 170:541–548, 1997

Kessler RC, McRae JA: Trends in sex and psychological distress. American Sociological Review 41:443–452, 1981

Kessler RC, McGonagle KA, Swartz M, et al: Sex and depression in the National Comorbidity Survey, I: lifetime prevalence, chronicity and recurrence. J Affect Disord 29:85–96, 1993

Kessler RC, McGonagle KA, Nelson CB, et al: Sex and depression in the National Comorbidity Survey, II: cohort effects. J Affect Disord 30:15–26, 1994

Kessler RC, Sonnega A, Bromet E, et al: Posttraumatic stress disorder in the National Comorbidity Survey. Arch Gen Psychiatry 52:1048–1060, 1995

Kessler RC, Nelson CB, McGonagle KA, et al: Comorbidity of DSM-III-R major depressive disorder in the general population: results from the US National Comorbidity Survey. Br J Psychiatry 168:17–30, 1996

Kessler RC, Zhao S, Blazer DG, et al: Prevalence, correlates, and course of minor depression and major depression in the National Comorbidity Survey. J Affect Disord 45:19–30, 1997

Kessler RC, Mroczek DK, Belli RF: Retrospective adult assessment of childhood psychopathology, in Assessment in Adolescent Child Psychopathology. Edited by Schaffer D, Richters J. New York, Guilford (in press)

Klerman GL, Hirshfeld RMA: Personality as a vulnerability factor: with special attention to clinical depression, in Handbook of Social Psychiatry. Edited by Henderson AS, Burrows JD. New York, Elsevier, 1988, pp 41–53

Lee CK, Han JH, Choi JO: The epidemiological study of mental disorders in Korea, IX: alcoholism, anxiety and depression. Seoul Journal of Psychiatry 12:183–191, 1987

McGrath E, Keita GP, Strickland BR, et al. (eds): Women and Depression: Risk Factors and Treatment Issues. Washington, DC, American Psychological Association, 1990

McLeod JD, Kessler RC, Landis RK: Speed of recovery from major depressive episodes in a community sample of married men and women. J Abnorm Psychol 101:277–286, 1992

Mirowsky J, Ross CE: Social Causes of Psychological Distress. New York, Aldine De Gruyter, 1989

Nazroo JY, Edwards AC, Brown GW: Gender differences in the onset of depression following a shared life event: a study of couples. Psychol Med 27:9–19, 1997

Nolen-Hoeksema S: Sex differences in unipolar depression: evidence and theory. Psychol Bull 101:259–282, 1987

Nolen-Hoeksema S, Morrow J, Fredrickson BL: Response styles and the duration of episodes of depressed mood. J Abnorm Psychol 102:20–28, 1993

Nolen-Hoeksema S, Parker LE, Larsen J: Ruminative coping with depressed mood following loss. J Pers Soc Psychol 67:92–104, 1994

Parker G, Tupling H, Brown LB: A parental bonding instrument. Br J Med Psychol 152:1–10, 1979

Phillips D, Segal B: Sexual status and psychiatric symptoms. American Sociological Review 34:58–72, 1969

Sherbourn CD, Wells KB, Hays RD, et al: Subthreshold depression and depressive disorder: clinical characteristics of general medical and mental health specialty outpatients. Am J Psychiatry 151:1777–1784, 1994

Simmons RG, Blythe DA: Moving Into Adolescence: The Impact of Pubertal Change and School Context. New York, Aldine De Gruyter, 1987

Simon GE, VonKorff M: Recall of psychiatric history in cross-sectional surveys: implications for epidemiologic research. Epidemiol Rev 17:221–227, 1995

Simon RW: Gender, multiple roles, role meaning, and mental health. J Health Soc Behav 36:182–194, 1995

Simpson HB, Nee JC, Endicott J: First-episode major depression: few sex differences in course. Arch Gen Psychiatry 54:633–639, 1997

Srole L, Fisher AK: The Midtown Manhattan Longitudinal Study vs. the Mental Paradise Lost doctrine: a controversy joined. Arch Gen Psychiatry 37:209–221, 1980

Weissman MM, Klerman GL: Sex differences and the epidemiology of depression. Arch Gen Psychiatry 34:98–111, 1977

Weissman MM, Klerman GL: Gender and depression. Trends Neurosci 8:416–420, 1985

Weissman MM, Klerman GL: Depression: current understanding and changing trends. Annu Rev Public Health 13:319–339, 1992

Weissman MM, Myers JK: Affective disorders in a U.S. urban community. Arch Gen Psychiatry 35:1304–1311, 1978

Weissman MM, Leaf PJ, Holzer CE III, et al: The epidemiology of depression: an update on sex differences in rates. J Affect Disord 7:179–188, 1984

Weissman MM, Bruce ML, Leaf PJ, et al: Affective disorders, in Psychiatric Disorders in America: The Epidemiologic Catchment Area Study. Edited by Robins LN, Regier DA. New York, Free Press, 1991, pp 53–80

Wells JE, Bushnell JA, Hornblow AR, et al: Christchurch Psychiatric Epidemiology Study, part I: methodology and lifetime prevalence for specific psychiatric disorders. Aust N Z J Psychiatry 23:315–326, 1989

Whiteley BE Jr: Sex role orientation and psychological well-being: two meta-analyses. Sex Roles 12:207–225, 1985

Wilhelm K, Parker G: Sex differences in lifetime depression rates: fact or artefact? Psychol Med 24:97–111, 1994

Wilhelm K, Parker G, Hadzi-Pavlovic D: Fifteen years on: evolving ideas in researching sex differences in depression. Psychol Med 27:875–883, 1997

Wittchen H-U, Essau CA, von Zerssen D, et al: Lifetime and six-month prevalence of mental disorders in the Munich Follow-Up Study. Eur Arch Psychiatry Clin Neurosci 241:247–258, 1992

Young MA, Fogg LF, Scheftner WA, et al: Sex differences in the lifetime prevalence of depression. J Affect Disord 18:187–192, 1990

CHAPTER 5

Pubertal Changes and Adolescent Challenges

Why Do Rates of Depression Rise Precipitously for Girls Between Ages 10 and 15 Years?

Ellen Frank, Ph.D.
Elizabeth Young, M.D.

An early memory, from fourth or fifth grade: I am walking down the hallway close to the walls, looking at the floor, because I feel I am not good enough to take up space or to look people in the eye. Why? I don't know. Another memory: sitting behind the toilet in the girls' restroom, my head on my knees and my arms wrapped around my legs. I am not crying. Nobody knows I am there. I am just wordlessly sad. . . .

On hot spring nights, I would wake up at 4 A.M. and lie sleepless until daylight, hearing the insistent song of a mockingbird over the frantic beating of my heart. Other times, I flew into rages over minor

This work was supported in part by National Institute of Mental Health (NIMH) grants 29618 (Dr. Frank), 49115 (Dr. Frank), 50030 (Dr. Young), and 00427 (Dr. Young), and by the MacArthur Foundation Network on Psychopathology and Development (Dr. Frank) and was initiated while the first author was a Fellow at the Center for Advanced Study in the Behavioral Sciences, where support was provided by the John D. and Catherine T. MacArthur Foundation. The authors are grateful for the thoughtful comments of Floyd Bloom, M.D., Thomas Boyce, M.D., Judith Cameron, Ph.D., William Durham, Ph.D., David J. Kupfer, M.D., and M. Katherine Shear, M.D., on the hypothesis proposed in this chapter.

> provocations. In my senior year of high school, crushed over an unrequited love, I swallowed half a bottle of aspirin, the first of a series of suicidal gestures. The aspirin only made me sick. . . .
>
> The most troublesome symptom was my inability to concentrate. It was as if my brain had a short circuit. One day I was beginning an interview, pen and paper in hand, and had to ask my interviewee's name three times before I could remember it long enough to write it down. . . .
>
> Tracy Thompson,
> *The Washington Post,*
> October 20, 1992, pp. Z10–Z14

Washington Post reporter Thompson's poignant description of her personal experience of depression makes several important points about this disorder: 1) it often begins in early adolescence; 2) many episodes of depression follow experiences of interpersonal loss or rejection; 3) it can have a devastating impact on one's ability to engage in the simplest tasks of everyday life; 4) it disproportionately targets females relative to males; and 5) it can be deadly. Often referred to as the "common cold" of mental illness, major depression is at least twice as likely to strike women as men at least once during their lifetimes (Kessler et al. 1993; Weissman et al. 1991, 1993).

Multiple reviews have been undertaken of the evidence for the existence of a gender difference in lifetime rates of depression as well as of the biological and psychosocial correlates of depressive conditions that differ in men and women (Nolen-Hoeksema 1991; Nolen-Hoeksema et al. 1993; Weissman and Klerman 1977; Wolk and Weissman 1995). However, all of these reviews have focused on the entire life span, and none has reached fully satisfactory explanations for the observed differences. In this chapter, we focus instead on the 5-year interval in development at which the gender difference in depression seems to manifest itself.

In their 1977 review of gender differences in depression, Weissman and Klerman devoted considerable attention to the issue of whether the apparent predominance of women among those with major depression was real or merely a function of the greater likelihood of treatment seeking on the part of women. There are now numerous well-designed studies of appropriately ascertained samples from the general community (Canino et al. 1987; Chen et al. 1993; Ernst and Angst 1992; Hwu et al. 1989; Karam 1991; Wittchen et al. 1992). All of these studies suggest that lifetime rates of major depression are higher in women.

As Wolk and Weissman (1995) point out in their recent review of this issue, we can now also turn to a series of well-designed epidemiological studies conducted outside the United States, including studies from the Far East and Africa, to examine the question of the validity of the observed gender difference in rates of depression. A cross-national collaborative group was formed and has reported on gender differences in depression for a total of 10 international sites. Although the female:male ratio varies from a high of 3.5:1 in Munich, Germany, to a low of 1.6:1 in Beirut and Taiwan, the consistent evidence for a female preponderance is striking. Indeed, the female:male ratios vary less than the overall lifetime prevalence rates, which range from a low of 1.5 in Taiwan to a high of 19.0 in Beirut.

It now seems clear that in broad-based community studies, women predominate among those with a lifetime history of major depression. Furthermore, this predominance obtains across a wide range of birth cohorts and diverse cultures.

What Might Account for the Gender Difference in Lifetime Risk?

As Weissman and Klerman pointed out in 1977, there are at least three ways in which a true predominance of females among those with major depression could occur: 1) by genetic transmission as an X-linked trait, 2) as a result of women's unique biology, and 3) as a consequence of women's unique psychosocial experiences. A possibility that these authors alluded to but did not address directly is that the predominance of depression among women could be a function of an *interaction* between women's unique biological endowment and their psychosocial experiences.

Genetic Transmission?

Merikangas et al. (1985) effectively demonstrated that intergenerational patterns of transmission of major depression are such as to preclude the possibility of a genetic explanation for women's greater risk. Examining risk of major depression in the first-degree relatives of male and female probands, they found the expected doubling of risk among female relatives but no difference whatever in the relative risk to relatives of females as opposed to males. If depression were an X-linked trait, the relatives of female probands would have demonstrated increased risk. Below we argue that women's unique biology is not *responsible* for women's greater vulnerability to depression; rather, that biology sets the stage upon which women's psychosocial experiences will be played, and this stage is quite different from the one upon which men's experiences unfold.

Women's Biology: Are Ovarian Steroids to Blame?

Although the data clearly indicate that lifetime rates of major depression increase around the time of menarche and that the gender bias is also established at that time, it is unlikely that ovarian steroids are directly responsible for mood changes. In women who suffer from depression, it is the periods of *withdrawal* from ovarian steroids that correlate with increased susceptibility to depression and not the periods of high estrogen and progesterone. Thus, in most depressed women we note exacerbations of symptoms during the premenstrual period, a time when hormones are falling, not rising. Premenstrual dysphoric disorder (PMDD), a cyclic mood disorder, is one of the best-studied mood disorders with regard to the influence of ovarian steroids on mood. If we examine PMDD as a model of hormonally induced depression, we find again that it is not the hormones themselves that cause depression; rather, depression occurs during the phase of hormone withdrawal. This finding previously led some individuals to propose that progesterone withdrawal was the cause of premenstrual syndrome (PMS) and to use progesterone as a treatment; however, all of the placebo-controlled blind trials with progesterone failed to find any effectiveness for progesterone treatment. The only agents that alleviate PMDD are antidepressants, particularly the selective serotonin reuptake inhibitors (SSRIs) (Steiner et al. 1995; Stone et al. 1991; Wood et al. 1992; Mortola 1993; Yonkers et al. 1997), or treatments that block menstrual cycling (e.g., leuprolide; C. S. Brown et al. 1994). Studies by Schmidt and Rubinow (1991) demonstrating that PMS could occur in the absence of a luteal phase and progesterone rise have led these investigators to hypothesize that PMS is a mood disorder "entrained" to the menstrual cycle rather than caused by ovarian steroid changes. Thus, even PMS is not clearly caused by ovarian steroids. Furthermore, studies in women without mood disorders (Montgomery et al. 1987) have demonstrated that estrogen improves mood and outlook on life, again suggesting that even if estrogen increases vulnerability to depression, this effect is not attributable to a depressogenic effect of ovarian steroids.

Other possible mechanisms include effects of estrogen and progesterone on brain norepinephrine and serotonin systems, systems that have been linked to depression. However, estrogen decreases norepinephrine uptake, thus increasing norepinephrine availability at the synapse, effects that form the therapeutic basis of a number of antidepressants. Estrogen increases the number of serotonin (5-hydroxytryptophan [5-HT]) receptors, particularly 5-HT_2 (Biegon and McEwen 1982)—again, an effect seen following treatment with antidepressant drugs. These data suggest that estrogen *does* modulate these neurotransmitter systems; however, its effects are in the direction observed with antidepressant treatment. Although this finding is in accord with clinical experience that the addition of estrogen to an antidepressant regimen can improve response, it argues against the hypothesis that ovarian steroids are in themselves depressogenic.

Psychosocial Experience: Are Women's Roles to Blame?

Those who have focused on psychosocial variables as explanatory of women's greater vulnerability to depression have generally pointed to four kinds of experiences that are more common in females than in males: childhood sexual abuse, adult experiences of sexual or physical victimization, marital dissatisfaction, and a subordinate social role associated with restricted financial and occupational opportunities. In 1991,

Cutler and Nolen-Hoeksema reviewed the literature on the prevalence of childhood sexual abuse. They concluded that in college students (Finkelhor 1979), probability samples of adults (Kercher and McShane 1984; Burnam et al. 1988), or probability samples of children (Finkelhor 1984), rates of childhood sexual abuse in females were estimated to be double that in males. In a 3-year prevalence study, Bifulco and colleagues (1991) convincingly demonstrated that women with a history of childhood sexual abuse have more than double the rate of major depression compared with women with no such history. With respect to the relationship between rape victimization and depression, our own research group (Frank and Stewart 1984) found that among women contacting a rape crisis center and assessed within 4 weeks of an assault, 43% met Research Diagnostic Criteria (RDC; Spitzer et al. 1978) for major depression. Kilpatrick et al. (1992) studied a nationally representative sample with respect to crime victimization and found that 30% of those who reported having been victims of rape met criteria for major depression at some point following the assault, and that 13% had made a suicide attempt at some time during that period.

Numerous studies have pointed to the relationship between marital dysfunction and depression in women, especially among those women who were not employed. One particularly striking example is Aneshensel's (1986) study of a random community sample of 590 Los Angeles women. Aneshensel found that married and employed women who reported marital strain but no work strain had a relative risk of 2.63 for depression as compared with married employed women who reported neither marital strain nor work strain. However, the most striking finding was the relative risk of depression among married, unemployed women reporting marital strain: their risk of depression was 5.47 times that of the women reporting neither marital nor work strain.

How Much of Women's Social Experience Is Relevant to Differences in Lifetime Rates of Depression?

If it were the case that a substantial proportion of the excess in lifetime rates of major depression resulted from first onsets during adulthood, the negative psychosocial experiences described above (with the exception of childhood sexual abuse) might well account for the gender difference in depression. Although these psychosocial experiences may indeed be related to the *maintenance* of depressive illness in adult women and to their *risk of recurrence* of depression, such negative events occurring in adult life cannot explain the emerging data suggesting that much of the excess in lifetime risk of depression for women can be attributed to onsets occurring in early adolescence.

Increasing evidence indicates that the excess in lifetime rates of major depression in women can be accounted for by a dramatic shift in relative lifetime prevalence between the ages of 10 and 15 years (Angold and Rutter 1992; Breslau et al. 1995; Kessler et al. 1993). Prior to age 10, there are no differences in lifetime rates for boys and girls. Shortly thereafter, rates begin to climb dramatically for girls. By age 15 years, the lifetime risk of major depression for males and females has achieved relative proportions that essentially do not change for at least the next 35–40 years (Kessler et al. 1993).

One of the major advances in our understanding of the epidemiology of depression in the last 20 years has been the recognition that children suffer from a clinical syndrome very similar, if not identical, to the major depression of adults. This recognition has led to studies examining the epidemiology of first onsets in children and adolescents. Angold and Rutter (1992), examining a clinical sample of more than 3,500 child psychiatric patients ranging in age from 8 to 16 years, found that both boys and girls showed increasing levels of depression across this age range; however, the rate of increase was significantly faster in girls once the children reached age 11. By age 16 years, girls were twice as likely as boys to evidence significant depressive symptomatology.

Examining data from their National Comorbidity Survey, Kessler and colleagues (1993, 1994) reported a similar finding for first onsets of major depression in a large, nationally representative community sample. Although boys and girls showed no evidence of differences in early childhood, by age 15 years there was a 2:1 ratio of females to males in first onsets. Kessler et al. argued that whereas lifetime rates of major depression continue to rise throughout the life cycle, the female:male ratio remains relatively constant at approximately 2:1 after age 15 years. This finding has now been replicated in two additional studies based on community samples (Breslau et al. 1995; B. R. Hinden, B. E. Compas, J. K. Connor, T. M. Achenbach, C. Hammen, G. Oppedisano, and C. A.

Gerhardt, "Gender Differences in Depressive Symptoms in Adolescence: Age Differences and Age Changes in a National Sample of Youth" [unpublished manuscript], August 1999).

Absolute rates of depression continue to rise until at least middle age for both men and women (Kessler et al. 1993; Weissman et al. 1991); however, almost all of the difference in relative lifetime risk can be accounted for by the changes that occur during the brief period when girls are making the pubertal/adolescent transition. Thus, examining this period between the ages of 10 and 15 years appears to be critical to understanding why females are more likely than males to experience depression.

This time period between ages 10 and 15 years is one of dramatic change in both the biological and the psychosocial spheres. The biological changes of puberty have multiple marked effects on brain function; likewise, the psychosocial challenges of adolescence call for a broad range of new behaviors and skills. Which of these changes should we blame for the rapid rise in incidence of depression in young women? Or is there some way in which these two developmental milestones interact to leave young women especially vulnerable to syndromal depression?

If a very substantial proportion of the difference between males and females in terms of lifetime risk of major depression occurs in the period between the ages of 10 and 15 years, any understanding of why females are more likely than males to experience depression should focus on understanding the interplay of risk and protective factors influencing girls and boys as they pass through the biological transition of puberty and confront the psychosocial challenges of adolescence. The fact that these two key life transitions overlap temporally suggests that we should look for possible synergy between the physiological changes associated with the pubertal transition and the psychosocial challenges associated with the transition into adolescence as they relate to the onset of depression.

What Is Occurring Between Ages 10 and 15 That Might Explain the Dramatic Rise in Depression Among Females?

In addition to dramatic changes in gonadal steroids occurring between 10 and 15 years of age, young women (and young men) undergo equally dramatic changes in social roles, social role expectations, and the structure of their school and social environments. Profound morphological changes and very pronounced changes are also taking place in hormones other than the gonadal steroids—hormones that, until recently, have largely been ignored in the search for explanations of the gender difference in major depression.

Oxytocin and Why It Might Be Important Between Ages 10 and 15 Years

Puberty is accompanied by increases in ovarian steroids and the onset of monthly cycling of these hormones in women. However, as we have previously argued, it seems unlikely that increases in the production of gonadal steroids or the onset of cycling of gonadal steroids are responsible for the dramatic rise of rates of depression among females relative to males between 10 and 15 years of age. This leads one to ask whether there are other hormonal events occurring at puberty that might play a role.

Oxytocin is a complex and multipurpose peptide that undergoes a fivefold increase at puberty (Chibbar et al. 1990). Involved in food satiety and inhibition of sodium appetite (Stricker and Verbalis 1993), oxytocin is also released at orgasm, leading both to penile and uterine contractions that facilitate sperm transport and to sexual satiety. In the context of childbearing, superphysiological amounts of oxytocin are released and appear to have a role in promoting both parturition and lactation. However, perhaps the most interesting of oxytocin's effects are related to behavior.

One of the richest areas of study in the physiological underpinnings of behavior in recent times is the biology of affiliative behavior in animals. The term *affiliative behavior* encompasses the range of behaviors that promote physical contact, sexual contact, nurturance of the young, and, in humans, emotional connectedness. In animals, oxytocin appears to promote not only pair bonding—that is, the bonding of the male and female of the species at least for a breeding season—but also parental behavior. In humans and nonhuman primates, oxytocin seems to be related to peer bonding as well as pair bonding. Early studies in sheep clearly established that oxytocin played a major role in attachment and bonding

(Keverne and Kendrick 1992a, 1992b; Klopfer 1971). In rats, injection of oxytocin into the brain ventricular system can stimulate maternal behavior in virgin females (Pedersen and Prange 1979). In a series of experiments, Insel, Carter, and colleagues (Carter et al. 1992; Insel 1992; Insel and Hulihan 1995; Insel and Shapiro 1992; Insel et al. 1995; Winslow et al. 1983) demonstrated that differences in degree of parental care between the prairie vole and the montane vole are mediated by differences in oxytocin receptor number and distribution in the brain, thus implicating oxytocin in the expression of these behaviors. Furthermore, these studies examining the biology of attachment in prairie voles have shown that 1) in females, blockade of brain oxytocin activation prevents both attachment to offspring and attachment to partner, and 2) in males, blockade of central vasopressin systems prevents both attachment to offspring and attachment to partner. It should be further noted that the effects of oxytocin and vasopressin antagonists on both partner and offspring attachment were tested in both genders. For the purposes of the argument we make below, it would be very useful to know more about how these systems operate in nonhuman primates. As far as we are aware, to date there has been only one such study, carried out it in squirrel monkeys (Winslow and Insel 1991), which did report findings similar to those found for the prairie vole. Thus, it appears that the biological mediator of pair bonding and mother–infant bonding is sexually dimorphic, utilizing different but closely related peptides—oxytocin and vasopressin—that are descended from the ancestral peptide vasotocin. Furthermore, all of these peptides show effects on sexual behavior.

Animal Evidence for Pubertal Changes in Oxytocin and Vasopressin Systems

Given the importance of brain oxytocin and vasopressin systems in sexual behavior (Arletti et al. 1992; DeVries et al. 1992), it is not surprising that these systems are regulated by gonadal steroids. Regulation of oxytocin receptors by estrogen and progesterone has been well described by a number of investigators and is believed to play the main role in regulating sexual receptivity in females, which varies across the estrus cycles in most mammals. Estrogen has also been demonstrated to regulate oxytocin receptor messenger RNA (mRNA) as well as receptor protein (Bale and Dorsa 1997). However, what is really striking is the 5- to 10-fold increase in hypothalamic oxytocin mRNA that accompanies puberty, thus initiating the biological drives for reproduction and pair bonding (Crowley et al. 1995). Combining behavioral data from rats and voles suggests that although this tremendous increase in oxytocin at puberty drives both sexual behavior and attachment in females, it increases sexual drive without increasing the drive for pair bonding in males. The brain vasopressin systems that regulate attachment in male voles are also regulated by testosterone, and thus puberty should be accompanied by increased attachment needs in males as well; however, the activation of an additional brain system (oxytocin) involved in increasing sexual drive in the absence of pair-bonding drives appears to lead simply to more activation of sexual drives rather than both sexual and pair-bonding drives in males relative to females. This finding suggests that the biological stage is set for adolescent male behavior that emphasizes sexual activity without pair bonding, while adolescent females find these two biological drives strongly linked.

What Does This Have To Do With Depression in Adolescents?

We argue that changes in hormonal milieu—specifically, changes in oxytocin production and receptor availability—that occur in human females during puberty serve to increase the intensity of desire for affiliation in general, for sex, for heterosexual pair bonding, and ultimately for mother–infant bonding. These changes in hormonal milieu, as they influence affiliative behavior, are adaptive for the individual and *have no direct effect on mood.* However, if and when the increasingly intense affiliative needs (and closely linked sexual needs) of the adolescent girl are frustrated through real or symbolic breaches in affiliative bonds, the hormonal changes of puberty can interact with the common interpersonal and romantic disappointments of adolescence in such a way as to produce depressive symptoms and, in many cases, syndromal depression.

Anthropologists call this reasoning a "correlated consequences" argument. The idea that depression is a correlated consequence of human affiliative need but leads to that consequence (depression) only when affiliative needs are challenged through real or imagined loss applies to both men and women. What we argue here is that a number of factors conspire to make females more vulnerable to such losses as they pass through the pubertal transition. Affiliative and sexual needs also "come on line" for males as they pass through puberty (Freedman 1967; Sorenson 1973; Weisfeld 1979); however, their need is for many partners, while what young females seek is a single stable partner. Of the two goals, the latter would seem more likely to lead to disappointment.

Does Affiliative Behavior Show Sexually Dimorphic Changes in Humans at Puberty?

Boys and girls begin to differ markedly in their affiliative behavior at adolescence. Girls become more intensely involved in their same-sex peer relations and, of course, "boy crazy" (Steinberg 1996). Boys, in contrast, become slightly more withdrawn, and, while beginning to evidence some interest in girls, are less likely to act on those interests. The validity of this folk wisdom has been documented in a well-designed time-sampling study of fifth through ninth grade students in two suburban Chicago school districts, one lower middle-class and one more affluent (Larson and Richards 1991). Over the five grade levels, girls were found to spend increasing amounts of time with peers, while time with family remained relatively constant and time alone decreased. Boys, in contrast, spent increasing amounts of time alone, decreasing their contact with both peers and family. All of the male:female differences observed in this investigation were highly significant.

The Link Between Breaches in Affiliative Bonds and Depression Onset

Over the last three decades, researchers both in the United Kingdom and in the United States have defined the nature of life circumstances that seem to put individuals in general, and women in particular, at risk for major depression. Stressful life events have long been implicated in the onset and maintenance of major depression (G. W. Brown and Harris 1978; Hammen 1992; Monroe and Depue 1991; Moos 1991). A careful review of the kinds of stressful life events that seem to be associated with the onset of depression suggests that many of these events represent real or symbolic breaches in affiliative bonds (G. W. Brown et al. 1995). Furthermore, among inner-city women in London, the kinds of more chronic difficulties most often associated with the onset or persistence of major depression also represent problems in the area of affiliation. Such events include chronic marital problems, social isolation, and, in earlier studies, lack of a confidante (G. W. Brown and Harris 1978).

Few sophisticated studies of stressful life events in relation to the onset of depression have been undertaken in adolescent populations. Our own research group has used the Life Events and Difficulties Schedule (LEDS; G. W. Brown and Harris 1978) to examine stressful life events and chronic difficulties in a group of adolescents with major depression and matched community controls (Frank et al. 1997). Depressed adolescents were significantly more likely than community controls to have experienced a severely stressful life event in the 6 months prior to the onset of their depression compared with a linked 6-month period in the control subjects. Contributing substantially to the differences between depressed subjects and controls were events such as the breakup of a romantic relationship, the disruption of an important friendship, or severe illness in a parent or other close relative. Furthermore, girls with major depression were significantly more likely to have experienced a severe event in the study period than were depressed boys, control boys, or control girls; however, when the analysis was restricted to "interpersonal events," the differences were even more striking. Sixty-eight percent of the depressed girls reported the occurrence of such an event in the 6 months prior to depression onset, in comparison with 30% of the control girls, 40% of the control boys, and a mere 14% of the depressed boys.

Conclusion

Among the changes that occur at puberty, one that might explain the marked increase in rates of major depression among girls compared with boys is the *interaction* between the hormonal changes and the psychosocial experiences to which young girls are exposed during this period. In all likelihood, increases in oxytocin drive the increase in affiliative behavior in girls at least as much as do the social influences around them. This increase in affiliative needs is not a problem per se. Indeed, as Lerner (1987) has argued, "the primary valuing of relationships (when relatedness does not come at the expense of self) is one of women's great strengths" (p. 219). However, not all affiliations, particularly in adolescence, are happy ones. In many cases, the powerful affiliative needs of the adolescent girl lead to disappointment and loss. When such loss occurs, it appears that major depression is frequently the result.

References

Aneshensel CS: Marital and employment role-strain, social support, and depression among adult women, in Stress, Social Support and Women. Edited by Hobfoll SE. New York, Hemisphere, 1986, pp 99–114

Angold A, Rutter M: Effects of age and pubertal status on depression in a large clinical sample. Dev Psychopathol 4:5–28, 1992

Arletti R, Benellt A, Bertolini A: Oxytocin involvement in male and female sexual behavior. Ann N Y Acad Sci 652:180–193, 1992

Bale TL, Dorsa DM: Cloning, novel promoter sequence, and estrogen regulation of a rat oxytocin receptor gene. Endocrinology 138:1151–1158, 1997

Biegon A, McEwen BS: Modulation by estradiol of serotonin receptors in brain. J Neurosci 2:199–205, 1982

Bifulco A, Brown GW, Adler Z: Early sexual abuse and clinical depression in adult life. Br J Psychiatry 159:115–122, 1991

Breslau N, Schultz L, Peterson E: Sex differences in depression: a role for preexisting anxiety. Psychiatry Res 58:1–12, 1995

Brown CS, Ling FW, Andersen RN, et al: Efficacy of depot leuprolide in premenstrual syndrome: effect of symptom severity and type in a controlled trial. Obstet Gynecol 84:779–786, 1994

Brown GW, Harris TO: Social Origins of Depression: A Study of Psychiatric Disorder in Women. London, Tavistock, 1978

Brown GW, Harris TO, Hepworth C: Loss, humiliation and entrapment among women developing depression: a patient and non-patient comparison. Psychol Med 25:7–21, 1995

Burnam MA, Stein JA, Golding JM, et al: Sexual assault and mental disorders in a community population. J Consult Clin Psychol 56:843–850, 1988

Canino GJ, Bird HR, Shrout PE, et al: The prevalence of specific psychiatric disorders in Puerto Rico. Arch Gen Psychiatry 44:727–735, 1987

Carter CS, Williams JR, Witt DM, et al: Oxytocin and social bonding. Ann N Y Acad Sci 652:204–211, 1992

Chen CN, Wong J, Lee N, et al: The Shatin community mental health survey in Hong Kong, II: major findings. Arch Gen Psychiatry 50:125–133, 1993

Chibbar R, Toma JG, Mitchell BF, et al: Regulation of neural oxytocin gene expression by gonadal steroids in pubertal rats. Mol Endocrinol 4:2030–2038, 1990

Crowley RS, Insel TR, O'Keefe JA, et al: Increased accumulation of oxytocin messenger ribonucleic acid in the hypothalamus of the female rat: induction by long term estradiol and progesterone administration and subsequent progesterone withdrawal. Endocrinology 136:224–231, 1995

Cutler SE, Nolen-Hoeksema S: Accounting for sex differences in depression through female victimization: childhood sexual abuse. Sex Roles 24:425–438, 1991

DeVries GJ, Crenshaw BJ, Ali Al-Shamma H: Gonadal steroids modulation of vasopressin pathways. Ann N Y Acad Sci 652:387–396, 1992

Ernst C, Angst J: The Zurich Study, XII: sex difference in depression—evidence from longitudinal epidemiological data. Eur Arch Psychiatry Clin Neurosci 241:222–230, 1992

Finkelhor D: What's wrong with sex between adults and children? Ethics and the problem of sexual abuse. Am J Orthopsychiatry 49:692–697, 1979

Finkelhor D: How widespread is child sexual abuse? Children Today 13:18–20, 1984

Frank E, Stewart BD: Depressive symptoms in rape victims: a revisit. J Affect Disord 7:77–85, 1984

Frank E, Hlastala S, Ritenour A, et al: Inducing lifestyle regularity in recovering bipolar disorder patients: results from the maintenance therapies in bipolar disorder protocol. Biol Psychiatry 41:1165–1173, 1997

Freedman DG: A biological view of man's social behavior, in Social Behavior From Fish to Man. Edited by Etkin W. Chicago, IL, University of Chicago Press, 1967, pp 152–299

Hammen C: Life events and depression: the plot thickens. Am J Community Psychol 20:179–193, 1992

Hwu HG, Yeh EK, Chang LY: Prevalence of psychiatric disorders in Taiwan defined by the Chinese Diagnostic Interview Schedule. Acta Psychiatr Scand 79:136–147, 1989

Insel TR: Oxytocin—a neuropeptide for affilitation: evidence from behavioral, receptor autoradiographic, and comparative studies. Psychoneuroendocrinology 17:3–35, 1992

Insel TR, Hulihan TJ: A gender-specific mechanism for pair bonding: oxytocin and partner preference formation in monogamous voles. Behav Neurosci 109:782–789, 1995

Insel TR, Shapiro LE: Oxytocin receptor distribution reflects social organization in monogamous and polygamous voles. Proc Natl Acad Sci U S A 89: 5981–5985, 1992

Insel TR, Winslow JT, Wang ZC, et al: Oxytocin and the molecular basis of monogamy. Adv Exp Med Biol 395:227–234, 1995

Karam E: War events and depression in Lebanon. Paper presented at a seminar of the International Traumatic Stress Society, Washington, DC, October 26, 1991

Kercher GA, McShane M: The prevalence of child sexual abuse victimization in an adult sample of Texas residents. Child Abuse Negl 8:495–501, 1984

Kessler RC, McGonagle KA, Swartz M, et al: Sex and depression in the National Comorbidity Survey, I: lifetime prevalence, chronicity and recurrence. J Affect Disord 29:85–96, 1993

Kessler RC, McGonagle KA, Nelson CB, et al: Sex and depression in the National Comorbidity Survey, II: cohort effects. J Affect Disord 30:15–26, 1994

Keverne EB, Kendrick KM: Oxytocin facilitation of maternal behavior in sheep. Ann N Y Acad Sci 652:83–101, 1992a

Keverne EB, Kendrick KM: Control of synthesis and release of oxytocin in the sheep brain. Ann N Y Acad Sci 652:102–121, 1992b

Kilpatrick DG, Edmunds CN, Seymour AK: Rape in America: A Report to the Nation. Arlington, VA, National Victim Center, 1992

Klopfer PH: Mother love: what turns it on? American Science 59:404–407, 1971

Larson R, Richards M: Daily companionship in late childhood and early adolescence: changing developmental contexts. Child Dev 62:284–300, 1991

Lerner HG: Female depression: self-sacrifice and self-betrayal in relationships, in Women and Depression: A Lifespan Perspective. Edited by Formanek R, Gurian A. New York, Springer, 1987, pp 200–221

Merikangas KR, Weissman MM, Pauls DL: Genetic factors in the sex ratio of major depression. Psychol Med 15:63–69, 1985

Monroe SM, Depue RA: Life stress and depression, in Psychosocial Aspects of Depression. Edited by Becker J, Kleinman A. Hillsdale, NJ, Lawrence Erlbaum, 1991, pp 101–130

Montgomery JC, Appleby L, Brincat M: Effect of estrogen and testosterone implants on psychological disorders of the climacteric. Lancet 1:297–299, 1987

Moos RH: Life stressors, social resources, and the treatment of depression, in Psychosocial Aspects of Depression. Edited by Becker J, Kleinman A. Hillsdale, NJ, Lawrence Erlbaum, 1991, pp 187–214

Mortola JF: Applications of gonadotropin-releasing hormone analogues in the treatment of premenstrual syndrome. Clin Obstet Gynecol 36:753–763, 1993

Nolen-Hoeksema S: Responses to depression and their effects on the duration of depressive episodes. J Abnorm Psychol 100:569–582, 1991

Nolen-Hoeksema S, Morrow J, Fredrickson BL: Response styles and the duration of depressed mood. J Abnorm Psychol 102:20–28, 1993

Pedersen CA, Prange AJ Jr: Induction of maternal behavior in virgin rats after intracerebroventricular administration of oxytocin. Proc Natl Acad Sci U S A 76:6661–6665, 1979

Schmidt PJ, Rubinow DR: Menopause-related affective disorders: a justification for further study. Am J Psychiatry 148:844–852, 1991

Sherrill JT, Anderson B, Frank E, et al: Is life stress more likely to provoke depressive episodes in women than in men? Depression and Anxiety 6:95–105, 1997

Sorenson RC: Adolescent Sexuality in Contemporary America. New York, World Publishing Company, 1973

Spitzer RL, Endicott J, Robins E: Research Diagnostic Criteria: rationale and reliability. Arch Gen Psychiatry 35:773–782, 1978

Steinberg L: Adolescence, 4th Edition. New York, McGraw-Hill, 1996

Steiner M, Steinberg S, Stewart D, et al: Fluoxetine in the treatment of premenstrual dysphoria. N Engl J Med 332:1529–1534, 1995

Stone AB, Pearlstein TB, Brown WA: Fluoxetine in the treatment of late luteal phase dysphoric disorder. J Clin Psychiatry 52:290–293, 1991

Stricker EM, Verbalis JG: Hormones and ingestive behaviors, in Behavioral Endocrinology. Edited by Becker JB, Breedlove SM, Crews D. Cambridge, MA, MIT Press, 1993, pp 451–472

Thompson T: Getting my self back: notes of a depression survivor. Washington Post, October 20, 1992, pp Z10–Z14

Weisfeld GE: An ethological view of human adolescence. J Nerv Ment Dis 167: 38–55, 1979

Weissman MM, Klerman GL: Sex differences and the epidemiology of depression. Arch Gen Psychiatry 34:98–111, 1977

Weissman MM, Bruce ML, Leaf PJ, et al: Affective disorders, in Psychiatric Disorders in America: The Epidemiologic Catchment Area Study. Edited by Robins LN, Regier DA. New York, Free Press, 1991, pp 53–80

Weissman MM, Bland R, Joyce PR, et al: Sex differences in rates of depression: cross-national perspectives. J Affect Disord 29:77–84, 1993

Winslow JT, Insel TR: Social status in pairs of male squirrel monkeys determines the behavioral response to central oxytocin administration. J Neurosci 11:2932–2938, 1991

Winslow JT, Hastings N, Carter CS, et al: A role for central vasopressin in pair bonding in monogamous prairie voles. Nature 356:545–548, 1983

Wittchen H-U, Essau CA, von Zerssen D, et al: Lifetime and six-month prevalence of mental disorders in the Munich Follow-Up Study. Eur Arch Psychiatry Clin Neurosci 241:247–258, 1992

Wolk SI, Weissman MM: Women and depression: an update, in American Psychiatric Press Review of Psychiatry, Vol 14. Edited by Oldham J, Riba M. Washington, DC, American Psychiatric Press, 1995, pp 227–259

Wood SH, Mortola JF, Chan YF, et al: Treatment of premenstrual syndrome with fluoxetine: a double-blind, placebo-controlled, crossover study. Obstet Gynecol 80 (3 part 1):339–344, 1992

Yonkers KA, Halbreich U, Freeman E, et al: Symptomatic improvement of premenstrual dysphoric disorder with sertraline treatment. JAMA 278:983–988, 1997

CHAPTER 6

Gender Differences in Response to Treatments of Depression

Michael E. Thase, M.D.
Ellen Frank, Ph.D.
Susan G. Kornstein, M.D.
Kimberly A. Yonkers, M.D.

The introduction of electroconvulsive therapy (ECT) in the 1940s and the tricyclic antidepressants (TCAs) and monoamine oxidase inhibitors (MAOIs) the following decade ushered in the modern era of treatment of the mood disorders. Women have a higher risk of suffering from nonbipolar mood disorders (Kessler et al. 1993; Nolen-Hoeksema 1990; Weissman et al. 1993), as well as a greater likelihood of seeking treatment (Nolen-Hoeksema 1990), and thus contribute disproportionately to what is known about these treatments. Yet, despite almost 50 years of accumulated experience, no clear consensus has emerged about the relationship between sex, or gender, and response to specific forms of antidepressant treatment. In this chapter, research addressing the response of men and

---

This work was supported in part by grants MH-30915 (Mental Health Clinical Research Center), MH-41884, MH-29618, and MH-48152 from the National Institute of Mental Health. Research cited in this chapter was also supported by a series of grants from Pfizer Pharmaceutical. The authors wish to thank Drs. Roger Haskett, Wilma Harrison, Harold Sackheim, and Alan Schatzberg for making unpublished data available for presentation.

women to different types of therapy is reviewed. Potential gender differences in illness pathophysiology that may account for differential treatment responses are also discussed.

Types of Therapy

The major classes of treatment for dysthymia and major depressive disorder include counseling and psychotherapy (both the more traditional psychodynamic and supportive approaches and the newer, structured, time-limited psychotherapies), antidepressant medication, and ECT. Antidepressant pharmacotherapy may be further subdivided: TCAs, MAOIs, a heterogeneous group of "second generation" compounds (e.g., trazodone, amoxapine, maprotiline, bupropion), the selective serotonin reuptake inhibitors (SSRIs; fluoxetine, sertraline, paroxetine, citalopram, and fluvoxamine), the serotonin-norepinephrine reuptake inhibitor (SNRI) venlafaxine, and two newer compounds that affect multiple pre- and postsynaptic mechanisms (nefazodone and mirtazapine). These classes differ with respect to their presumed modes of action and their side-effect profiles, which may be different in men and women.

Before turning to specific classes of treatment, consideration of the importance of placebo-expectancy factors is warranted. Nonspecific placebo-expectancy factors account for at least 50% of the therapeutic benefit of outpatient antidepressant therapy (Depression Guideline Panel 1993). Moreover, placebo response rates vary widely among studies, ranging from as low as 10% to as high as 70%, with an average of about 40% in outpatient studies (Depression Guideline Panel 1993). The placebo response rate thus provides an estimate of the short-term prognosis of the patients enrolled in a particular study, against which the efficacy of antidepressants can be gauged.

Placebo response rates also help to calibrate differences across diagnostic or sociodemographic subgroups. For example, if a particular antidepressant yielded response rates of 50% for women and 70% for men, knowing the corresponding placebo response rates would greatly influence interpretation of this finding. If, on one hand, women were less responsive to placebo than men (e.g., 20% versus 40%), there would be main effects for Gender (i.e., men are more likely to improve than women) and Treatment (i.e., Drug > Placebo), but there would be *no* gender difference in response to that specific antidepressant (see Figure 6–1A). On the other hand, if both men and women had 30% placebo response rates, a Drug × Gender interaction would be observed, and interpretation of this finding would supersede the main effects (see Figure 6–1B). In another scenario, a treatment could appear equally effective for men and women, yet a difference in placebo response rates would reveal that one gender was actually more specifically treatment responsive than the other (Figure 6–1C).

The proportion of placebo-controlled studies conducted over the past few decades has decreased, largely because of ethical concerns about withholding active treatments from depressed people. Unfortunately, only a minority of the studies reviewed here include a placebo control group, and thus specific and nonspecific elements of response cannot be uncoupled. The necessity of a placebo control in contemporary studies is now a controversial topic (Rothman and Michels 1994), and it is unlikely that this circumstance will change in the near future.

Counseling and Psychotherapy

Although supportive counseling is used widely to treat depression, such counseling has not been studied extensively (Depression Guideline Panel 1993) and it is not known whether there are gender differences in response rates. Similarly, despite a storied clinical tradition, there are insufficient data from controlled studies to comment on the efficacy of psychodynamic psychotherapy in depressed men and women.

By contrast, a number of studies of the newer time-limited psychotherapies have been conducted, and potential gender differences in outcome can begin to be assessed. This task is not, however, as easy as it might seem. Several of the "depression specific" psychotherapies, including social skills training (Hersen et al. 1984) and interpersonal psychotherapy (IPT) (DiMascio et al. 1979), were initially developed for treatment of women, and men were not enrolled in the initial randomized clinical trials. Most other psychotherapy studies have enrolled fewer than 30 patients per treatment cell and, typically, at least 75% of the participants are female (Thase et al. 1994). Thus, any particular study may enter only 5 to 8 men per treatment condition. Even the multicenter National Institute of Mental Health Treatment of Depression Collaborative Research Program (TDCRP) (Elkin et al. 1989), which enrolled 239 sub-

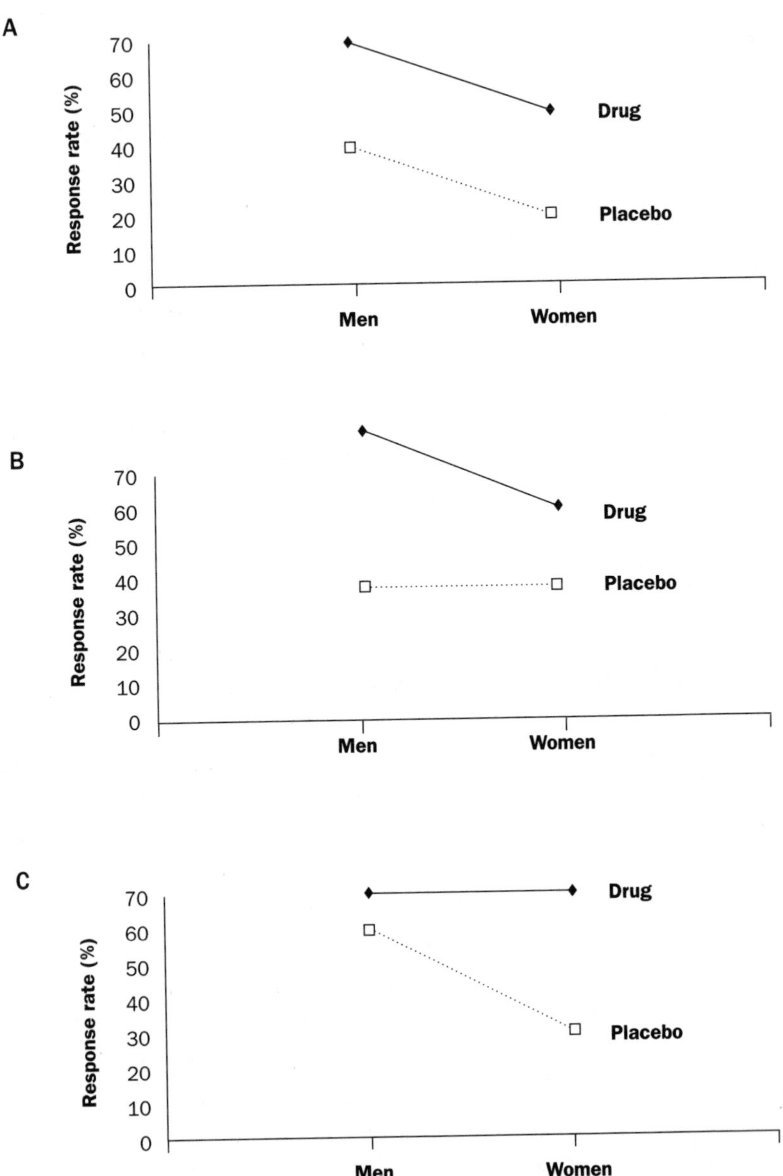

FIGURE 6–1. Hypothetical examples illustrating the impact of placebo response rate on interpretation of gender differences in treatment response. Panel A illustrates main effects for Gender and Treatment, but no interaction. Panel B illustrates a Gender × Treatment interaction attributable to a gender difference in response to active medication. Panel C illustrates another Gender × Treatment interaction, this time explained by a gender difference in placebo response.

jects, included only about 18 men per treatment condition. Thus, no single study has adequate statistical power to detect more moderate—yet still clinically relevant—gender differences in response rates.

Several larger studies of depressed patients treated with cognitive-behavior therapy (CBT) or IPT have been conducted by investigators at the University of Pittsburgh. These studies did not employ randomized comparison groups but did have the power to detect 20%–30% of the between-group differences. One report by Thase et al. (1994)compared the responses of men (n = 40) and women (n = 44) with acute major depressive disorder treated with CBT. Overall, outcomes of men and women did not differ in terms of symptomatic improvement or remission rates. There was a significant interaction between pretreatment severity and gender, however, such that the subgroup of women with more severe depression (i.e., pretreatment Hamilton Rating Scale for Depression (HAMD; M. Hamilton 1960) scores of ≥20) was significantly *less* responsive to CBT than were the other three subgroups (women/less severe, men/more severe, and men/less severe). This gender difference was found even though men attended significantly fewer sessions of therapy. A subsequent report from Thase et al. (1997a) compared men (n = 25) and women (n = 66) with recurrent major depressive disorder treated with IPT. Men and women were found to have comparable symptomatic responses and remission rates, irrespective of initial HAMD scores. Pooling the samples of these studies suggests a three-way interaction: higher levels of symptom severity adversely affected only the depressed women treated with CBT (see Figure 6–2).

These provocative findings obviously require replication, and no other existing data set may be large enough to serve this purpose. However, a parallel finding was observed in the TDCRP (Elkin et al. 1989), which included 71 men and 168 women. Specifically, CBT was again less effective in more severe depression, whereas IPT was equally effective in both severity groups. It remains to be seen if this difference was mediated by gender.

We suspect that the less-structured methods used in IPT, which focus on transitions in social roles, role disputes, unresolved grief, or social deficits, may be a more relevant approach for women with more severe symptomatology. By contrast, we are concerned that the structure, homework, and Socratic analysis of thought and behavior patterns employed in CBT may be less suitable for some severely depressed women—in partic-

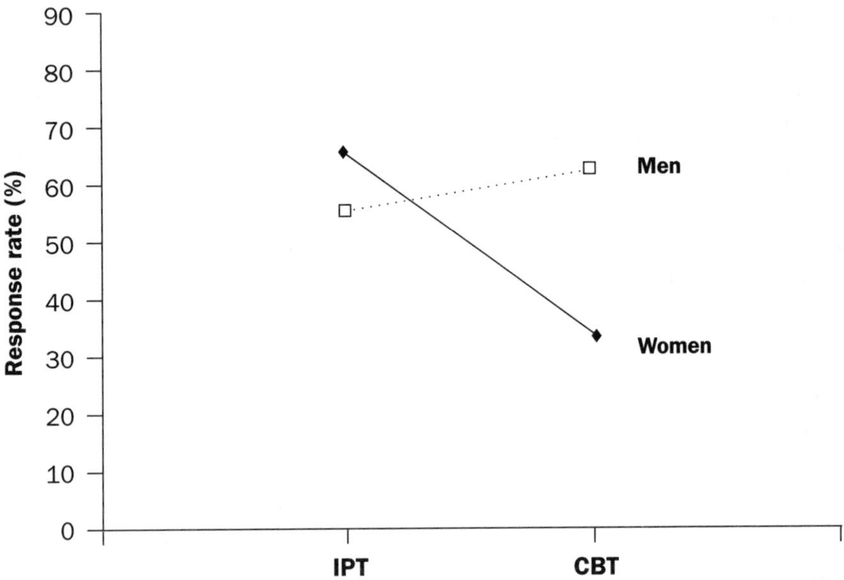

FIGURE 6–2. Cognitive-behavior therapy (CBT) may be a less effective treatment than interpersonal therapy (IPT) for more severely depressed women. All patients scored ≥20 on the Hamilton Rating Scale for Depression (M. Hamilton 1960). CBT and IPT were equally effective for severely depressed men as well as for less severely depressed patients of both genders.
Source. Data from Thase et al. 1994, 1997a.

ular, those who use emotion-focused coping strategies (Nolen-Hoeksema 1990). Consistent with this notion, recent reanalyses of therapy transcripts of 30 patients (about 75% female) treated with CBT found better outcomes when therapists emphasized interpersonal or developmental issues (Castonguay et al. 1996), whereas a predominantly cognitive focus appeared to weaken therapeutic alliances (Hayes et al. 1996).

Antidepressant Pharmacotherapy

Tricyclic Antidepressants and Monoamine Oxidase Inhibitors

These older compounds have been studied extensively in both milder and more severe episodes of major depression, dysthymia, and other chronic depressions (Depression Guideline Panel 1993). Although possible gender differences in treatment responsivity have been suspected for quite some time (West and Dally 1959), data documenting such an effect conclusively have been slow to emerge.

In 1959, West and Dally described a form of early-onset, chronic depression characterized by panic attacks, phobic anxiety, and reverse neurovegetative symptoms (e.g., overeating or oversleeping) that appeared to be less responsive to TCAs *and* more responsive to MAOIs. West and Dally considered these nonmelancholic depressions to be "atypical," although they are now known to be relatively common among younger women (Thase et al. 1991). Furthermore, given the progressive reduction in age at onset of depression since 1940 (Klerman and Weissman 1989), reverse vegetative symptoms can no longer be considered atypical.

In 1974, Raskin (1974) published a reanalysis of data from two large inpatient clinical trials suggesting that the response of women, but not men, to imipramine and phenelzine may differ in an age-dependent fashion. These studies included 880 depressed inpatients stratified by gender (268 men, 612 women) and age (<40 years and ≥40 years). Fortuitously, for women this stratification approximated pre- and postmenopausal status. In study 1, the treatments compared were chlorpromazine, imipramine, and placebo. Raskin found that imipramine was significantly more effective than placebo for men, regardless of age. However, imipramine was no more effective than placebo for women under age 40, and it actually worsened scores on a measure of hostility. By contrast, the older women were as responsive to imipramine as the men. In study 2, phenelzine and diazepam were compared with placebo. Overall, phenelzine was relatively ineffective, although it did show some advantage for younger women relative to both placebo and phenelzine response among younger men. The rather low dose of phenelzine (45 mg/day) used in this study limits confidence in the conclusions, but the results are consistent with the observations of West and Dally (1959).

Subsequently, Davidson and Pelton (1985) analyzed data from five clinical trials to compare treatment response rates between "typical" and "atypical" depressive syndromes. The data set included the results of 151 patients (40 men, 111 women) who were treated with either MAOIs (phenelzine or isocarboxazid, $n = 84$) or TCAs (imipramine or amitriptyline, $n = 67$). One analysis focused on the response of patients with panic attacks. A significant Gender × Treatment × Diagnosis interaction was observed. Women with panic attacks (*n* = 16) had poorer responses to TCAs than did either men with panic attacks treated with TCAs (*n* = 6) or women with panic attacks treated with MAOIs (*n* = 19) (*P* < .01). Another analysis focused on patients with hypersomnia and hyperphagia. Unfortunately, only 19 women (17%) with both of these reverse vegetative symptoms were identified, yielding too small a sample for a meaningful comparison of response to MAOIs (*n* = 13) and TCAs (*n* = 6). Among the patients with more "typical" depression, women (*n* = 45) were less responsive to TCAs than were men (*n* = 16), although the 14% difference in improvement scores did not quite reach statistical significance.

J. A. Hamilton, Grant, and Jensvold (1996) conducted a meta-analysis of 35 studies that reported imipramine response rates separately for men (*n* = 342) and women (*n* = 711). These studies accounted for only 19% of the imipramine trials published between 1957 and 1991, illustrating the short shrift given to gender differences in pharmacotherapy response in the treatment literature. Across studies, there was an 11% difference in imipramine response rates favoring the men (62% versus 51%), which was highly significant in this large sample (P < .001). That J. A. Hamilton et al. were not able to take age into account, however, might have obscured an even larger difference in imipramine response rates.

Investigators at the University of Pittsburgh reported the acute-phase outcome of a protocol in which patients were treated first with the combination of IPT and imipramine and then, if necessary, with a trial of an MAOI (Frank et al. 1988; Thase et al. 1991, 1992). All patients (*n* = 201) had recurrent major depressive disorder and more than half had reverse neurovegetative features (Thase et al. 1991). As noted previously, women (*n* = 159) were significantly more likely to manifest reverse neurovegetative symptoms than were men (*n* = 45) (69% versus 56%; *P* < .05).

During the initial IPT + imipramine treatment period, women had significantly slower remissions (Frank et al. 1988), as did patients with reverse neurovegetative features (Thase et al. 1991). The slower response associated with reverse vegetative symptoms was not statistically significant when gender was covaried in the analysis, suggesting that it was the greater prevalence of vegetative reversal that mediated poorer TCA response in women.

Following unsuccessful treatment with the IPT + imipramine combination, 42 patients were withdrawn from the TCA and treated with either phenelzine ($n = 4$) or tranylcypromine ($n = 38$) (Thase et al. 1992). Among the 40 completers, the proportion of responders was significantly higher among the patients with prominent reverse neurovegetative features (67% versus 31%; $P < .05$). Response to MAOI therapy was inversely proportional to the percentage of improvement experienced during the initial imipramine trial. Women and men benefited equally from MAOI therapy, which indicates that it may be the reverse neurovegetative profile, and not gender per se, that accounts for their more favorable MAOI response. Consistent with this notion, a recent reanalysis of a published study (Himmelhoch et al. 1991) comparing imipramine and tranylcypromine in a sample of 52 bipolar depressed patients with reverse vegetative features revealed that men and women responded equally well to the MAOI and equally poorly to the TCA.

The MAOIs differ from the TCAs in many respects, including fewer anticholinergic and antihistaminergic side effects and more potent effects on serotonergic (5-hydroxytryptophan [5-HT]) neurotransmission (Thase et al. 1995). However, it is the need for dietary precautions, the potential for serious pharmacodynamic interactions, and several common vexing side effects (e.g., edema, weight gain, and orthostasis) that limit the utility of the older nonselective and irreversible MAOIs. The reversible and selective inhibitor of MAO type A, moclobemide, which is not available for use in the United States, has several advantages vis-à-vis phenelzine or tranylcypromine, but we were not able to find any studies reporting outcome for age and gender. Moreover, in countries where moclobemide is available, there is concern that it is not as effective as the older MAOIs (Thase et al. 1995).

Selective Serotonin Reuptake Inhibitors

The SSRIs now account for the vast majority of new prescriptions of antidepressants. This success is usually attributed to convenience, relative safety, and fewer "nuisance" side effects, in addition to vigorous marketing (Thase and Kupfer 1996). Like the MAOIs, the SSRIs have few antihistaminic and anticholinergic effects and potent effects on serotonergic neurotransmission (Thase and Kupfer 1996). Thus, we hypothesized that the success of the SSRIs also may reflect a heretofore unappreciated advantage for treatment of younger women.

Extensive databases from Phase II and Phase III clinical trials exist for the first three SSRIs approved for the treatment of depression in the United States: fluoxetine, sertraline, and paroxetine. Similar databases exist in Europe for fluvoxamine and citalopram. These studies include placebo and/or active comparators (usually TCAs), and age and gender are undeniably reliable variables that can be retrieved easily from archival sources. It is hoped that these potential "gold mines" can be tapped fully in the near future.

In an early report, Reimherr et al. (1984) found that diagnoses of atypical and chronic depression predicted a more favorable response to fluoxetine than to the TCA comparator. Subsequently, Pande et al. (1996) compared fluoxetine and phenelzine in a prospective randomized clinical trial of atypical depression and found them to be equally effective. However, although both studies enrolled a majority of female subjects, gender differences were not reported in either.

Recently, investigators at Eli Lilly (Lewis-Hall et al. 1997) reported on the efficacy of fluoxetine and TCAs in 850 women drawn from their clinical trials database. The authors found that fluoxetine was better tolerated than the TCAs but was no more effective for treatment of depressed women. Data were presented neither for the placebo comparison groups nor for the men treated with fluoxetine or TCAs. The possibility of Age × Gender × Drug interactions thus remains to be explored.

Steiner et al. (1993) presented an analysis of gender differences in SmithKline Beecham's paroxetine clinical trials database. Although these data have not been published, it appears that paroxetine was somewhat more effective than imipramine in women and that the converse was true in men. Further analyses of these data are needed, particularly analyses that take into account age and possible gender differences in placebo response rates.

To date, no published reports of gender differences in treatment response have used the Pfizer database for sertraline. However, analyses are under way from two large multicenter studies that compared the efficacy of sertraline and imipramine in the treatment of chronic depressive syndromes (Keller et al. 1998; Thase et al. 1996). Like the episodic major depressive disorders, chronic depressive disorders are significantly more common in women than in men, and their onset typically occurs earlier in women (Weissman et al. 1988). We predicted that chronically depressed patients would also show a relatively poorer response to a TCA than to an SSRI and that this difference would be determined by gender.

In the first of these two multicenter studies (Thase et al. 1996), 410 patients with "pure" dysthymia (i.e., onset before age 21 years, a continuous duration greater than 5 years, and no major depressive episodes within the preceding 6 months) were randomly assigned to 12 weeks of double-blind treatment with placebo, imipramine, or sertraline. The study group included 144 men and 266 women. Both active compounds were significantly more effective than placebo, and, although not different in efficacy, sertraline was significantly better tolerated than imipramine.

Kimberly Yonkers is taking the lead in studying gender differences in treatment response rates and tolerability in this data set. In preliminary analyses, sertraline was significantly better tolerated by women than imipramine, and, in fact, this difference accounted for almost the entire effect observed in Thase et al.'s analysis of the main study. A significant Gender × Treatment interaction also was observed for placebo-adjusted response rates (Figure 6–3). There was a 22% gender difference in sertraline response rates (men 42%; women 64%; $P = .02$). Imipramine response rates were not significantly different between men and women. Ongoing analyses of these data will address the potential moderating effects of age and reverse neurovegetative features.

In the second of the two multicenter studies (Keller et al. 1998), 635 patients (235 men, 400 women) with either chronic major depression (i.e., index episode of greater than 2 years' duration) *or* a current major depressive episode superimposed on antecedent dysthymia (i.e., "double" depression) were randomly assigned to 12 weeks of double-blind therapy with either sertraline ($n = 424$) or imipramine ($n = 211$). Nonresponders to acute-phase therapy were "crossed over" to the other medication for a second 12-week double-blind trial (Thase et al. 1997c). Overall, imipramine and sertraline were equally effective in both chronic major and double depressions (Keller et al. 1998). As in the study of "pure" dysthymia (Thase et al. 1996), there were significant tolerability differences favoring the SSRI.

Susan Kornstein is leading the analyses of the relationship between gender and treatment response in the Keller et al. (1998) study. In preliminary analyses, a gender difference in antidepressant tolerability has

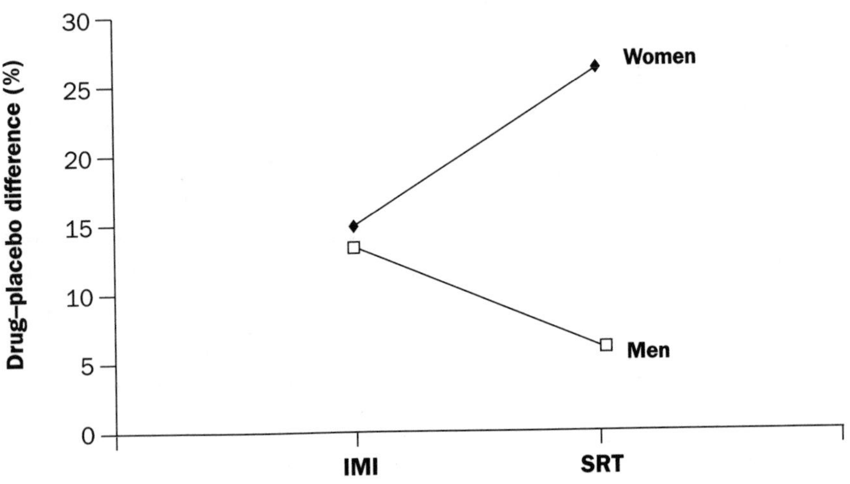

FIGURE 6–3. Gender differences in placebo-adjusted rates of response to sertraline (SRT) and imipramine (IMI) treatment of dysthymic disorder.
Source. Unpublished data provided by Drs. Wilma Harrison (Pfizer Pharmaceuticals) and Kimberly Yonkers, April 1997.

been observed: 19.8% of the women withdrew from imipramine because of side effects, compared with only 9.5% of men (see Figure 6–4). Moreover, premenopausal women were more than three times as likely to drop out of imipramine therapy as postmenopausal women (29% versus 8%; $P < .05$). Thus, postmenopausal women ($n = 72$) tolerated the TCA as well as men. Attrition due to side effects from sertraline also was identical for men and women (4.9% from each group). With respect to intent-to-treat response rates, there was a significant Gender × Drug interaction (Figure 6–4). Women were more likely to respond to sertraline (57%) than to imipramine (46%), whereas men had a 17% greater response rate when receiving the TCA (i.e., 62% versus 45%).

An additional analysis compared the response of women to sertraline and imipramine as a function of menopause status (Figure 6–5). The TCA and SSRI were equally effective for the 72 postmenopausal women (imipramine: 14/25, 56%; sertraline: 27/47, 57%). By contrast, sertraline was significantly more effective for treatment of the premenopausal women (imipramine: 41/96, 43%; sertraline: 115/201, 57%; $P = .007$).

Similar results were observed during the crossover phase (Thase et al. 1997c). Women constituted 78% (40/51) of the imipramine non-

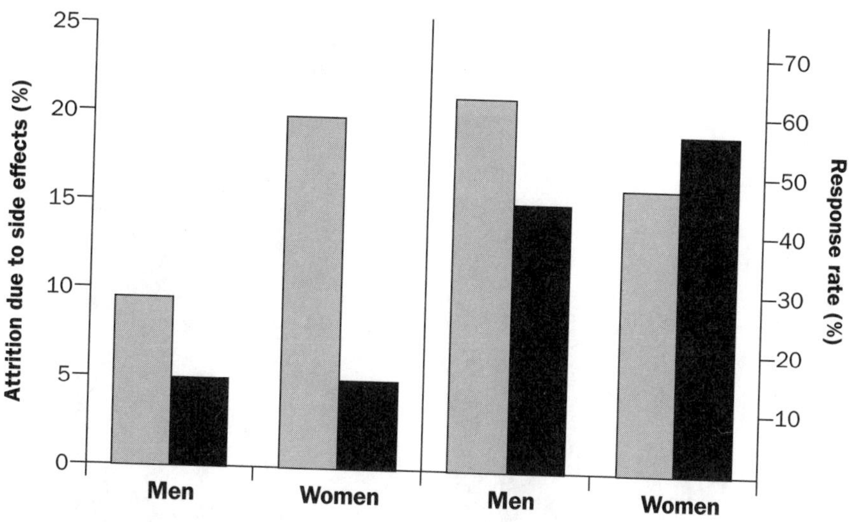

FIGURE 6–4. Chronically depressed men and women showed differential tolerability and responsivity to imipramine *(dark bars)* and sertraline *(lighter bars)*.
Source. Unpublished data provided by Drs. Wilma Harrison (Pfizer Pharmaceuticals) and Susan Kornstein, April 1997.

responder group, compared with 62% (72/117) of the sertraline nonresponders ($P < .05$). Sertraline was again better tolerated than imipramine, and among the patients crossed over to sertraline, intention-to-treat response rates were 49% for men and 62% for women. Among the sertraline nonresponders, 55% of the men but only 33% of the women responded to imipramine. These gender differences in response rates resulted in a significant two-way interaction. Moreover, patients who obtained the least benefit from the first drug tended to be the most likely to respond to crossover to another class of medication.

Combined Treatment

Many psychiatrists prefer to treat major depressive episodes with a combination of psychotherapy and pharmacotherapy, although surprisingly little evidence from controlled studies supports the practice of routinely using both modalities (Persons et al. 1996). Generally, an adequate trial of either an antidepressant *or* a form of contemporary psychotherapy re-

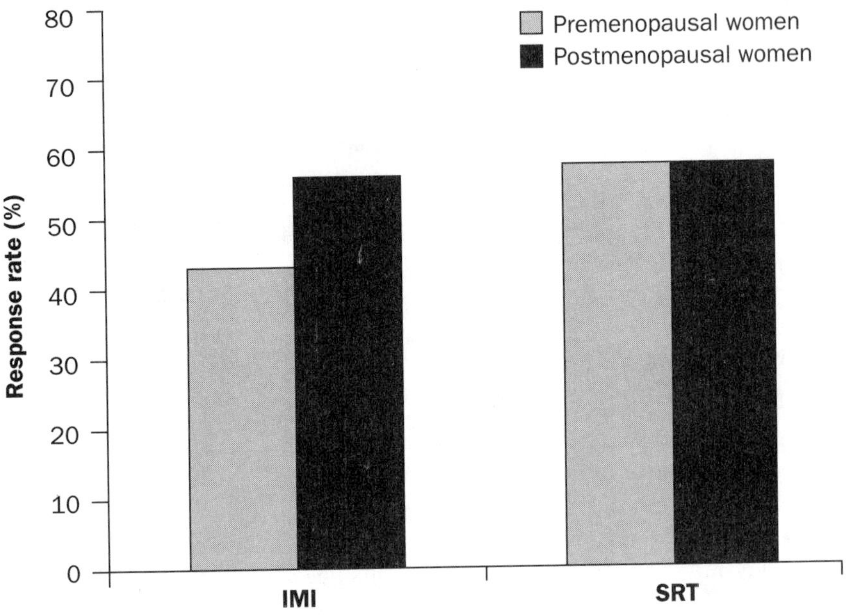

FIGURE 6–5. The poorer response of chronic depressive disorders to TCAs was observed specifically in premenopausal women's lower response rates with imipramine (IMI). Postmenopausal women were equally responsive to sertraline (SRT) and imipramine.

sults in response rates comparable to those found for combined therapy within the confines of a randomized clinical trial. Methodological factors (i.e., a "ceiling effect," inadequate statistical power, or exclusion of more complicated cases) might account for the discrepancy between practice preferences and empirical results, but it also now seems possible that the use of TCAs in studies enrolling a large proportion of younger women might help to explain the disappointing performance of combined treatment regimens. No controlled trials of major depressive disorder published to date have studied the combination of an SSRI and psychotherapy.

Having identified gender and age as correlates of differential treatment response, existing data sets can be reexamined to test the following predictions: 1) younger men will be more responsive to the combination of a TCA and psychotherapy than will younger women; 2) older women will be relatively more responsive to such a combination than will younger women; and 3) combined treatment will be no more effective than psychotherapy alone for younger women.

These predictions have been tested in the University of Pittsburgh data set by using a meta-analysis of original data (Thase et al. 1997b). Patients (*n* = 595) were drawn from six studies; all were outpatients, and they were treated with either IPT or CBT alone (*n* = 243) or IPT plus TCA (*n* = 352). There were 187 men and 408 women in the study group, ranging in age from 18 to 79 years. As predicted, there was no difference between response to psychotherapy alone and response to combined treatment among women under age 40. Men, on the other hand, had a more favorable response to combined treatment (compared with psychotherapy alone) across all age groups. The response to combined treatment among women over age 50 also was comparable to that observed in men. Thus, prior studies of combined treatment probably have underestimated the potential for additive benefit because of younger women's poorer response to TCAs. Future research on combined treatment would be more productive if classes of antidepressants that are better tolerated by and/or more effective in younger women were studied.

Maintenance Pharmacotherapy

Only two clinical trials have examined gender differences in prophylaxis against recurrent depressive episodes. In the study of Frank et al. (1990), 125 patients who responded to acute-phase therapy with imipramine plus IPT and remained well throughout 16 weeks of continuation therapy were enrolled in a 3-year placebo-controlled study of maintenance-phase treatment. Patients were randomly assigned to one of five maintenance-treatment conditions: placebo alone, IPT alone, IPT plus placebo, IPT plus imipramine, or imipramine alone. Imipramine was more effective than IPT, which in turn was more effective than placebo. There was no evidence of gender differences in survival time (i.e., well-time prior to relapse) or recurrence risk during the maintenance trial. However, with cell numbers of 25 and an approximately 3:1 (female:male) preponderance of women in this study, only large gender differences in outcome could be detected with adequate statistical power. Perhaps more importantly, the study design had already "sieved out" the disproportionately female subgroup of imipramine-nonresponsive patients (Thase et al. 1991).

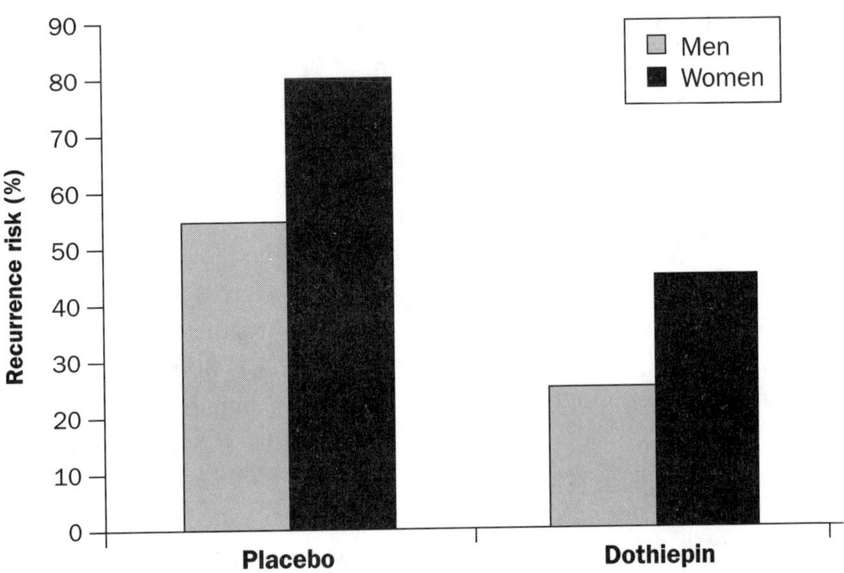

FIGURE 6–6. Gender differences in recurrence risk during placebo or dothiepin prophylactic therapy of depressed elderly patients.
Source. Adapted from Old Age Depression Interest Group 1993.

The Old Age Depression Interest Group (1993) conducted a multicenter clinical trial of 69 elderly patients who had responded to treatment with dothiepin (a TCA much like amitriptyline or doxepin that is not available in the United States). A post hoc analysis suggested that this group of older men and women responded equally well to acute-phase treatment. During the 2-year, double-blind, placebo-controlled maintenance trial, dothiepin was significantly more effective than placebo. However, women were significantly more likely to suffer recurrent depressive episodes than were men, whether treated with dothiepin or placebo (see Figure 6–6).

Electroconvulsive Therapy

Despite the fact that ECT is the oldest somatic treatment of depression still in use, relatively little attention has been given to the possibility of gender differences in ECT response. However, a wealth of clinical research has documented a number of clinical correlates of ECT non-response, including chronicity, Axis II personality disorders, and anxiety or other "neurotic" symptoms. These associations indicate that many of the same patients who might respond better to an MAOI or SSRI also would have a poorer response to ECT. Consistent with this speculation, Prudic et al. (1996) observed that failure to respond to an adequate trial of a TCA predicted a poorer response to ECT, whereas an unsuccessful SSRI trial did not.

We were able to identify four studies that examined gender differences in ECT response (Coryell and Zimmerman 1984; M. Hamilton 1982; Herrington et al. 1974; Medical Research Council 1965). In three of these (Coryell and Zimmerman 1984; Herrington et al. 1974; Medical Research Council 1965), women had a *more* favorable acute-phase response to ECT than did men. Careful patient selection may account for these unexpected findings by excluding younger women with anxiety or reverse neurovegetative features. It is also possible that women respond better to acute-phase ECT because men have, on average, a 50% higher seizure threshold (thicker skin, thicker skulls, and a longer distance between electrodes) (Sackeim et al. 1987). Thus, if stimulus intensity is not routinely determined or subsequently titrated to ensure adequacy, as was the case in early studies, men may be more likely than women to receive subtherapeutic courses of ECT.

Investigators at the New York State Psychiatric Institute, the University of Iowa, the Carrier Clinic (New Jersey), and the University of Pittsburgh are conducting a two-stage protocol to examine initial ECT response and subsequent outcome during a controlled trial of continuation pharmacotherapy. During the acute treatment phase, patients received a course of up to 20 ECT treatments administered according to "state of the art" methodology (Prudic et al. 1996). The patients were typically older than those in the earlier studies (mean age 60 years), and about one-half had failed to respond to multiple antidepressant trials. Patients usually received an initial course of unilateral ECT (titrated to 150% above seizure threshold), and nonresponders were switched to bilateral treatments after 6 unsuccessful treatments. The past treatment history of each patient was assessed carefully, and the study group was stratified according to level of treatment resistance documented during the index episode. Following completion of the course of ECT, consenting responders were randomized to one of three continuation treatment strategies: the combination of nortriptyline and lithium carbonate,

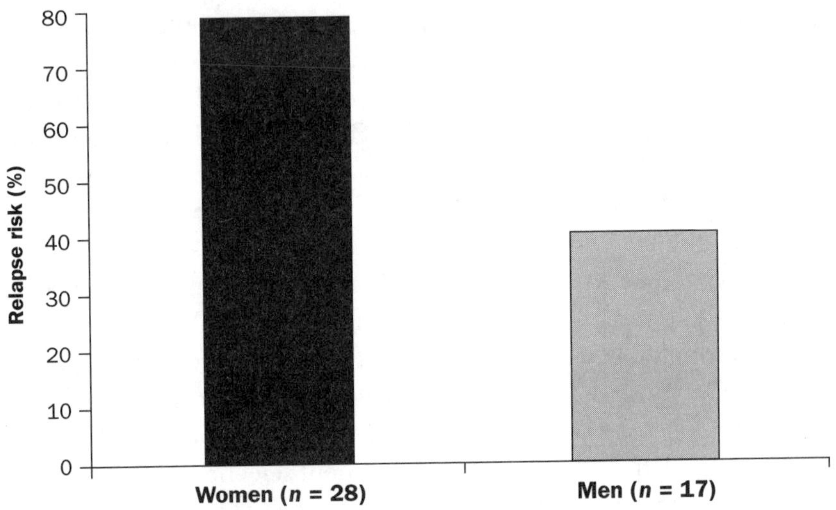

FIGURE 6–7. Gender differences in relapse risk during the first 6 months following electroconvulsive therapy (ECT) for depression.
Source. Unpublished data provided by Drs. Harold Sackeim (New York State Psychiatric Institute), Roger Haskett, and Michael E. Thase, April 1997.

nortriptyline plus placebo, or a "double" placebo control group.

This study is still in progress, and the treatment-specific outcomes of the second, preventive phase remain blinded. However, gender differences in acute-phase ECT response and relapse risk can be examined without jeopardizing the double-blind study. As in previous studies, acute-phase therapy with ECT was significantly more effective for women than for men (Prudic et al. 1996). A reexamination of prior treatment history suggested that this difference was attributable to the fact that the men had received more numerous and vigorous pharmacotherapy trials than had the women.

Post-ECT outcomes of 17 men and 28 women were then compared during continuation treatment, with the blind maintained. The men had significantly longer survival times and a lower risk of relapse than did the women (Figure 6–7). Until Treatment × Gender interactions can be examined, the most plausible explanation is that women with severe affective disorders have a poorer prognosis than do men with such disorders, consistent with the results of the longer-term study of depressed elderly patients reviewed previously (Old Age Depression Interest Group 1993).

Summary of Treatment Data

There are gender differences in tolerability and response to specific antidepressant therapies. Younger women are significantly less tolerant of the side effects of the TCA imipramine in comparison with men, and typically have response rates that are 10%–20% lower. Younger women are, however, responsive to MAOIs and the SSRIs. It remains to be seen whether these differences are mediated by premenopausal status, a predominance of reverse neurovegetative features, or an additive interaction of these factors.

There are also clinically significant gender differences in response to psychotherapy and ECT. In the case of psychotherapy, women with more severe depressive symptoms appear to be significantly more responsive to IPT than to CBT. The advantage favoring IPT in more severely depressed women may be attributable to the greater focus of this form of therapy on gender-relevant issues, to severity-linked differences in information processing that interfere with women's ability to use the therapeutic techniques of CBT, or to some combination of the two. Women are more responsive to acute-phase treatment with ECT than are men. Differences in seizure thresholds are a potentially relevant factor, as are prior treatment histories. Despite having a better initial response to ECT, women appear to be at greater subsequent risk of recurrent depression. Preventive pharmacotherapy may not fully offset this higher risk, particularly among older women.

Proposed Mechanisms of Differential Effects

Antidepressant Mechanisms

If younger women require antidepressants with greater serotonergic potency, one would expect them to show similarly poorer responses in studies of desipramine or nortriptyline. However, we could not identify any relevant data. If serotonergic potency is important, clomipramine also should be a significantly more effective antidepressant for younger women than imipramine. One might also predict gender differences in response to bupropion, a novel aminoketone antidepressant that is virtually devoid of serotonergic effects. Again, relevant data have not been published. In our group's experience, bupropion appears to be an effective treatment for younger women. Goodnick and Extein (1989) have also suggested that bupropion may be more effective than fluoxetine for treatment of depressions characterized by reverse neurovegetative features. Existing data sets can be reanalyzed to test each of these predictions.

Separating the effects of reverse neurovegetative symptoms from those of gender and premenopausal status will be a more difficult matter. Such an investigation will require a very large group of women, including a subset who are postmenopausal with reverse neurovegetative features and another who are premenopausal with more "typical" or melancholic features. The fact that such phenomenological subtypes are not prevalent in these demographic groups will make such a study daunting. Perhaps the data set of the Columbia group (i.e., Quitkin et al. 1993) holds the answers to these questions. This group has treated a large number of men and women with TCAs, MAOIs, and placebo, including more than 300 patients with reverse neurovegetative features.

Neurobiological Correlates of Depression

Establishing the existence of gender differences in treatment response heightens interest in questions about more fundamental differences in brain function and depressive pathophysiology. These differences, in turn, appear to be moderated by age, severity (in the case of response to CBT versus IPT), and menopausal status (in the case of response to MAOIs or SSRIs versus TCAs). Thus, understanding the neurobiological basis for gender differences in antidepressant response may be informed by surveying three related areas of research, as discussed below.

Age-Dependent Changes

Depression appears to accelerate certain neurophysiological and neuroendocrine changes associated with normal aging (Thase and Howland 1995). Specifically, there is a premature loss of slow-wave sleep and an age-related increase in sleep continuity disturbances in depression. An early onset of the first rapid eye movement (REM) sleep period, also referred to as reduced REM latency, accompanies the loss of slow-wave sleep. These changes probably reflect increased nocturnal arousal (Gillin et al. 1995), an abnormality also suggested by hypercortisolism, increased peripheral levels of catecholamine metabolites, and a blunting of the circadian nadir in body temperature (Gillin et al. 1995; Thase and Howland 1995). Clinically, this constellation of neurobiological disturbances is most common in patients with melancholic features (Feinberg and Carroll 1984; Gillin et al. 1995; Thase and Howland 1995). A deficit of inhibitory serotonergic neurotransmission, coupled with increased levels of corticotropin-releasing hormone and increased noradrenergic "drive," has been implicated in the genesis of these abnormalities (Gillin et al. 1995; Thase and Howland 1995). Protracted hypercortisolism may accelerate this age-dependent process by decreasing the number of glucocorticoid receptors in the hippocampus and inducing cortical atrophy (Thase and Howland 1995). Young (1995) proposes that premenopausal women are "protected" against overactivation of the hypothalamic-pituitary-adrenal (HPA) axis by estrogens, although it appears that such protection may come at the expense of an increased incidence of reverse neurovegetative symptoms.

State-Dependent Changes

The neurobiological disturbances associated with depression can be sorted into state-independent (trait-like) and state-dependent abnormalities (Kupfer and Ehlers 1989; Thase and Howland 1995). The latter disturbances, also called *episode markers,* include increased phasic REM sleep, hypercortisolism, sleep continuity disturbances, and alterations in cerebral metabolism (Drevets and Botteron 1997; Kupfer and Ehlers 1989). Patients manifesting such abnormalities tend to be more severely depressed and less responsive to attention-placebo interventions (Thase and Howland 1995). As noted previously, these severity-linked disturbances are also more common among older patients.

Younger patients with reverse neurovegetative symptoms generally do not manifest these state-dependent abnormalities (Thase and Howland 1995). These patients, more commonly women, have relatively normal polysomnograms (Thase 1998) and are usually eucortisolemic (Feinberg and Carroll 1984). It appears that inhibitory serotonergic neurotransmission may be functionally intact in reverse neurovegetative depressions. Although pure conjecture, hypersomnolence may be viewed as an adaptive, homeostatic response that facilitates restorative slow-wave sleep during times of stress (Thase 1998). Hyperphagia may similarly be viewed as a compensatory response that results in increased dietary intake of L-tryptophan, the precursor of brain 5-HT levels (Wurtman 1993). Antidepressants that principally enhance serotonergic neurotransmission may be particularly well suited for patients without pervasive disturbances in 5-HT neuronal function.

Gender-Dependent Differences

Depressed women have more normal levels of slow-wave sleep than do age-matched depressed men (Reynolds et al. 1990). Prior to menopause, women also have relatively normal neuroendocrine responses to noradrenergic (Halbreich and Lumley 1993) and serotonergic (McBride et al. 1990) probes when compared with either older women or age-matched men. After menopause, and particularly in the context of recurrent depression, the polysomnographic and neuroendocrine profiles of depressed women and men are, at the least, comparable (Thase and Howland 1995). Some evidence suggests that older women with recurrent depression have an even higher incidence of hypercortisolism than do age-matched men (Meador-Woodruff et al. 1987).

Estrogen and naturally circulating estradiols have subtle yet manifold psychoactive effects (Halbreich 1997). Of greatest importance, estrogen modulates or upregulates 5-HT_2 receptors. This effect may explain the relative sparing of slow-wave sleep in younger depressed women, as well as their more normal responses to serotonergic agonists such as fenfluramine. Menopause thus appears to be a crucial event in understanding gender differences in the phenomenology and treatment of depression.

When used therapeutically, estrogens have a modest beneficial effect on mood for peri- and postmenopausal women as well as for those whose menopause is surgically induced (Halbreich 1997). The addition of estrogen also may augment or enhance antidepressant response in some postmenopausal women (Klaiber et al. 1979; Schneider et al. 1997). The underutilization of hormone replacement therapy might even account for the poorer prognosis of some women with recurrent depression.

Summary

Men and women respond differently to a number of treatments for depression. Although the gender differences in antidepressant response are often modest in statistical terms, they can be clinically significant. Interpersonal psychotherapy, for example, may be more broadly effective for depressed women than cognitive therapy, whereas depressed men do equally well with either therapy. The principal gender difference in medication responsivity is seen in younger women, particularly among those with reverse neurovegetative symptoms. For this group, the SSRIs have clearly become the treatment of first choice, and when they are ineffective, MAOIs such as phenelzine have well-established value. When a TCA must be used, clomipramine might be considered on theoretical grounds. Men and postmenopausal women appear to be equally responsive to SSRIs, TCAs, and MAOIs. There may be an advantage for women, compared with men, for ECT response. In later life, women also appear to be at greater risk for recurrent depression, even when receiving maintenance pharmacotherapy. The value of estrogen replacement therapy in the treatment of the postmenopausal depressed woman should not be overlooked. Recognition of gender differences in response to antidepressant treatments is long overdue, and, if confirmed, these differences may inform a more rational and effective selection of treatments.

References

Castonguay LG, Goldfried MR, Wiser S, et al: Predicting the effect of cognitive therapy for depression: a study of unique and common factors. J Consult Clin Psychol 64:497–504, 1996

Coryell W, Zimmerman M: Outcome following ECT for primary unipolar depression: a test of newly proposed response predictors. Am J Psychiatry 141:862–867, 1984

Davidson J, Pelton S: Forms of atypical depression and their response to antidepressant drugs. Psychiatry Res 17:87–95, 1985

Depression Guideline Panel: Clinical Practice Guideline Number 5. Depression in Primary Care, Vol 2. Treatment of Major Depression (AHCPR Publ No 93-0551). Rockville, MD, U.S. Department of Health and Human Services Agency for Health Care Policy and Research, 1993

DiMascio A, Weissman MM, Prusoff BA, et al: Differential symptom reduction by drugs and psychotherapy in acute depression. Arch Gen Psychiatry 36: 1450–1456, 1979

Drevets WC, Botteron K: Neuroimaging in psychiatry, in Adult Psychiatry. Edited by Guzé SB. New York, Mosby, 1997, pp 53–82

Elkin I, Shea MT, Watkins JT, et al: National Institute of Mental Health Treatment of Depression Collaborative Research Program: general effectiveness and treatments. Arch Gen Psychiatry 46:973–983, 1989

Feinberg M, Carroll BJ: Biological "markers" for endogenous depression: effect of age, severity of illness, weight loss, and polarity. Arch Gen Psychiatry 41: 1080–1085, 1984

Frank E, Carpenter LL, Kupfer DJ: Sex differences in recurrent depression: are there any that are significant? Am J Psychiatry 145:41–45, 1988

Frank E, Kupfer DJ, Perel JM, et al: Three-year outcomes for maintenance therapies in recurrent depression. Arch Gen Psychiatry 47:1093–1099, 1990

Gillin JC, Ho AC, Buchsbaum MS, et al: Functional brain imaging, sleep, and sleep deprivation: contributions to the "overarousal" hypothesis of depression. Acta Neuropsychiatr 7:33–34, 1995

Goodnick PJ, Extein IL: Bupropion and fluoxetine in depressive subtypes. Ann Clin Psychiatry 1:119–122, 1989

Halbreich U: Hormonal interventions with psychopharmacological potential: an overview. Psychopharmacol Bull 33:281–286, 1997

Halbreich U, Lumley LA: The multiple interactional biological processes that might lead to depression and gender differences in its appearance. J Affect Disord 29:159–173, 1993

Hamilton JA, Grant M, Jensvold MF: Sex and treatment of depression, in Psychopharmacology and Women. Sex, Gender, and Hormones. Edited by Jensvold MF, Halbreich U, Hamilton JA. Washington, DC, American Psychiatric Press, 1996, pp 241–260

Hamilton M: A rating scale for depression. J Neurol Neurosurg Psychiatry 23: 56–62, 1960

Hamilton M: Prediction of the response of depressions to ECT, in Electroconvulsive Therapy: Biological Foundations and Clinical Applications. Edited by Abrams R, Essman WB. New York, Spectrum Publications, 1982, pp 113–128

Hayes AM, Castonguay LG, Goldfried MR: Effectiveness of targeting the vulnerability factors of depression in cognitive therapy. J Consult Clin Psychol 64:623–627, 1996

Herrington RM, Bruce A, Johnstone EEC: Comparative trial of L-tryptophan and ECT in severe depressive illness. Lancet 2:731–734, 1974

Hersen M, Bellack AS, Himmelhoch JM, et al: Effects of social skill training, amitriptyline, and psychotherapy in unipolar depressed women. Behavior Therapy 15:21–40, 1984

Himmelhoch JM, Thase ME, Mallinger AG, et al: Tranylcypromine versus imipramine in anergic bipolar depression. Am J Psychiatry 148:910–916, 1991

Keller MB, Gelenberg AJ, Hirschfeld RM, et al: The treatment of chronic depression, part 2: a double-blind, randomized trial of sertraline and imipramine. J Clin Psychiatry 59:598–607, 1998

Kessler RC, McGonagle KA, Swartz M, et al: Sex and depression in the National Comorbidity Survey, I: lifetime prevalence, chronicity and recurrence. J Affect Disord 29:85–96, 1993

Klaiber EL, Broverman DM, Vogel W, et al: Estrogen therapy for severe persistent depressions in women. Arch Gen Psychiatry 36:550–554, 1979

Klerman G, Weissman M: Increasing rates of depression. JAMA 261:2229–2235, 1989

Kupfer DJ, Ehlers CL: Two roads to rapid eye movement latency. Arch Gen Psychiatry 46:945–948, 1989

Lewis-Hall FC, Wilson MG, Tepner RG, et al: Fluoxetine vs. tricyclic antidepressants in women with major depressive disorder. J Womens Health 6: 337–343, 1997

McBride PA, Tierney H, DeMeo M, et al: Effects of age and gender on CNS serotonergic responsivity in normal adults. Biol Psychiatry 27:1143–1155, 1990

Meador-Woodruff JH, Gurguis G, Grunhaus L, et al: Multiple depressive episodes and plasma post dexamethasone cortisol levels. Biol Psychiatry 22: 583–592, 1987

Medical Research Council: Clinical trial of the treatment of depressive illness. BMJ 5439:881–886, 1965

Nolen-Hoeksema S: Sex Differences in Depression. Palo Alto, CA, Stanford University Press, 1990

Old Age Depression Interest Group: How long should the elderly take antidepressants? A double-blind placebo-controlled study of continuation/prophylaxis therapy with dothiepin. Br J Psychiatry 162:175–182, 1993

Pande A, Birkett M, Fechner-Bates S, et al: Fluoxetine versus phenelzine in atypical depression. Biol Psychiatry 40:1017–1020, 1996

Persons JB, Thase ME, Crits-Christoph P: The role of psychotherapy in the treatment of depression. Arch Gen Psychiatry 53:283–290, 1996

Prudic J, Haskett RF, Mulsant B, et al: Resistance to antidepressant medications and short-term clinical response to ECT. Am J Psychiatry 153:985–992, 1996

Quitkin FM, Stewart JW, McGrath PJ, et al: Columbia atypical depression: a subgroup of depressive with better response to MAOI than to tricyclic antidepressants or placebo. Br J Psychiatry 163:30–34, 1993

Raskin A: Age-sex differences in response to antidepressant drugs. J Nerv Ment Dis 159:120–130, 1974

Reimherr FW, Woods DR, Byerley B, et al: Characteristics of responders to fluoxetine. Psychopharmacol Bull 20:70–72, 1984

Reynolds CF III, Kupfer DJ, Thase ME, et al: Sleep, gender, and depression: an analysis of gender effects on the electroencephalographic sleep of 302 depressed outpatients. Biol Psychiatry 28:673–684, 1990

Rothman KH, Michels KB: The continuing unethical use of placebo controls. N Engl J Med 331:394–398, 1994

Sackeim HA, Decina P, Prohovnik I, et al: Seizure threshold in electroconvulsive therapy: effects of sex, age, electrode placement, and number of treatments. Arch Gen Psychiatry 44:355–360, 1987

Schneider LS, Small GW, Hamilton SH, et al: Estrogen replacement and response to fluoxetine in a multicenter geriatric depression trial. Am J Geriatr Psychiatry 5:97–106, 1997

Steiner M, Wheadon D, Kreider M, et al: Antidepressant response to paroxetine by gender (NR462), in New Research Program and Abstracts: American Psychiatric Association 146th Annual Meeting, San Francisco, CA, May 22–27, 1993, p 274

Thase ME: Depression, sleep, and antidepressants. J Clin Psychiatry 59 (suppl 4):55–65, 1998

Thase ME, Howland RH: Biological processes in depression: an updated review and integration, in Handbook of Depression. Edited by Beckham EE, Leber WR. New York, Guilford, 1995, pp 213–279

Thase ME, Kupfer DJ: Recent developments in the pharmacotherapy of mood disorders. J Consult Clin Psychol 64:646–659, 1996

Thase ME, Carpenter L, Kupfer DJ, et al: Clinical significance of reversed vegetative subtypes of recurrent major depression. Psychopharmacol Bull 27: 17–22, 1991

Thase ME, Frank E, Mallinger A, et al: Treatment of imipramine-resistant recurrent depression, III: efficacy of monoamine oxidase inhibitors. J Clin Psychiatry 53:5–11, 1992

Thase ME, Reynolds CF III, Frank E, et al: Do depressed men and women respond similarly to cognitive behavior therapy? Am J Psychiatry 151:500–505, 1994

Thase ME, Trivedi MH, Rush AJ: MAOIs in the contemporary treatment of depression. Neuropsychopharmacology 12:185–219, 1995

Thase ME, Fava M, Halbreich U, et al: A placebo-controlled randomized clinical trial comparing sertraline and imipramine for the treatment of dysthymia. Arch Gen Psychiatry 53:777–784, 1996

Thase ME, Buysse DJ, Frank E, et al: Which depressed patients will respond to interpersonal psychotherapy? The role of abnormal EEG sleep profiles. Am J Psychiatry 154:502–509, 1997a

Thase ME, Greenhouse JB, Frank E, et al: Treatment of major depression with psychotherapy or psychotherapy–pharmacotherapy combinations. Arch Gen Psychiatry 54:1009–1015, 1997b

Thase ME, Keller MB, Gelenberg A, et al: Double-blind crossover antidepressant study: sertraline vs. imipramine (abstract). Biol Psychiatry 42:230S, 1997c

Weissman MM, Leaf PJ, Bruce ML, et al: The epidemiology of dysthymia in five communities: rates, risks, comorbidity, and treatment. Am J Psychiatry 145:815–819, 1988

Weissman MM, Bland R, Joyce PR, et al: Sex differences in rates of depression: cross-national perspectives. J Affect Disord 29:77–84, 1993

West ED, Dally PJ: Effects of iproniazid in depressive syndrome. BMJ 1:1491–1494, 1959

Wurtman JJ: Depression and weight gain: the serotonin connection. J Affect Disord 29:183–192, 1993

Young EA: Glucocorticoid cascade hypothesis revisited: role of gonadal steroids. Depression 3:20–27, 1995

CHAPTER 7

Gender Differences in Major Depression

The Role of Anxiety

Naomi Breslau, Ph.D.
Howard D. Chilcoat, Sc.D.
Edward L. Peterson, Ph.D.
Lonni R. Schultz, Ph.D.

One of the most consistent findings in psychiatric epidemiology is the higher rate of depression in women compared with men (Bland et al. 1988; Canino et al. 1987; Faravelli et al. 1990; Kessler et al. 1993; Lee et al. 1990; Robins et al. 1991; Weissman et al. 1993; Wittchen et al. 1992). This gender difference is consistently found despite marked variations in the lifetime prevalence across studies (Weissman et al. 1993). In contrast with the gender difference in the *rates* of major depression, various aspects of the *course* of the disorder (i.e., age at onset, chronicity, or recurrence) have been found to be similar in both genders (Frank et al. 1988; Kessler et al. 1993; Weissman et al. 1993; Young et al. 1990). In addition, there is no consistent evidence supporting gender differences in the phenomenology of depressive episodes. The gender difference in the rate of major depression emerges early in life, that is, at age 15 years or even earlier (Burke et al. 1990; Kessler et al. 1993; McGee et al. 1990). Furthermore, there is evidence from previous studies that females continue to be at higher risk for depression beyond adolescence, when the gender difference is observed for the first time (Eaton et al. 1989, 1997; Kessler et al. 1993), although there are exceptions to this general pattern.

The finding of gender differences in depression has received considerable scientific attention, and both biological and social explanations have been proposed. Although it is now well accepted that the gender difference is not an artifact, there is little agreement on the mechanisms that might account for it (Merikangas et al. 1985; Nolen-Hoeksema 1987; Nolen- Hoeksema and Girgus 1994; Weissman and Klerman 1977). The observation that females are at increased risk for first onset of major depression beyond adolescence and into the adult years suggests that factors specific to one stage in the life span—say, early adolescence—could not provide a full explanation. Explanations might be sought in biological or social factors that have their origins in adolescence but continue to exert an influence in later years. It might also be the case that the set of factors implicated in the emergence of the gender difference in adolescence is different from the factors implicated in females' relatively greater risk for depression in later years.

Anxiety Disorders and Major Depression

Epidemiological studies have documented high rates of comorbidity between major depression and anxiety disorders (Maser and Cloninger 1990). Comorbidity of major depression with other psychiatric disorders, such as substance use disorders, is far weaker (Kessler et al. 1996; Merikangas et al. 1996). The rate of anxiety disorders in persons with major depression is markedly higher than the rate of major depression in persons with anxiety disorders, and "pure" major depression—that is, major depression without a history of anxiety—is relatively rare (Alloy et al. 1990; Regier et al. 1990). There is evidence of a predominant temporal sequence between major depression and anxiety, with anxiety disorders predating the onset of major depression (Angst et al. 1990; Kendell 1974; Kessler et al. 1996). The association between major depression and anxiety disorders might be relevant to the gender difference in major depression in two ways:

1. Females' higher risk for major depression might reflect their greater propensity to become depressed following an anxiety disorder (an interaction between gender and prior anxiety).

2. Even if females did not differ from males in their propensity to become depressed after the onset of an anxiety disorder, their higher rates of anxiety disorders (Blazer et al. 1991; Breslau et al. 1991; Eaton et al. 1997; Kessler et al. 1994; Weissman et al. 1984) might explain their greater risk for major depression.

In this chapter we examine the role of anxiety disorders in the gender difference in major depression. Data were from a longitudinal epidemiological study of young adults in the Detroit metropolitan area (Breslau et al. 1991). The analysis proceeds as follows: First, we describe the gender difference in major depression. Second, we focus on the gender difference in anxiety disorders. Third, we test two hypotheses regarding the role of prior anxiety in the gender difference in major depression: 1) gender might modify the relationship between prior anxiety and subsequent major depression (the interaction hypothesis); and 2) the gender difference in major depression might be explained by the gender difference in earlier anxiety. Finally, we extend the analysis and consider also the role of prior alcohol abuse or dependence in this relationship. The question we address is as follows: Does controlling for prior alcohol abuse or dependence, a disorder in which males predominate, alter the results of our analysis? That is, since controlling for anxiety disorders might reduce the gender difference in major depression, controlling additionally for alcohol abuse or dependence might reverse that effect and reestablish the initial gender difference in major depression.

Methods

Sample and Data

A random sample of 1,200 persons was drawn from all 21- to 30-year-old members of a 400,000-member health management organization (HMO) in southeast Michigan, which includes the city of Detroit and surrounding communities. A total of 1,007 individuals (84% of sample) were interviewed in person in 1989. Follow-up personal interviews were conducted in 1992 with 979 subjects and in 1994 with 974 subjects, in each case exceeding 97% of the target sample, excluding 3 who died during the follow-up intervals. Telephone follow-up interviews were conducted with subjects who moved out of the geographic area. At baseline, the median age was 26 years. Approximately 80% of the subjects were white, and 62% were female; 29% had completed college.

The National Institute of Mental Health Diagnostic Interview Schedule (NIMH DIS), revised to cover DSM-III-R disorders (Robins et al. 1989), was used at baseline to measure lifetime history of psychiatric disorders. Follow-up interviews assessed psychiatric disorders during the interval periods. Detailed descriptions of the NIMH DIS and information on its reliability and validity have been previously reported (Anthony et al. 1985; Helzer et al. 1985; Robins et al. 1982). The NIMH DIS is a structured interview designed to be administered by professional interviewers without clinical training. An extensive training program was used to ensure close adherence to the questionnaire and the sequence of follow-up probes. Diagnoses were made with computer algorithms, following DSM-III-R (American Psychiatric Association 1987) diagnostic definitions.

The DSM-III-R disorders covered in this chapter are major depression and anxiety disorders—specifically, panic disorder, generalized anxiety disorder (GAD), obsessive-compulsive disorder (OCD), posttraumatic stress disorder (PTSD), agoraphobia, social phobia, and simple phobia. In the analysis of the role of prior anxiety in the gender–major depression relationship, we used a single composite variable—Any Anxiety—and defined age at onset as the age at which the earliest anxiety disorder first occurred.

Statistical Analysis

The analysis was conducted on the combined data gathered at baseline and at the two follow-up interviews. At baseline, lifetime psychiatric history ascertained disorders up to the time of the interview; new cases of disorders, ascertained at follow-up interviews, were added to form the combined data. Compared with the prospective follow-up data, which covered 5 years in young adulthood, the combined longitudinal data provided lifetime information up to age 35 years, the upper age limit of the sample at the last follow-up. History of Any Anxiety, defined as the occurrence of any of the specific anxiety disorders, was used. We first display the cumulative incidence curves of major depression and of Any Anxiety in males and females. Kaplan-Meier survival analysis (Kaplan and Meier 1958), with time defined as respondent's age, was used to estimate the cumulative incidence of each disorder from the earliest to the latest case, up to approximately 35 years of age. Cox proportional hazards regressions were used to estimate female-to-male hazard ratios and 95% confidence intervals (CIs) for first-onset major depression and first-onset Any Anxiety. Standard life-table methods were used to estimate *age-specific* hazard rates of first-onset major depression and Any Anxiety.

Cox proportional hazards models for censored survival data with Any Anxiety as a time-dependent covariate were used to examine the role of prior anxiety in the gender–major depression relationship (Breslow 1974; Cox 1972; Kay 1977). The censored subjects were those who had not developed major depression at the time of the last interview. Age at earliest anxiety disorder was used as the time of occurrence of Any Anxiety. The parameter estimates in the proportional hazards model are regression coefficients from which hazard ratios can be obtained. An advantage of the Cox proportional hazards model with time-dependent covariates is that it permits us to take into account the age at onset of major depression in relation to the age at onset of Any Anxiety. We first estimated the interaction between gender and Any Anxiety in relation to subsequent major depression in a model that included gender, prior occurrence of Any Anxiety, and their interaction term. To estimate the effect of prior anxiety on the gender–major depression relationship, we used two successive models, the first without and the second with prior anxiety disorder. A comparison of the regression coefficients for major depression associated with gender in the first and second models can be used to estimate the impact of prior anxiety disorder on the relationship between gender and major depression. Cases in which the onset of major depression and the onset of Any Anxiety were reported to have occurred in the same year were censored just prior to the year in which the two events occurred. This procedure avoids assumption of a temporal sequence where none could be observed in the data.

Results

Incidence of Major Depression by Gender

Figure 7–1 displays the cumulative incidence of major depression in males and females up to age 35 years, estimated via Kaplan-Meier sur-

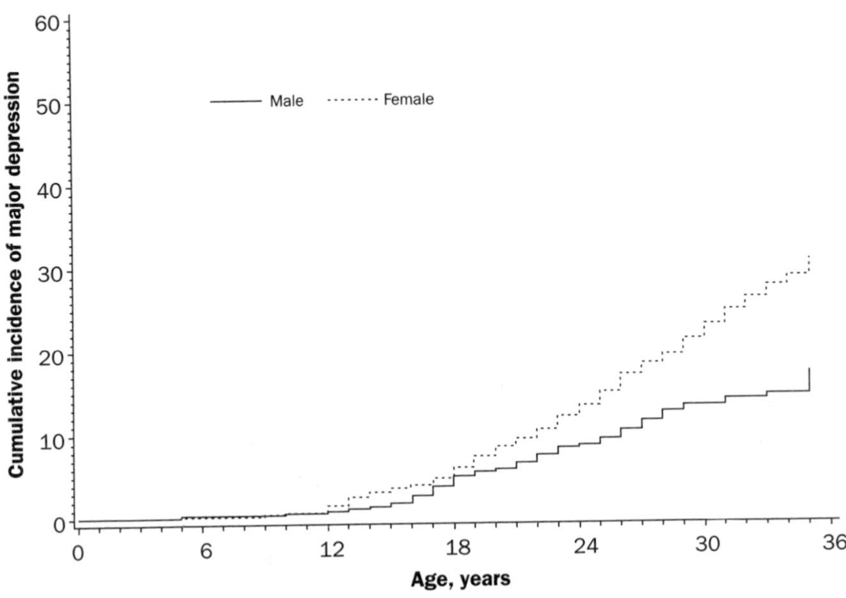

FIGURE 7–1. Cumulative incidence of major depression by gender (n = 1,007).

vival analysis. As can be seen, the females' curve was significantly higher than the males' (log-rank test = .0001). The female-to-male hazard ratio, estimated in a Cox proportional hazards model, was 1.9 (95% CI = 1.4–2.6). A comparison of the two curves reveals that the cumulative percentages of major depression began to diverge for males and females at about age 12 years. The gap between the genders continued to increase with increasing age throughout the period of observation, up to age 35 years. In other words, females' higher cumulative incidence of major depression in the 20s and early 30s is not just a reflection of their higher rate of major depression in adolescence. Compared with males, females have both an early excess of major depression and an excess of first-onset cases of major depression.

Table 7–1 presents estimates of the age-specific female-to-male hazard ratios for first-onset major depression from early childhood through age 35 years. The gender difference in the hazard rates begins at the 5-year period of age 10–14 years. The hazard ratio at that age was 2.7. In the third decade of life, between 20 and 29 years of age, the female-

TABLE 7–1.
Age-specific female-to-male hazard ratios (HRs) for first-onset major depression (n = 1,007)

Age group (years)	HR
0–9	1.2
10–14	2.7
15–19	1.0
20–24	2.0
25–29	1.8
30–34	6.2

to-male hazard ratio was about 2.00. The data suggest that this ratio might be higher in the mid-30s. These findings are consistent with previous findings from both retrospective and prospective studies showing that females' higher risk for first-onset major depression in adolescence continues into adulthood.

Incidence of Any Anxiety by Gender

Figure 7–2, displaying the cumulative incidence of Any Anxiety in males and females up to age 35 years, shows a higher cumulative percentage in females than in males (log-rank test = 0.0001). The female-to-male hazard ratio of Any Anxiety, estimated in a Cox proportional hazards model, was 2.1 (95% CI = 1.6–2.6). A comparison of the two curves reveals that from early childhood, the cumulative percentage of Any Anxiety was higher in females than in males.

The female-to-male hazard ratios for lifetime prevalence of *specific anxiety disorders* appear in Table 7–2. For five of the seven specific anxiety disorders examined, the hazard ratios were 2 and above. Social phobia and OCD showed smaller gender differences, and in the case of OCD the gender difference was not significant.

Figure 7–3 depicts the age-specific hazard rates of first onset of Any Anxiety in females and males. It shows that females' higher risk for first onset of Any Anxiety characterizes the entire period of observation in this study, up to age 35 years.

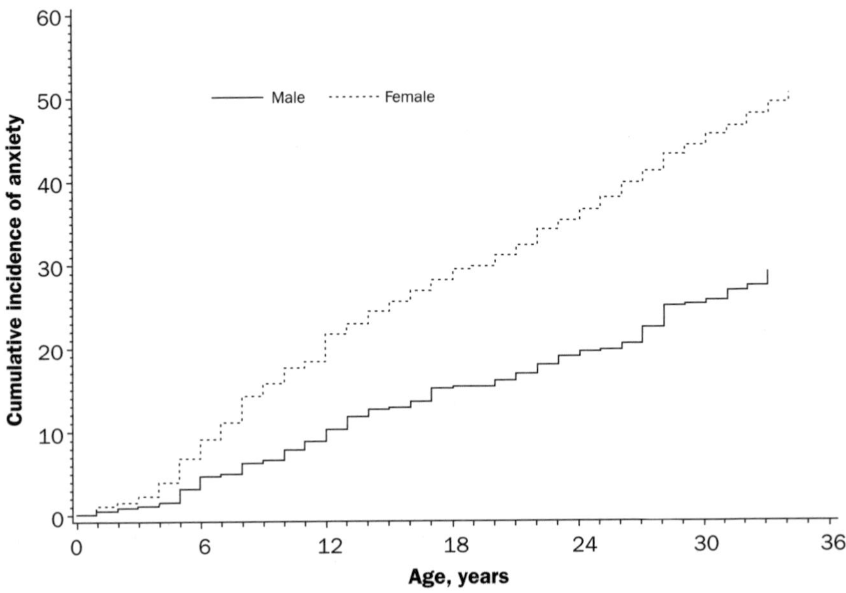

FIGURE 7–2. Cumulative incidence of Any Anxiety by gender (*n* = 1,007).

TABLE 7–2.
Female-to-male lifetime hazard ratios (HRs) and 95% confidence intervals (CIs) for specific anxiety disorders (*n* = 1,007)

	HR (95% CI)	*P*
Simple phobia	2.6 (1.8–3.7)	.0001
Social phobia	1.4 (1.0–2.0)	.035
Agoraphobia	3.4 (1.7–6.7)	.0004
Posttraumatic stress disorder	2.1 (1.4–3.2)	.0007
Generalized anxiety disorder	2.0 (1.2–3.4)	.005
Panic disorder	2.7 (1.4–5.4)	.005
Obsessive-compulsive disorder	1.4 (0.6–3.3)	.406

Comorbidity Among the Anxiety Disorders

In our study, anxiety disorders were comorbid with one another, and the majority of persons with a history of any specific anxiety disorder also reported a history of one or more other anxiety disorders. Rates of co-

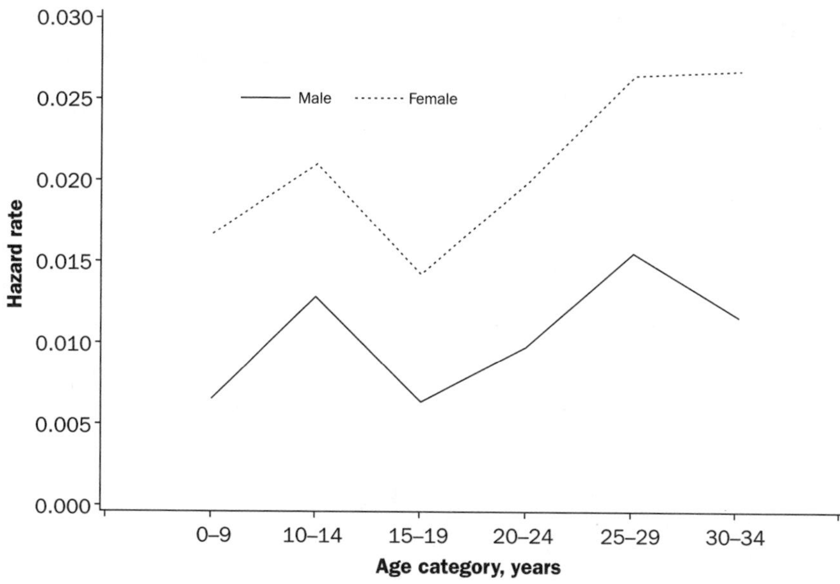

FIGURE 7–3. Age-specific hazard rates of first onset of Any Anxiety by gender (n = 1,007).

morbidity with other anxiety disorders ranged from a low of 54% for social phobia to a high of 88% for OCD. In Table 7–3, we present the proportions of persons with each specific anxiety disorder in whom the disorder was either pure (in the sense of being unaccompanied by a history of any other anxiety disorders) or—if comorbid with other anxiety disorders—primary or secondary in onset. As can be seen in the table, simple and social phobia were mostly primary or pure anxiety disorders, whereas generalized anxiety disorder and OCD were chiefly secondary to other anxiety disorders, with 60% or more of individuals with these disorders reporting a history of a prior anxiety disorder.

Each specific anxiety disorder was more likely to occur in persons with a prior history of other anxiety disorders (Table 7–4). For example, social phobia and PTSD were 2.5 times more likely to occur in persons with a prior history of another anxiety disorder, compared with persons with no prior anxiety. Apart from these relationships, females were found to be at greater risk than males for experiencing a first onset of each anxiety disorder *in the absence of* a history of another anxiety disorder (Table 7–5). Significant female-to-male hazard ratios were observed for first

TABLE 7–3.
Lifetime comorbidity and temporal order among specific anxiety disorders

	N	"Pure," %	Primary, %	Secondary, %
Simple phobia	173	39	38	23
Social phobia	158	46	26	28
Posttraumatic stress disorder	117	36	26	38
Panic disorder	53	24	25	51
Agoraphobia	63	17	31	52
Generalized anxiety disorder	83	26	14	60
Obsessive-compulsive disorder	26	12	23	65

TABLE 7–4.
Hazard ratios (HRs) and 95% confidence intervals (CIs) for specific anxiety disorders in the presence of prior anxiety disorders

	HR (95% CI)
Simple phobia	3.1 (2.1–4.6)
Social phobia	2.5 (1.7–3.6)
Posttraumatic stress disorder	2.6 (1.8–3.8)
Panic disorder	4.1 (2.3–7.5)
Agoraphobia	5.6 (3.3–9.5)
Generalized anxiety disorder	4.9 (3.0–7.9)
Obsessive-compulsive disorder	10.9 (4.4–26.9)

Note. Estimated in seven univariate Cox proportional hazard models, with prior onset of any other anxiety disorder as a time-dependent covariate.

onset of simple phobia (3.1), PTSD (2.0), agoraphobia (3.3), and GAD (2.7) in the absence of any other prior anxiety disorder.

Major Depression and Prior Anxiety Disorders

We examined the hypothesis that the gender difference in major depression might reflect females' greater propensity to become depressed fol-

TABLE 7–5.

Female-to-male hazard ratios (HRs) and 95% confidence intervals (CIs) for specific anxiety disorders in the absence of prior anxiety disorders

	HR (95% CI)
Simple phobia	3.1 (1.9–4.8)
Social phobia	1.4 (0.9–2.1)
Posttraumatic stress disorder	2.0 (1.2–3.3)
Panic disorder	1.2 (0.5–2.8)
Agoraphobia	3.3 (1.3–8.8)
Generalized anxiety disorder	2.7 (1.1–6.7)
Obsessive-compulsive disorder	1.8 (0.4–9.3)

Note. Estimated in seven univariate Cox proportional hazard models that included gender, prior occurrence of Any Anxiety as a time-dependent covariate, and an interaction term.

lowing an anxiety disorder—the interaction hypothesis—in a Cox proportional hazards model with gender, preexisting Any Anxiety (as a time-dependent covariate), and their interaction term. The results, which appear in Table 7–6, showed that the interaction between gender and preexisting anxiety was not significant ($P = .670$). Moreover, from the negative sign of the coefficient of the interaction term, it can be inferred that females might be *less* vulnerable than males to depression after an anxiety disorder, rather than the reverse. The hazard ratio for major depression associated with prior Any Anxiety in males was 5.9 (95% CI = 3.4–10.1), whereas in females it was 3.9 (95% CI = 2.8–5.6). The analysis in Table 7–6 also indicates that in the absence of preexisting Any Anxiety, the hazard ratio for major depression in females versus males is significantly greater than one (beta = 0.49, hazard ratio = 1.56). We will return to this finding later in more detail.

To test the hypothesis that the gender difference in major depression might be explained by a gender difference in preexisting Any Anxiety, two successive Cox proportional hazards models were used: the first estimates the risk for major depression associated with gender, and the second reestimates that risk, controlling for preexisting Any Anxiety as a time- dependent covariate (Table 7–7). In the first model, the coefficient of gender, which estimates the risk for major depression in females rela-

TABLE 7–6.

Testing for an interaction between gender and preexisting Any Anxiety

	Beta	*P*
Gender (female)	0.49	.04
Preexisting anxiety	1.77	.0001
Interaction	0.40	.670

TABLE 7–7.

Gender difference in major depression, controlling for preexisting Any Anxiety

	Model 1			Model 2		
	Beta	*P*	HR	Beta	*P*	HR
Gender (female)	.56	.0006	1.75	.28	.087	1.33
Preexisting anxiety		–		1.48	.0001	4.41

Note. Results from two successive Cox proportional hazard models, with and without Any Anxiety as a time-dependent covariate. HR = hazard ratio.

tive to males, was equal to 0.56. When preexisting Any Anxiety was controlled in the second model, the coefficient of gender was reduced to 0.28, a 50% reduction. Expressed in terms of hazard ratios, the reduction is from 1.75 to 1.33. (It should be noted that the 1.75 *unadjusted* female-to-male hazard ratio in Table 7–6 is lower than the 1.90 reported initially, because of the deletion from this analysis of cases with same-year onset of major depression and Any Anxiety, cases that are censored in the second model. Failure to correct for these same-year cases in the first model would have resulted in overstating the reduction in the coefficient of gender from the first to the second model.)

To more clearly illustrate the results of the analysis depicted in Table 7–6, we present in Figure 7–4 the gender-specific cumulative incidence curves of major depression, according to the presence or absence of preexisting Any Anxiety. As can be seen, at each age, the cumulative percentage of major depression in both genders was higher among those with preexisting Any Anxiety than among those without. Differences between males and females, when prior Any Anxiety was held constant, were small.

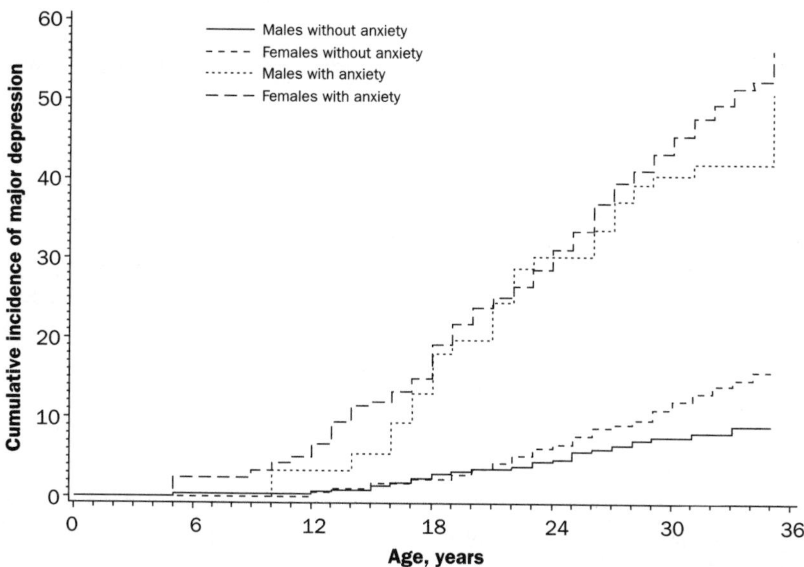

FIGURE 7–4. Cumulative incidence of major depression by prior Any Anxiety and gender (n = 1,007).

Additional Analysis: Prior Alcohol Abuse or Dependence and Gender Differences in Major Depression

To address the concern that the observed effect on the gender difference in major depression of controlling for prior Any Anxiety might be reversed when prior alcohol abuse or dependence (A/D) is controlled, we extended the model shown in Table 7–6 to include prior alcohol A/D. Before presenting these results, we should note that the lifetime comorbidity of alcohol A/D in persons with major depression was far lower than the lifetime comorbidity of Any Anxiety in these individuals: 32.7% versus 74.4%. Furthermore, the temporal sequence between major depression and alcohol A/D did not show the typical pattern seen in relation to anxiety. Whereas the onset of major depression rarely preceded the onset of any anxiety disorder, the onset of major depression preceded the onset of alcohol A/D in 40% of the comorbid cases. The hazard ratio for major depression in persons with prior alcohol A/D was 1.02 (95% CI = 0.71–1.46). No interaction between gender and prior alcohol A/D was detected (P = .315).

TABLE 7–8.
Gender difference in major depression, controlling for prior Any Anxiety and prior alcohol abuse or dependence

	Beta	SE	*P*	HR (95% CI)
Gender (female)	0.33	0.17	.06	1.39 (0.99–1.95)
Anxiety first/only	1.52	0.16	.0001	4.55 (3.31–6.27)
Alcohol first/only	0.49	0.26	.06	1.63 (0.98–2.72)

Note. CI = confidence interval; HR = hazard ratio.

In Table 7–8, we present the results of a Cox proportional hazards model that estimated the gender difference in major depression, controlling for prior Any Anxiety *and* prior alcohol A/D. In persons with a history of both disorders, Any Anxiety was coded as present if it occurred first, and prior alcohol A/D was coded as present if it preceded Any Anxiety. In this analysis, 21 cases of major depression and either Any Anxiety or alcohol A/D with onset at the same age were censored just prior to that age. As shown in Table 7–8, when preexisting Any Anxiety was controlled, the hazard ratio for major depression in persons with prior alcohol A/D was 1.63 (95% CI = 0.98–2.72; *P* = .06). However, controlling for alcohol A/D had no effect on the earlier results. The reduction in the coefficient of gender when prior Any Anxiety *and* prior alcohol A/D were controlled in the same model was from 0.57 to 0.33. In terms of hazard ratios, the excess risk for major depression in females was reduced from 1.78 to 1.39, a 50% reduction. This analysis supports the unique role of prior anxiety in females' increased risk for major depression. Anxiety disorders not only are more common in females than in males but also hold a uniquely strong relationship with major depression in both genders and, as a rule, precede the onset of major depression. In contrast, alcohol A/D is relatively weakly associated with major depression and is nearly as likely to precede as to follow the onset of that illness.

Gender Differences in Pure Major Depression

The finding that preexisting Any Anxiety explained a large part of the gender difference in the lifetime risk for major depression does not imply that if we were to exclude cases of major depression comorbid with Any

Anxiety, the rates of pure major depression in the two genders would be equal. Our analysis suggested, rather, that in the absence of preexisting Any Anxiety, females had a higher risk for major depression than males. Figure 7–5 shows the age-specific female-to-male hazard ratios of major depression in the presence of preexisting Any Anxiety and in its absence. In the presence of preexisting Any Anxiety, the female-to-male hazard ratios for major depression rarely exceed the null value of one, indicating no excess in females compared with males. In contrast, in the absence of preexisting Any Anxiety, the female-to-male hazard ratios for major depression are greater than one beginning at about age 15 years. This finding is not incompatible with our key finding—namely, that females' higher lifetime risk for major depression is considerably reduced when prior anxiety is controlled. The reason is that only a small fraction of cases of major depression occur in the absence of preexisting anxiety. The preponderance of cases of major depression in both genders are those with preexisting anxiety, and with respect to the cases with preexisting anxiety, no gender difference was observed.

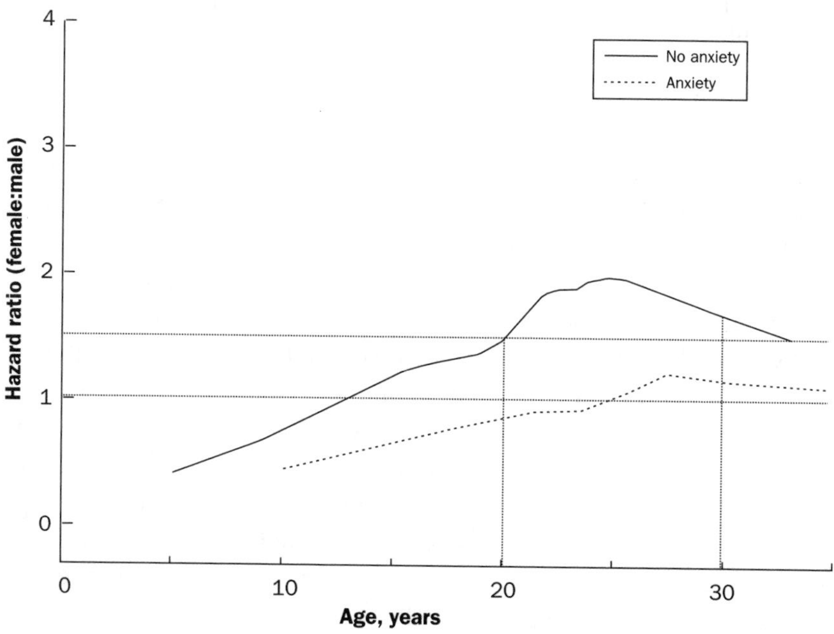

FIGURE 7–5. Age-specific female-to-male hazard ratios of major depression in the presence and absence of preexisting Any Anxiety (n = 1,007).

Discussion

The results of our analysis can be summarized as follows:

1. The lifetime risk for major depression was approximately two times higher in females than in males.
2. The gender difference in the rate of first-onset major depression that emerged in adolescence continued into adulthood.
3. The lifetime risk for one or more anxiety disorders was approximately two times higher in females than in males.
4. Females were at increased risk for first onset of an anxiety disorder throughout the age span covered in the study (i.e., up to 35 years).
5. Prior anxiety was associated with an increased risk for major depression in both genders, and females were not more vulnerable than males to becoming depressed following an anxiety disorder.
6. Prior anxiety disorders accounted for a considerable part of the observed gender difference in depression.
7. Additionally controlling for prior alcohol A/D did not alter these results.

Our analysis suggests that females' higher rates of anxiety disorders might play a part in their higher risk for major depression. Although major depression is often a secondary disorder in relation to a variety of mental and substance use disorders, its link with prior anxiety disorders is unique. In both genders, major depression is strongly comorbid with anxiety disorders, which, as a rule, precede the onset of major depression. The lifetime association between major depression and alcohol A/D is relatively weak, and alcohol A/D is as likely to follow as to precede the onset of major depression. Our findings on the relationship between major depression, on the one hand, and anxiety disorders or alcohol A/D, on the other, are consistent with previous reports (Merikangas et al. 1996). Furthermore, they support the unique role of anxiety in the gender difference in major depression. Our analysis indicated that alcohol A/D was not males' counterpart to anxiety, in terms of its potential role in the gender difference in major depression. Although far more prevalent in males than in females, alcohol A/D appears to have little effect on the gender difference in major depression.

It should be noted that our finding that the association between major depression and anxiety disorders is not stronger in females than in males does not imply that the rate of anxiety disorders in depressed females is not higher than that in depressed males. On the contrary, depressed females are more likely than depressed males to report a history of one or more anxiety disorders. The higher rates of anxiety disorders in depressed females reflect the overall gender difference in anxiety: both depressed and nondepressed females have higher rates of anxiety disorders than do their male counterparts. In other words, the difference in the rate of anxiety disorders between depressed females and depressed males reflects the main effect of gender on anxiety disorder and should not be interpreted as a gender difference in the expression of major depression.

Our findings of high rates of comorbidity among the anxiety disorders is consistent with previous reports (Blazer et al. 1991; Boyd et al. 1984; Breier et al. 1986; Breslau et al. 1991; Eaton et al. 1997; Weissman et al. 1994). Specific anxiety disorders rarely occur as pure anxiety disorders across the life span. Furthermore, each specific anxiety disorder is more likely to occur in persons who have already experienced another anxiety disorder. Given the proportion of cases involving comorbid other anxiety disorders among persons with each specific anxiety disorder, findings of studies that focus on the relationship between major depression and a single anxiety disorder—say, panic disorder—should be interpreted with caution if the studies do not exclude the contribution to that relationship of other co-existing anxiety disorders.

The results of this analysis raise an important question for future research—namely, why are females at greater risk for anxiety disorders beginning early in life and continuing in adulthood? The results also suggest that anxiety disorders in both genders, especially early in life, deserve clinical attention, not only in their own right but also for their strong association with an increased liability for subsequent major depression.

References

Alloy LB, Kelly KA, Mineka S, et al: Comorbidity of anxiety and depressive disorders: a helplessness-hopelessness perspective, in Comorbidity of Mood and Anxiety Disorders. Edited by Maser JD, Cloninger CR. Washington, DC, American Psychiatric Press, 1990, pp 499–543

American Psychiatric Association: Diagnostic and Statistical Manual of Mental Disorders, 3rd Edition, Revised. Washington, DC, American Psychiatric Association, 1987

Angst J, Vollrath M, Merikangas KR, et al: Comorbidity of anxiety and depression in the Zurich cohort study of young adults, in Comorbidity of Mood and Anxiety Disorders. Edited by Maser JD, Cloninger CR. Washington, DC, American Psychiatric Press, 1990, pp 123–137

Anthony JC, Folstein M, Romanoski AJ, et al: Comparison of the lay Diagnostic Interview Schedule and a standardized psychiatric diagnosis. Arch Gen Psychiatry 42:667–675, 1985

Bland RC, Orn H, Newman SC: Lifetime prevalence of psychiatric disorders in Edmonton. Acta Psychiatr Scand Suppl 338:24–32, 1988

Blazer DG, Hughes D, George LK, et al: Generalized anxiety disorder, in Psychiatric Disorders in America: The Epidemiologic Catchment Area Study. Edited by Robins LN, Regier DA. New York, Free Press, 1991, pp 180–203

Boyd JH, Burke JD, Gruenberg E, et al: Exclusion criteria of DSM-III: a study of co-occurrence of hierarchy-free syndromes. Arch Gen Psychiatry 41:983–989, 1984

Breier A, Charney DS, Heninger GR: Agoraphobia with panic attacks: Development, diagnostic stability, and course of illness. Arch Gen Psychiatry 43: 1029–1036, 1986

Breslau N, Davis GC, Andreski P, et al: Traumatic events and posttraumatic stress disorder in an urban population of young adults. Arch Gen Psychiatry 48:216–222, 1991

Breslow N: Covariance analysis of censored survival data. Biometrics 30:89–99, 1974

Burke JD Jr, Wittchen H-U, Regier DA, et al: Extracting information from diagnostic interviews on co-occurrence of symptoms of anxiety and depression, in Comorbidity of Mood and Anxiety Disorders. Edited by Maser JD, Cloninger CR. Washington, DC, American Psychiatric Press, 1990, pp 649–667

Canino GJ, Bird HR, Shrout PE, et al: The prevalence of specific psychiatric disorders in Puerto Rico. Arch Gen Psychiatry 44:727–735, 1987

Cox DR: Regression models and life tables. Journal of the Royal Statistical Society Series B 34:187–220, 1972

Eaton WW, Kramer M, Anthony JC, et al: The incidence of specific DIS/DSM-III Mental Disorders: data from the NIMH Epidemiologic Catchment Area Program. Acta Psychiatr Scand 79:163–178, 1989

Eaton WW, Anthony JC, Gallo J, et al: Natural history of Diagnostic Interview Schedule/DSM-IV major depression: The Baltimore Epidemiologic Catchment Area follow-up. Arch Gen Psychiatry 54:993–999, 1997

Faravelli C, Degl'Innocenti BG, Aiazzi L, et al: Epidemiology of mood disorders: a community survey in Florence. J Affect Disord 20:135–141, 1990

Frank E, Carpenter LL, Kupfer DJ: Sex differences in recurrent depression: are there any that are significant? Am J Psychiatry 145:41–45, 1988

Helzer JE, Robins LN, McEvoy LT, et al: A comparison of clinician and diagnostic interview schedule diagnoses. Arch Gen Psychiatry 42:657–666, 1985

Kaplan EL, Meier P: Nonparametric estimation from incomplete observations. Journal of the American Statistical Association 53:457–481, 1958

Kay R: Proportional hazard regression models and the analysis of censored survival data. Applied Statistics 26:227–237, 1977

Kendell RE: The stability of psychiatric diagnosis. Br J Psychiatry 124:352–356, 1974

Kessler RC, McGonagle KA, Swartz M, et al: Sex and depression in the National Comorbidity Survey, I: lifetime prevalence, chronicity and recurrence. J Affect Disord 29:85–96, 1993

Kessler RC, McGonagle KA, Zhao S, et al: Lifetime and 12-month prevalence of DSM-III-R psychiatric disorders in the United States: results from the National Comorbidity Study. Arch Gen Psychiatry 51:8–19, 1994

Kessler RC, Nelson CB, McGonagle KA, et al: Comorbidity of DSM-III-R major depressive disorder in the general population: results from the US National Comorbidity Survey. Br J Psychiatry 168:17–30, 1996

Lee CK, Kwak YS, Yamamoto J, et al: Psychiatric epidemiology in Korea, Part 1: gender and age differences in Seoul. J Nerv Ment Disord 178:242–246, 1990

Maser JD, Cloninger CR (eds): Comorbidity of Mood and Anxiety Disorders. Washington, DC, American Psychiatric Press, 1990

McGee R, Feehan M, Williams S, et al: DSM-III disorders in a large sample of adolescents. J Am Acad Child Adolesc Psychiatry 29:611–619, 1990

Merikangas KR, Weissman MM, Pauls DL: Genetic factors in the sex ratio of major depression. Psychol Med 15:63–69, 1985

Merikangas KR, Angst J, Eaton W, et al: Comorbidity and boundaries of affective disorders with anxiety disorders and substance misuse: results of an international task force. Br J Psychiatry 168:58–67, 1996

Nolen-Hoeksema S: Sex differences in unipolar depression: evidence and theory. Psychol Bull 101:259–282, 1987

Nolen-Hoeksema S, Girgus JS: The emergence of gender differences in depression during adolescence. Psychol Bull 115:424–443, 1994

Regier DA, Burke JD Jr, Burke KC: Comorbidity of affective and anxiety disorders in the NIMH Epidemiologic Catchment Area Program, in Comorbidity of Mood and Anxiety Disorders. Edited by Maser JD, Cloninger CR. Washington, DC, American Psychiatric Press, 1990, pp 113–122

Robins LN, Helzer JE, Ratcliff KS, et al: Validity of the Diagnostic Interview Schedule, Version II: DSM III diagnoses. Psychol Med 12:855–870, 1982

Robins LN, Helzer JE, Cottler L, et al: NIMH Diagnostic Interview Schedule, Version III, Revised. St Louis, MO, Washington University, 1989

Robins LN, Locke BZ, Regier DA: An overview of psychiatric disorders in America, in Psychiatric Disorders in America: The Epidemiologic Catchment Area Study. Edited by Robins LN, Regier DA. New York, Free Press, 1991, pp 328–366

Weissman MM, Klerman GL: Sex differences and the epidemiology of depression. Arch Gen Psychiatry 34:98–111, 1977

Weissman MM, Leckman JF, Merikangas KR, et al: Depression and anxiety disorders in parents and children. Arch Gen Psychiatry 41:845–852, 1984

Weissman MM, Bland R, Joyce PR, et al: Sex differences in rates of depression: cross-national perspectives. J Affect Disord 29:77–84, 1993

Weissman MM, Bland RC, Canino GJ, et al: The Cross-National Epidemiology of Obsessive Compulsive Disorder. J Clin Psychiatry 55:5–10, 1994

Wittchen H-U, Essau CA, von Zerssen D, et al: Lifetime and six-month prevalence of mental disorders in the Munich Follow-Up Study. Eur Arch Psychiatry Clin Neurosci 241:247–258, 1992

Young MA, Scheftner WA, Fawcett J, et al: Gender differences in the clinical features of unipolar major depressive disorder. J Nerv Ment Dis 178:200–203, 1990

CHAPTER 8

Gender Differences in Anxiety Disorders

Clinical Implications

M. Katherine Shear, M.D.
Ulrike Feske, Ph.D.
Catherine Greeno, Ph.D.

The majority of persons seeking treatment for anxiety disorders are women. In addition, data from the most recent large-scale epidemiological study, the National Comorbidity Survey (Kessler et al. 1994), show anxiety disorders to be almost twice as prevalent among women in the community as among men. The fact that gender differences are found in community samples suggests that the overrepresentation of women in clinical settings is not due to women's greater tendency to seek help for their problems (Bourdon et al. 1988).

Nor do gender differences appear to be the result of a verbal report bias. Although there is some evidence that men's conformance to male gender stereotypes leads to an underreporting of fears (e.g., Pierce and Kirkpatrick 1992), these findings are not consistent (e.g., Arrindell et al. 1993). In several laboratory studies with college students fearful of small

This work was supported in part by National Institute of Mental Health grant MH-53817.

The authors thank Ms. Barbara Kumer, Mrs. Miyako Hanekamp, and Ms. Nancy Will for technical assistance with manuscript preparation.

animals, women showed higher rates of avoidance than men, suggesting that women truly are more phobic (e.g., Huber and Altmeier 1983; Speltz and Bernstein 1976). Moreover, results from the large-scale Epidemiologic Catchment Area (ECA) Study (Robins and Regier 1991) failed to demonstrate that men are less likely than women to report fears or to seek treatment for their phobias (Bourdon et al. 1988).

Are men more likely to mask their anxiety through the excessive use of alcohol? Men with anxiety disorders are more likely to abuse or depend on alcohol than women (e.g., Bibb and Chambless 1986; Kessler et al. 1995), raising the possibility that the percentage of men with hidden anxiety disorders may exceed that of women (Barlow 1988). On the other hand, researchers have not yet systematically examined the extent to which women mask their anxiety by using alcohol, anxiolytic medication, or other substances, or by using coping strategies such as binge eating (Bekker 1996; Root 1989). It is quite likely that the number of hidden anxiety disorders among women is rather similar to that among men, once coping strategies that are specific to women are taken into account.

Gender differences in psychological disorders are not limited to anxiety. Major depression and dysthymia occur about twice as often among women as among men (Kessler et al. 1994). An important study examining the role of anxiety disorders in the development of gender differences in major depression was conducted by Breslau et al. (1995). These investigators found that anxiety was a significant risk factor for major depression in both men and women. Women's higher risk for depression was explained by the higher prevalence of anxiety disorders in females beginning early in life, a finding that emphasizes the need for further studies to elucidate the underpinnings of gender differences in anxiety across the life span.

We conclude that gender ratios of anxiety disorders presented in the literature are reasonably accurate and that women are indeed more vulnerable to these disorders. The obvious question then becomes "Why is this the case?" Even in the meager existing literature, researchers have approached this question in different ways, some emphasizing biological, others psychological, and still others sociocultural explanations. In this brief review we focus on aspects of psychosocial functioning that appear to influence the development or expression of anxiety disorders. Although we believe that vulnerability to anxiety involves biological as well as psychosocial factors, in this paper we focus on four areas in which gender differences in psychosocial functioning are know to exist: 1) gender roles, 2) gender-role stress, 3) social relationships, and 4) gender differences in exposure to social adversity (e.g., women have more adversity). We discuss the possible relationship of each of these differences to anxiety disorders.

Gender Role

Fodor (1974; Brehony 1983; Chambless 1989; Wolfe 1984) was among the first to assert that traditional gender roles predispose women to become anxious and phobic. She argued that women are systematically taught to be fearful, dependent, submissive, and passive, whereas men are encouraged to be courageous, autonomous, achievement oriented, and active. Subsequent work by Chambless and Mason (1986) clarified the relationship between gender role and anxiety. This group found that conforming to a male gender-role stereotype appeared to have a prophylactic effect on anxiety, whereas female gender-role adherence had little effect. A large body of treatment outcome literature demonstrates that exposure to feared stimuli leads to a decrease in anxiety. It is very plausible that an assertive, goal-oriented, competitive style would lead a person to be less avoidant and therefore less anxious.

Current research on gender role, building on Bem's pioneering work (1974, 1977), includes both the independent traits of masculinity and femininity and the combination traits of androgynous and undifferentiated. The trait *masculinity* is characterized by instrumental and aggressive behaviors (e.g., being assertive and active), whereas *femininity* is characterized by expressive and affiliative behaviors (e.g., being kind and nurturing) (Spence and Helmreich 1978). *Androgyny* describes a trait reflecting both high masculinity and high femininity (Bem 1977); *undifferentiated* denotes a trait low in both. Clinical studies exploring the relationship between gender-role stereotypes and (mostly agoraphobic) anxiety provide support for the hypothesis that low masculinity, rather than high femininity, is associated with symptoms of anxiety and avoidance (Chambless and Mason 1986; Gournay 1989). Our own data, from an anxiety disorders clinic sample, again confirms that scores on the masculinity scale of the Bem Sex-Role Inventory (Bem 1981) are negatively correlated with scores on ratings of depression, agoraphobia, social pho-

TABLE 8–1.
Relationship between masculinity/femininity and symptomatology: Pearson correlations between the Bem Sex-Role Inventory and measures of anxiety and depression among outpatients in an open anxiety disorders clinic

Measure	Bem—Masculinity	Bem—Femininity
Fear Questionnaire—Agoraphobia	–.27*	.10
Fear Questionnaire—Social Phobia	–.46**	–.09
Penn State Worry Questionnaire	–.34**	.01
Beck Depression Inventory	–.30*	–.12

Note. Sample sizes ranged from 97 to 109. Beck Depression Inventory (Beck and Steer 1987); Bem Sex-Role Inventory (Bem 1981); Fear Questionnaire (Marks and Mathews 1979); Penn State Worry Questionnaire (Meyer et al. 1990).
*$P < .01$; **$P < .001$ (all P values are two-tailed).

bia, and worry (Table 8–1). Studies in nonclinical populations also support the hypothesis that lower levels of masculinity are associated with higher levels of anxiety, whereas femininity bears little relationship to anxiety (Arrindell et al. 1993; Brehony 1983).

Of interest, recent epidemiological data suggest that a decline in gender differences in anxiety disorders may have been occurring over the past decade. For instance, a study conducted in the 1970s showed that women with agoraphobia outnumbered men 4:1 (Robins et al. 1984), whereas a study conducted in the early 1990s found the gender ratio to be about 2:1 (Kessler et al. 1994). Although there were substantial methodological differences between these two studies, the decline in sex ratio would be consistent with changing roles of women over this period. Women's greater social equality and increased participation in the labor force (Bekker 1996) may mean that women are becoming more self-reliant. As this occurs, we may see a decrease in phobias among women.

Gender-Role Stress

Although a masculine gender-role orientation appears to be protective against anxiety, some interesting research suggests that rigid adherence to a masculine stance may also be a problem. Eisler and colleagues (Eisler and Skidmore 1987; Wethington et al. 1987) suggest that certain types of common, everyday life stresses may cause psychological distress in individuals who are rigidly committed to a masculine gender-role position. Distress occurs because self-esteem, influenced by overvalued masculinity, is challenged or threatened by certain kinds of events. For instance, a challenge to his authority or autonomy may be particularly threatening to a man whose self-esteem is dependent on masculine imperatives of successful competitiveness and independence (Eisler and Skidmore 1987).

Eisler and colleagues (Eisler and Blalock 1991; Eisler and Skidmore 1987; Eisler et al. 1988) contend that masculine gender-role stress (MGRS) occurs when individuals rely excessively on masculine gender-role schemata. Such reliance increases the threat valence of some types of daily life hassles and limits coping strategies to those that match masculine gender-role schemata. Eisler et al. have identified five types of stressful situations that threaten masculine gender-role schemata: those that 1) reveal physical inadequacy, 2) evoke emotional expressiveness, 3) require subordination to women, 4) expose intellectual inferiority, or 5) elicit performance failure. Individuals with overreliance on the masculine gender role tend to react to these stresses with dysfunctional coping strategies such as aggressive/violent behavior or substance abuse/dependence.

MGRS should not be confused with a masculine gender-role orientation, as the latter reflects traits that are socially desirable and adaptive (Bem 1974; Spence and Helmreich 1978). Instead, MGRS results when adherence to such traits is excessive and rigid. Consistent with this theoretical distinction, correlations between MGRS and masculinity tend to be near zero (Eisler et al. 1988). Also of note, women as well as men may score highly on measures of MGRS.

On the other hand, certain stressors—such as not being able to remain cheerful and friendly no matter what happens—may be especially salient for women who overvalue femininity. Gillespie and Eisler (1992) have begun to examine feminine gender-role stress (FGRS). In an initial study, the authors developed the FGRS scale, intended to assess a range of situations that are perceived as stressful by women with a rigid feminine gender-role orientation. The FGRS scale consists of five factor-analytically derived subscales: 1) fear of unemotional relationships (e.g., feeling pressured to engage in sexual activity), 2) fear of physical unattractiveness (e.g., being perceived as overweight by others), 3) fear of victimization (e.g., hearing a strange noise while being home alone), 4) fear of behaving assertively (e.g., bargaining with a salesperson when buying a car), and 5) fear of not being nurturing (e.g., having someone else raise one's children). Similar to the relationship between MGRS and masculinity, FGRS was found to be unrelated to femininity, thus providing evidence for the distinction between these two constructs (Gillespie and Eisler 1992). Potentially maladaptive female strategies for coping with FGRS have yet to be determined, but such strategies might involve self-denigration or other self-destructive behaviors.

How does the concept of gender-role stress relate to anxiety? Research on gender roles has demonstrated that masculinity (i.e., instrumentality) serves as protection against anxiety and depression. Research on gender-role stress, on the other hand, has revealed that rigid adherence to masculine gender-role schemata causes masculinity to lose its adaptive function. Interestingly, men with high levels of MGRS are more likely to experience anger, whereas women with high MGRS are more likely to experience anxiety (Eisler et al. 1988). Men experience higher levels of MGRS than do women, and high MGRS predicts increased anger, increased anxiety, and poorer health behaviors (e.g., use of alcohol or tobacco). The fact that epidemiological data show men to be twice as likely as women to be diagnosed with substance abuse or dependence and four to five times as likely to be diagnosed with antisocial personality disorder (Kessler et al. 1994) may be related to these differences.

Social Relationships

Men and women differ in the goals of interpersonal relationships. Whereas men's relationships tend to focus on instrumental behaviors, such as activities and interests, women's relationships tend to focus on affective aspects, such as mutual understanding and emotional intimacy. Women are thus more likely to be supportive (Eisler and Blalock 1991) and to need supportive social relationships. Women tend to rely on the support of their social networks to help manage problems. When interpersonal relationships are troubled, therefore, women experience more distress than do men.

Initial findings from our research seem to provide support for this hypothesis. In a sample of nonpsychotic patients in a rural community mental health center, we found men and women to report comparable (and low) levels of social support. However, in women (but not in men), social support bore a strong negative relationship to the number of current DSM-IV (American Psychiatric Association 1994) diagnoses. Similarly, although there were no gender differences in reports of verbal or physical abuse from partners, in women such reported abuse was moderately correlated with the number of current psychological disorders, whereas in men no correlation was found. Likewise, in patients presenting to our anxiety disorders clinic, we observed gender differences in the relationship between interpersonal problems and anxiety symptoms. Again, men and women obtained similar scores on the Inventory of Interpersonal Problems (Horowitz et al. 1988; see Table 8–2). However, for women interpersonal problems were consistently related to symptoms of somatic anxiety, anxiety sensitivity, worry, and agoraphobic avoidance, such that more severe interpersonal problems were associated with more severe anxiety. This was much less true for men, in whom interpersonal problems tended to show little relationship to anxiety. These data from clinical groups suggest that lack of social support combined with the presence of interpersonal problems is more likely to have adverse affects on women's than on men's mental health. Because these studies cannot tell us about the causal direction of these relationships, it is also possible that having more symptoms is more likely to lead to interpersonal problems in women than it is in men. In either case, the gender differences have potential clinical significance.

Gender-Specific Social Adversity

Women's participation in the workforce and enrollment in institutions of higher education have increased dramatically over the past decades. Yet, on average, women are still poorer and less educated than men. Data from our open anxiety disorders clinic document this difference in a clinical group. Male patients were twice as likely as female patients to have had a college education (Table 8–3). Our male patients also had considerably higher household incomes (see Table 8–3). Of note, such gender

TABLE 8–2.

Gender differences in anxiety disorder symptomatology among outpatients in an open anxiety disorders clinic

	Men		Women		
	n	Mean (SD)	*n*	Mean (SD)	*P* <
Bem—Masculinity	29	4.59 (0.87)	71	4.0 (1.16)	.007
Bem—Femininity	32	4.69 (0.51)	77	5.06 (0.74)	.004
FQ—Agoraphobia	63	7.52 (8.21)	134	12.58 (11.11)	.0005
FQ—Social Phobia	63	13.46 (7.90)	135	15.84 (9.30)	.09
PSWQ	68	58.22 (13.0)	150	60.07 (14.20)	.37
BDI	79	17.07 (9.8)	167	20.56 (12.28)	.02
IIP—Total	74	1.42 (0.60)	157	1.41 (0.70)	.88
IIP—H Assertive		1.68 (0.82)		1.80 (0.96)	.37
IIP—H Intimate		1.10 (0.69)		0.89 (0.72)	.05
IIP—H Sociable		1.86 (0.94)		1.70 (1.02)	.27
IIP—H Submissive		1.33 (0.74)		1.13 (0.76)	.07
IIP—T Responsible		1.54 (0.75)		1.74 (0.97)	.09
IIP—T Controlling		0.88 (0.49)		0.91 (0.70)	.74
ASI	83	32.71 (13.10)	166	1.78 (14.42)	.63
BAI	77	20.09 (10.74)	151	24.89 (13.95)	.005

Note. Bem = Bem Sex-Role Inventory (Bem 1981); FQ = Fear Questionnaire (Marks and Mathews 1979); PSWQ = Penn State Worry Questionnaire (Meyer et al. 1990); BDI = Beck Depression Inventory (Beck and Steer 1987); IIP = Inventory of Interpersonal Problems (Horowitz et al. 1988)—H = Hard to be; T = Too; ASI = Anxiety Sensitivity Index (Peterson and Reiss 1987); BAI = Beck Anxiety Index (Beck et al. 1988).

TABLE 8–3.

Gender differences in demographic variables among outpatients in an open anxiety disorders clinic

	Men (%)	Women (%)	χ^2	*P*
Education				
High school graduate	25.5	36.7		
Some college	52.1	51.5		
College graduate or beyond	22.3	11.7	13.16	.001
Yearly income, $				
<20,000	43.9	48.9		
20,000–50,000	31.6	37.8		
>50,000	24.6	13.4	6.64	.040

Note. Sample sizes ranged from 115 to 188 for men and from 215 to 324 for women.

differences in demographic variables were not found in a recently completed multicenter collaborative treatment study of panic disorder (D. H. Barlow, J. M. Gorman, M. K. Shear, and S. W. Woods, "A Randomized Controlled Trial of Cognitive Behavioral Treatment vs. Imipramine and Their Combination for Panic Disorder: Primary Outcome Results [unpublished study], August 1999), suggesting that women with more psychosocial adversity may not be adequately represented in clinical treatment trials. Results from the National Comorbidity Survey (Kessler et al. 1994) show that the rates of almost all psychological disorders decline monotonically with education and income. Lower socioeconomic status is typically associated with increased risk for both onset and chronicity of a disorder. A link between poverty and both depression and anxiety has also been documented (Brown and Moran 1997). It is noteworthy that in the National Comorbidity Survey, socioeconomic status proved to be even more strongly related to anxiety disorders than to affective disorders. Low educational attainment and financial hardship are associated with high levels of chronic stress and limited resources for obtaining professional help, both of which can increase worry and anxiety. Even if a woman is successful in obtaining treatment for anxiety, chronic life stress is likely to reduce her chances of recovery (Wade et al. 1993).

Brown and colleagues' studies (e.g., Brown and Moran 1997) focus on low-income single mothers, a population often found to be at high risk for depression. In our anxiety disorders clinic, mothers with one or more children living at home were less well educated and had more severe symptoms of anxiety compared with women without children and compared with men. Perhaps not surprisingly, mothers were at least six times as likely as fathers to be single parents. Single mothers, in turn, tended to be less well educated and poorer than their married counterparts (also see Weissman et al. 1987). Parenthood clearly has different implications for women than it does for men. More often than not, mothers are responsible for taking care of their children, whereas fathers are usually under more pressure to provide the needed financial support. These different role-expectations may in part explain our finding that parenthood was associated with an increase in agoraphobia among female anxiety disorder patients but a decrease among male patients (Figure 8–1).

Approximately 27% of adult women are survivors of childhood sexual abuse (Finkelhor et al. 1990), 7% of women are in relationships with physically abusive partners (Hyde 1985), and 12.5% are survivors of rape in adulthood (Kilpatrick et al. 1992). Child sexual abuse, domestic violence, and rape are disproportionately experienced by girls and women. Psychological sequelae of these traumatic experiences include symptoms

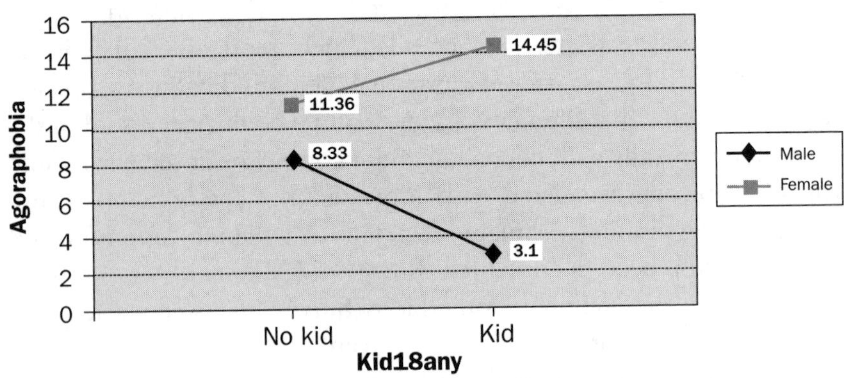

FIGURE 8–1. Parenthood (Kid18any) and agoraphobic symptoms among anxiety disorder outpatients. Depicted are Fear Questionnaire—Agoraphobia scores for women and men with children (Kid) and without children (No kid). Kid18any: F = 0.30; *P* = .588. Gender: F = 13.35; *P* = .000. Kid18any × Gender: F = 4.48; *P* = .036.

of posttraumatic stress disorder (PTSD), generalized anxiety, agoraphobia, and depression. Once a girl or woman has been victimized, her likelihood of being victimized again increases dramatically (Kilpatrick et al. 1992). There is some evidence that men and women are equally likely to experience traumatic events. However, more girls than boys are exposed to childhood sexual abuse, and childhood sexual abuse is far more likely than childhood physical abuse to cause symptoms of PTSD (Deblinger et al. 1989). Similarly, of the different types of traumatic stressors encountered by civilians, sexual assault is the one most likely to result in psychological problems, especially PTSD (Kilpatrick et al. 1992). We therefore contend that girls and women are more frequently exposed to civilian trauma leading to severe psychological symptoms.

Conclusion

We have reviewed four areas of sociocultural gender differences that may be related to gender differences in anxiety disorders. We conclude by asking the following question: Do gender differences have any implications for the treatment of anxiety disorders? The few studies in which researchers examined and reported results on gender differences in symptom presentation and response to treatment generally yielded few differences between female and male anxiety disorder patients. Does this mean that we should ignore the types of differences we have identified here? We think not.

Even if men and women do not differ with respect to symptom severity before or after treatment, the processes contributing to the onset, persistence, and reduction of anxiety may still differ significantly. For example, preliminary results from our multicenter comparative treatment trial for panic disorder showed virtually no gender differences in demographic characteristics, baseline symptom severity, or outcome in response to treatment with cognitive-behavior therapy or medication (D. H. Barlow, J. M. Gorman, M. K. Shear, and S. W. Woods, "A Randomized Controlled Trial of Cognitive Behavioral Treatment vs. Imipramine and Their Combination for Panic Disorder: Primary Outcome Results [unpublished study], August 1999). However, correlational analyses of baseline symptoms showed different patterns of relationships among symptoms in men and women.

Studies are needed to test hypotheses that attempt to explain differential treatment effects in men and women. For example, treatment may need to target different areas in male and female patients. Therapists may need to consider gender-role functioning when presenting treatment plans and explaining symptoms. Men may respond better to a more physical and less emotion-based view of symptoms and a more instrumental presentation of therapy (see Thase et al. 1994). Women may value the personal relationship and support and be very willing to explore emotionality. They are therefore more likely to feel that therapy is not something to be ashamed of. Further research is needed to examine gender-specific constructs of stereotypes, stress, and coping mechanisms and to explore how these gender differences affect the etiology and treatment of anxiety disorders.

There is ample evidence that effective psychosocial treatments have been developed for all of the DSM anxiety disorders. However, a significant number of patients drop out of treatment, fail to benefit from treatment, or stop short of recovery. Long-term follow-up studies demonstrate that short-term cognitive-behavioral treatments often lead to insufficient or unstable improvement. Accordingly, researchers are beginning to focus their attention on how to improve the effects of cognitive-behavioral treatments, frequently by adding additional components to a treatment package. We suggest that a comprehensive treatment approach would do well to include treatment strategies that are sensitive to the effects of gender stereotypes, gender-specific stress, and gender-specific coping styles. Because the majority of persons seeking treatment for anxiety disorders are women, we need to pay particular attention to women's needs in psychotherapy. This might include addressing interpersonal conflicts with interpersonal psychotherapy or training in interpersonal problem solving, teaching women the skills they need to compete with men in the workplace, and accommodating the special needs of mothers with small children by providing childcare services and skills to cope with the stress of being a parent.

References

American Psychiatric Association: Diagnostic and Statistical Manual of Mental Disorders, 4th Edition. Washington, DC, American Psychiatric Association, 1994

Arrindell WA, Kolk AM, Pickersgill MJ, et al: Biological sex, sex role orientation, masculine sex role stress, dissimulation and self-reported fears. Advances in Behaviour Research and Therapy 15:103–146, 1993

Barlow DH: Anxiety and Its Disorders: The Nature and Treatment of Anxiety and Panic. New York, Guilford, 1988

Beck AT, Steer RA: Manual for the Revised Beck Depression Inventory. San Antonio, TX, Psychological Corporation, 1987

Beck AT, Epstein N, Brown G, et al: An inventory for measuring clinical anxiety: psychometric properties. J Consult Clin Psychol 56:893–897, 1988

Bekker MHJ: Agoraphobia and gender: a review. Clin Psychol Rev 16:129–146, 1996

Bem SL: The measurement of psychological androgyny. J Consult Clin Psychol 42:155–162, 1974

Bem SL: On the utility of alternative procedures for assessing psychological androgyny. J Consult Clin Psychol 45:196–205, 1977

Bem SL: The Bem Sex-Role Inventory—Professional Manual. Palo Alto, CA, Consulting Psychologists Press, 1981

Bibb JL, Chambless DL: Alcohol use and abuse among diagnosed agoraphobics. Behav Res Ther 24:49–58, 1986

Bourdon KH, Boyd JH, Rae DS, et al: Gender differences in phobias: results from the ECA community survey. J Anxiety Disord 2:227–241, 1988

Brehony KA: Women and agoraphobia: a case for the etiological significance of the feminine sex-role stereotype, in The Stereotyping of Women: Its Effects on Mental Health. Edited by Franks V, Rothblum ED. New York, Springer, 1983, pp 112–128

Breslau N, Schultz L, Peterson E: Sex differences in depression: a role for preexisting anxiety. Psychiatry Res 58:1–12, 1995

Brown GW, Moran PM: Single mothers, poverty and depression. Psychol Med 27:21–33, 1997

Chambless DL: Gender and phobia, in Fresh Perspectives on Anxiety Disorders. Edited by Emmelkamp PMG, Everaerd WTAM, Kraaimaat F, et al. Amsterdam, The Netherlands, Swets & Zeitlinger, 1989, pp 133–141

Chambless DL, Mason J: Sex, sex-role stereotyping and agoraphobia. Behav Res Ther 24:231–235, 1986

Deblinger E, McLeer SV, Atkins MS, et al: Post-traumatic stress in sexually abused, physically abused, and nonabused children. Child Abuse Negl 13: 403–408, 1989

Eisler RM, Blalock JA: Masculine gender role stress: implications for the assessment of men. Clin Psychol Rev 11:45–60, 1991

Eisler RM, Skidmore JR: Masculine gender role stress: scale development and component factors in the appraisal of stressful situations. Behav Modif 11:123–136, 1987

Eisler RM, Skidmore JR, Ward CH: Masculine gender role stress: predictor of anger, anxiety, and health risk behaviors. J Pers Assess 52:133–141, 1988

Finkelhor D, Hotaling G, Lewis IA, et al: Sexual abuse in a national survey of adult men and women: prevalence, characteristics, and risk factors. Child Abuse Negl 14:19–28, 1990

Fodor IG: The phobic syndrome in women, in Women in Therapy. Edited by Franks V, Burtle V. New York, Brunner/Mazel, 1974, pp 132–168

Gillespie BL, Eisler RM: Development of the Feminine Gender Role Stress Scale: a cognitive-behavioral measure of stress, appraisal, and coping for women. Behav Modif 16:426–438, 1992

Gournay K: The behavioural treatment of agoraphobia: the impact of sex role, in Fresh Perspectives on Anxiety Disorders. Edited by Emmelkamp PMG, Everaerd WTAM, Kraaimaat F, et al. Amsterdam, The Netherlands, Swets & Zeitlinger, 1989, pp 143–150

Horowitz LM, Rosenberg SE, Baer BA, et al: Inventory of Interpersonal Problems: psychometric properties and clinical applications. J Consult Clin Psychol 56:885–892, 1988

Huber JW, Altmeier EM: An investigation of the self-statement systems of phobic and nonphobic individuals. Cognitive Therapy and Research 7:355–362, 1983

Hyde JS: Half the Human Experience: The Psychology of Women. Lexington, MA, Heath, 1985

Kessler RC, McGonagle KA, Zhao S, et al: Lifetime and 12-month prevalence of DSM-III-R psychiatric disorders in the United States: results from the National Comorbidity Study. Arch Gen Psychiatry 51:8–19, 1994

Kessler RC, Sonnega A, Bromet E, et al: Posttraumatic stress disorder in the National Comorbidity Survey. Arch Gen Psychiatry 52:1048–1060, 1995

Kilpatrick DG, Edmunds CN, Seymour AK: Rape in America: A Report to the Nation. Charleston, SC, Crime Victims Research and Treatment Center, 1992

Marks IM, Mathews AM: Brief standard self-rating for phobic patients. Behav Res Ther 17:263–267, 1979

Meyer TJ, Miller RL, Metzger RL, et al: Development and validation of the Penn State Worry Questionnaire. Behav Res Ther 28:487–495, 1990

Peterson RA, Reiss S: Anxiety Sensitivity Index Manual. Palos Heights, IL, International Diagnostic Systems, 1987

Pierce KA, Kirkpatrick DR: Do men lie on fear surveys? Behav Res Ther 30:415–418, 1992

Reiss S, Peterson RA, Gursky DM, et al: Anxiety sensitivity, anxiety frequency, and the prediction of fearfulness. Behav Res Ther 24:1–8, 1986

Robins LN, Regier DA: Psychiatric Disorders in America: The Epidemiologic Catchment Area Study. New York, Free Press, 1991

Robins LN, Helzer JE, Weissman MM, et al: Lifetime prevalence of specific psychiatric disorders in three sites. Arch Gen Psychiatry 41:949–958, 1984

Root MPP: Treatment failures: the role of sexual victimization in women's addictive behavior. Am J Orthopsychiatry 59:542–549, 1989

Speltz ML, Bernstein DA: Sex differences in fearfulness: verbal report, overt avoidance and demand characteristics. J Behav Ther Exp Psychiatry 7:117–122, 1976

Spence JT, Helmreich RL: Masculinity and Femininity: Their Psychological Dimensions, Correlates, and Antecedents. Austin, TX, University of Texas Press, 1978

Thase ME, Reynolds CF III, Frank E, et al: Do depressed men and women respond similarly to cognitive behavior therapy? Am J Psychiatry 151:500–505, 1994

Wade SL, Monroe SM, Michelson LK: Chronic life stress and treatment outcome in agoraphobia with panic attacks. Am J Psychiatry 150:1491–1495, 1993

Weissman MM, Leaf PJ, Livingston-Bruce M: Single parent women: a community study. Social Psychiatry 22:29–36, 1987

Wethington E, MacLeod JD, Kessler RC: The importance of life events for explaining sex differences in psychological distress, in Gender and Stress. Edited by Barnett RC, Beiner L, Baruch GK. New York, Free Press, 1987, pp 144–154

Wolfe BE: Gender ideology and phobias in women, in Sex Roles and Psychopathology. Edited by Spatz Widom C. New York, Plenum, 1984, pp 51–72

SECTION III

Schizophrenia

CHAPTER 9

Gender and Schizophrenia

An Overview

Steven O. Moldin, Ph.D.

Although distinctions between men and women in the clinical expression and incidence of schizophrenia were observed nearly 80 years ago by Kraepelin (1919/1971), systematic empirical research on such distinctions has been pursued for only about the last 15 years. The determination of robust gender differences may have important implications both in future research on the pathophysiology and etiology of schizophrenia and in clinical practice. In this chapter I review empirical studies of gender differences in schizophrenia and briefly discuss explanatory theories that have relevance to neurobiological models of etiology.

Lifetime Prevalence/Incidence

Male:female ratios greater than one for first hospital admissions for schizophrenia were observed in Norwegian and Danish psychiatric case registers (Munk-Jorgensen 1987; Ødegaard 1971), leading the authors of these studies to conclude that schizophrenia has a higher incidence in men than in women. A review of the literature on gender differences in

The views expressed here are the personal scientific opinions of the author and do not necessarily represent the views of the National Institutes of Health or the Department of Health and Human Services.

incidence through 1983 found essentially equal lifetime morbid risks for men and women (Hambrecht et al. 1994). Male:female ratios in annual incidence rates for schizophrenia ranged from 0.70 to 3.47, although the authors of the review noted several problematical design characteristics (i.e., small catchment areas, small samples, long observation periods, narrow screening criteria, nonrepresentative samples, lack of operationalized criteria and/or standardized interviewing, and misdiagnosis) that limit the quality of the studies. Hambrecht and colleagues (1992a) have discussed several potential sources of gender bias in previous epidemiological studies that would contribute to the underrepresentation of women in studies of schizophrenic individuals: disease-related factors, sociocultural influences, service-related factors, and research design characteristics.

The ABC (Age, Beginning, Course) Schizophrenia Study (Häfner et al. 1993; also see Chapter 10 in this volume), a large-scale epidemiological investigation in a defined western German catchment area of 1.5 million, was designed to overcome the methodological limitations of previous studies. No significant gender differences in schizophrenia incidence were found in this study, regardless of which diagnostic definition the investigators used (Hambrecht et al. 1994). Gender differences were likewise not detected on operationalized diagnoses in the pooled data of the World Health Organization (WHO) Determinants of Outcome Study (Hambrecht et al. 1992b), although male:female ratios varied considerably among centers around the world (Sartorius et al. 1986). A very well-designed epidemiologically based family study in western Ireland found that about 65% of all schizophrenia cases were in men (Kendler and Walsh 1995), which was consistent with results from a comparable study of first admissions in three Irish counties (Ni Nuallain et al. 1987).

A number of studies have reported recent declines in the incidence of schizophrenia in developed countries (e.g., Waddington and Youssef 1994), but numerous sources of bias may account for the observed drop in first hospital admission rates (Kendell et al. 1993). In an age-period-cohort analysis, Takei and colleagues (1996) found evidence for a cohort effect. After adjustment for the effects of age and period, the incidence of schizophrenia in men and in women was decreased by 55% and 39%, respectively, over a 50-year birth period. A tendency for declines in admission rates to be relatively greater in younger versus older age groups, especially for women, has also been reported for other birth periods

(Geddes et al. 1993). Although interesting, these findings require replication in other studies.

Age at Onset

Dating the exact onset of schizophrenia is not easy, and a variety of methodological approaches have been developed (Häfner et al. 1992; Hambrecht and Häfner 1997; Maurer and Häfner 1995). Regardless of how onset is defined, the earlier appearance of symptoms in men than in women has been reported in numerous studies; in fact, gender differences in age at onset are currently assumed to be among the few robust, well-replicated findings in the entire field of schizophrenia research. Kraepelin (1919/1971) reported that women with a diagnosis of dementia praecox were admitted an average of 5–10 years later than men. More than 50 studies have found a gender difference in age at first admission (Angermeyer and Kühn 1988). However, many of the older studies had considerable design shortcomings.

Three very large and methodologically rigorous epidemiologically based studies have examined gender differences in age at onset. The ABC Schizophrenia Study found age at onset to be between 3.2 and 4.1 years greater (depending on the operationalized definition of onset) in women than in men (Häfner et al. 1994). In the WHO Determinants of Outcome Study (Jablensky et al. 1992), a difference of 3.4 years in mean age at onset was observed (Hambrecht et al. 1992b), and the mean onset ages (men = 26.7 years; women = 30.1 years) were very similar to those reported in the ABC Schizophrenia Study (men = 26.5 years; women = 30.6 years). In addition, late-onset schizophrenia is significantly more common in women than in men (Häfner, Chapter 10 in this volume). Analysis of the Danish and the Mannheim, Germany, case registers (Riecher et al. 1991) showed about a 4- to 5-year difference in mean ages at onset, with men having a younger age at first hospitalization.

The ages at onset observed in a series of patients may of course be biased by the underlying age distribution in the general population (Heimbuch et al. 1980). Excess gender-specific mortality could also lead to artifactual differences in age at onset. Faraone and colleagues (1994) applied a nonparametric method to correct the male and female age-at-onset distributions for gender-specific age distributions. Analysis of uncorrected data showed that men's mean age at onset was 4 years earlier than that of women; after correction, the age-at-onset distribution shifted slightly toward older ages, but the difference between men and women remained statistically significant.

Some inconsistencies in the literature exist, given that at least five studies have failed to find gender differences in age at onset. Shimizu and colleagues found that male schizophrenic patients were less than 1 year younger than female schizophrenic patients (Shimizu et al. 1988). No significant differences were found in a study of 679 schizophrenic individuals in Croatia (Folnegovic and Folnegovic-Smalc 1994) or in a series of 113 Canadian schizophrenic inpatients (Addington et al. 1996). No significant gender differences in age at onset were observed in the Roscommon Family Study (Kendler and Walsh 1995), and a recent reanalysis of data in the WHO Determinants of Outcome Study showed that the observed male:female difference was significantly attenuated when gender was unconfounded from marital status, cultural variation, premorbid personality traits, and family history of a mental disorder (Jablensky and Cole 1997).

Earlier age at onset in schizophrenia is assumed to index familial liability to illness (Häfner, Chapter 10 in this volume). Two reports have found an inverse relationship between age at onset and risk in relatives (Kendler and MacLean 1990; Pulver et al. 1990). However, based on the previous literature (reviewed in Kendler et al. 1987) and the absence of such a relationship in the Roscommon Family Study (Kendler and Walsh 1995), Kendler and colleagues (1996) concluded that environmental or random developmental factors probably account for much of the variation in the age at onset of schizophrenia. Chance findings or true population differences might account for the discrepancies between the findings of Kendler et al. and those of the two studies reporting a relationship between age at onset and familial liability (Kendler and MacLean 1990; Pulver et al. 1990).

Familial Risk

Seven studies have examined the relationship between the gender of a schizophrenic proband and the risk of illness in relatives. Four found that the risk for schizophrenia was significantly lower in relatives of male versus female schizophrenic probands (Bellodi et al. 1986; Goldstein et al. 1990; Maier et al. 1993; Sham et al. 1994; Wolyniec et al. 1992). Shimizu and colleagues (1987) found similar results using parental but not sibling data. Analysis of family data collected in the 1950s and 1960s in Sweden did not reveal a difference in the risk of schizophrenia among the relatives of male versus female probands (Sham et al. 1993). Likewise, the risks for schizophrenia and schizophrenia-related spectrum disorders were similar in relatives of male and female schizophrenic probands in the Roscommon Family Study (Kendler and Walsh 1995).

The results of the two studies that failed to find gender differences in familial risk (Kendler and Walsh 1995; Sham et al. 1993) are consistent with those of earlier family studies (Bleuler 1978; Kallmann 1938). Twin studies have produced contradictory findings, but gender differences in twin concordance may reflect sampling bias: no such differences have been observed in twins ascertained from population-based case registers (Kendler and Walsh 1995).

Liability-threshold models of multifactorial inheritance (Falconer 1965, 1967; Reich et al. 1972) predict that if a disease is more common in one gender, familial risks will be greater for relatives of the less commonly affected gender. The failure to observe gender differences in familial risk, given the gender differences in population prevalence, may reflect the fact that a greater proportion of schizophrenia in women than in men is attributable to nonfamilial environmental risk factors (Kendler and Walsh 1995).

Premorbid Functioning

Abnormalities in social functioning that precede the clinical onset of schizophrenia have been well described. Follow-back studies of school reports, retrospective studies, and prospective high-risk studies have found a consistent pattern of more severe premorbid deficits in social competence and occupational functioning for men than for women (McGlashan and Bardenstein 1990). Premorbid IQ has also been found to be lower for men in some (Offord 1974) but not all (McGlashan and Bardenstein 1990) studies.

Season of Birth

The observation that schizophrenic patients are more likely to be born in the winter and early spring in comparison with individuals from the general population has been reported in numerous studies (Bradbury and Miller 1985), but gender differences have not been consistently found. Pulver and colleagues (1992) examined the risk for schizophrenia among first-degree relatives of male and female schizophrenic probands. The results showed that the relatives of probands born in the months February to May (winter to spring) had the highest risk, although the association between month of birth and familial risk among male probands was present only for relatives whose onset of schizophrenia occurred before age 30 years; for relatives with an onset after age 30, there was no association between proband birth month and risk in relatives. A study of computer records of inpatient admissions showed a significant excess of winter births for female schizophrenic patients with no family history of mental disorder (Dassa et al. 1996).

Given that influenza and other viruses are most prevalent in winter or spring, it has been argued that women with schizophrenia have greater susceptibility to early environmental effects (Castle et al. 1995). Several studies have investigated the relationship between prenatal exposure to influenza and risk of schizophrenia (reviewed in Castle et al. 1995); five showed that the effect reached significance only for women. However, controversy exists. Some studies find no relationship between prenatal influenza or other infectious disease exposure and later schizophrenia (Crow and Done 1992; O'Callaghan et al. 1994); others find no evidence of a season-of-birth effect in schizophrenia (Chen et al. 1996; Hettema et al. 1996). Furthermore, it has been argued that the observed season-of-birth differences may represent an age-incidence effect artifact resulting from errors in interpretation of seasonal studies (M. S. Lewis 1989; M. S. Lewis and Griffin 1981).

Eagles and colleagues (1995) analyzed the ratio of winter/spring to summer/autumn births for individuals with schizophrenia across seven decades. The results showed that the incidence of schizophrenia decreased in both genders, but the proportion of winter/spring births increased only in schizophrenic men. The authors concluded that women are more susceptible than men to environmental effects such as prenatal virus exposure, and that the frequency of such factors is declining; thus, the observed increased proportion of winter/spring births in men actually reflects the decrease of winter/spring births in women who develop schizophrenia (which accompanies a decrease in exposure to the putative environmental agents).

Obstetric Complications

Five studies have found a history of pre- or perinatal insults to be more common in male than in female schizophrenic patients (Foerster et al. 1991; O'Callaghan et al. 1992; Owen et al. 1988; Pearlson et al. 1985; Wilcox and Nasrallah 1987). Two studies found that age at onset was significantly earlier in men whose mothers experienced obstetric complications versus those whose mothers did not (Kirov et al. 1996; O'Callaghan et al. 1992). However, other studies found no such gender differences (Done et al. 1991; McCreadie et al. 1992).

Symptomatology

Based on their own work and reviews of the literature, several authors have concluded that there are gender differences in schizophrenic symptomatology (Bardenstein and McGlashan 1990; Castle and Murray 1991; Goldstein and Link 1988; S. Lewis 1992). Males are more prone to exhibit the more typical positive symptoms of hallucinations and delusions, antisocial behavior, and negative symptoms such as blunted affect and avolition, whereas women are more prone to show an atypical presentation of affective symptoms such as dysphoria and depression. However, other studies have failed to find comparable gender differences (Fennig et al. 1995; Häfner et al. 1994; Kendler and Walsh 1995). Analyses conducted in the ABC Schizophrenia Study identified socially negative behaviors (e.g., self-neglect, social inattentiveness) as being more common in men and socially positive behaviors (conformity) as being more common in women during the first episode of illness (Häfner, Chapter 10 in this volume). These results are consistent with the premorbid gender differences discussed earlier.

Neuroanatomy

Castle and Murray (1991) reviewed the results from several imaging studies and concluded that structural brain abnormalities have been reported more commonly in male than in female schizophrenic patients. However, many of these studies had small sample sizes, and thus the Type I error rate may have been elevated. Other studies either failed to find such gender differences or reported inconsistent results. For example, as pointed out by S. Lewis (1992), methodologically sophisticated magnetic resonance imaging (MRI) studies have reported reduced coronal brain area (Marsh et al. 1991), enlarged lateral ventricles (Andreasen et al. 1990), and small left hippocampal formation (Bogerts et al. 1990) in male but not female schizophrenic patients. Other groups using comparably rigorous methods have found ventricular enlargement in both male and female schizophrenic patients, and at least two studies have reported ventricular enlargement in women but not men (Gur et al. 1991; Nasrallah et al. 1990). Gender differences in structural pathology have disappeared in some studies when the effects of other confounding factors such as height, ethnicity, and social class were controlled (Harvey et al. 1991).

Course/Outcome

There has been a strong recent interest in gender and schizophrenia as related to outcome and treatment response (Angermeyer 1989; Goldstein 1988; Seeman 1986). Such effects are arguably of clinical relevance. Angermeyer and colleagues (1990) found that about half of the studies they reviewed showed statistically significant gender differences, with women having more favorable outcomes. In general, however, there were marked methodological differences across studies. Analyses conducted in the ABC Schizophrenia Study show marked gender differences in early social course (much worse for men) that persisted 5 years after first admission but had disappeared by 14 years after first admission (Häfner, Chapter 10 in this volume). It was hypothesized by the authors of this study that the initial differences leveled out over time because of the age-related decrease in men's socially negative behaviors. It also has been suggested by other investigators that gender differences are eliminated (Opjordsmoen 1991) or become diluted (Goldstein 1988) over longer periods of follow-up. Harrison and colleagues (1996) reported a gender effect sustained over a 13-year period that remained after adjustment for sociodemographic covariates and type of early course. Few studies have specifically addressed gender differences in therapeutic drug response. Female schizophrenic patients appeared to respond more favorably than male patients and required lower doses of neuroleptics in at least one study (Seeman 1986). A more recent study of gender differences in neuroleptic-nonresponsive clozapine-treated schizophrenic patients (Szymanski et al. 1996) failed to show an equivalent antipsychotic treatment response in women and men. Other carefully designed studies have failed to find gender differences in daily antipsychotic medication doses (Jeste et al. 1996) or in course/outcome of schizophrenia (Häfner et al. 1994; Kendler and Walsh 1995). Clearly, more work is needed regarding gender differences in new-onset cases and in response to new therapeutic compounds.

Summary of Past Research

Consideration of the positive results previously reported across all substantive domains reviewed thus far may lead to the following conclusions: compared with female schizophrenic patients, male schizophrenic patients are more common; confer less familial risk to their relatives; are more frequently born in the winter/spring; are more likely to exhibit negative symptoms and to have suffered obstetric or other birth complications; and have worse courses/outcomes, a greater incidence of structural brain changes, an earlier age at onset, and worse premorbid functioning.

Unfortunately, the results across studies are far from being this clear. For each of the areas reviewed, at least one well-designed and methodologically rigorous study has failed to find gender differences. Likewise, no single study has found the full pattern of gender differences, and one well-designed epidemiologically based study (Kendler and Walsh 1995) failed to find gender differences in multiple domains (age at onset, course/outcome, symptoms, familial risk). The aggregate of results suggests that the similarities between men and women considerably outweigh the reported differences, with a large overlap between men and women (S. Lewis 1992). If one looks at each of the domains of variables for which gender differences have been reported, a hierarchy can be assembled according to the strength of empirical evidence (Table 9–1).

Gender differences in premorbid adjustment (including marital status, social functioning, and occupational attainment)—with schizophrenic women having higher premorbid functioning—have been replicated in many studies. This observation probably accounts for gender differences in symptomatology during the first illness episode and the early social course (Häfner, Chapter 10 in this volume). Schizophrenic women have been found to have an onset about 3–5 years later than that of men in several studies, but this is not a universal finding. It is not possible to determine whether methodological differences or true population differences are responsible for the discrepancies. Gender differences with regard to obstetric complications, familial risk, and symptomatology have been reported in several studies, but the results have not been consistently replicated; methodological differences among studies make it hard

TABLE 9–1.

Gender differences in schizophrenia

Variable	Strength of empirical evidence	Directionality in women
Premorbid adjustment (including early social course and early symptomatology)	Strong	Higher
Age at onset	Strong	Later
Obstetric complications	Moderate	Less frequent
Familial risk	Moderate	Higher
Symptomatology	Moderate	Atypical symptoms (depression, dysphoria) more common
Lifetime risk	Controversial	Lower
Long-term course/outcome	Controversial	Better
Neuropathology	Controversial	Absent
Season of birth	Controversial	Increased winter/spring births

to draw definitive conclusions. Finally, findings of gender differences with regard to lifetime risk, long-term course/outcome, neuropathology, and season of birth are more controversial. The failure to convincingly replicate these results across several studies suggests that reported gender differences on these variables may be attributable to methodological biases or Type I error.

Theoretical Integration

Several authors have developed theories to explain the range of gender differences. My discussion here focuses on two of these theories in particular. Seeman (Seeman 1982; Seeman and Lang 1990) and others (Häfner et al. 1991) have proposed that neuroendocrine characteristics may confer protection on women. Specifically, it has been argued that estrogens directly or indirectly modify symptom expression and account for many of the reported gender differences. The possible effects at the neurochemical and molecular level of estrogen on dopamine (Riecher-Rössler and Häfner 1993), serotonin (Sumner and Fink 1997), and glutamate (Woolley and McEwen 1994) receptors have been described. The primary focus of the estrogen theory has generally been to explain gender differences in age at onset, treatment response, and course/outcome as manifestations of different hormonal subtypes; however, the primary disease etiology in men and women is assumed to be the same. An absence of gender differences on variables related to the illness process has been interpreted as being consistent with the same pathophysiological mechanism in schizophrenic men and women, with gender differences in age at onset, social course, and early illness symptomatology attributable to nonspecific biological factors, differences in genetic liability, differences in social and cognitive stages of development at onset, and age-dependent, gender-specific behavior and cognitive patterns (Häfner, Chapter 10 in this volume).

Castle and colleagues (Castle and Murray 1991; Castle et al. 1994, 1995) have proposed a neurodevelopmental theory to explain gender differences in schizophrenia. This theory essentially postulates two different disease processes. Schizophrenia in men is hypothesized to reflect greater susceptibility to a neurodevelopmental disorder, with accompanying early onset and worse premorbid functioning, abnormalities in brain structure/function, poor treatment response and course, and lesser genetic contribution. Women predisposed to affective disorders who have been subjected to maternal viral infections during gestation develop a more limited neurodevelopmental injury that lends a "schizophrenia-like" flavor to their psychosis; thus, their illness is characterized by later onset, better premorbid functioning, better treatment response and course, prenatal exposure to infectious agents, lesser occurrence of neuropathology, greater occurrence of spring/winter births, and a greater familial risk of affective illness. The essential distinction between these theories concerns whether there are one or two disease etiologies for schizophrenic psychosis.

The inherent difficulty of using the data reviewed in this chapter to test etiological hypotheses is that a variety of factors entirely unrelated to primary etiology (e.g., social differences in behavioral expression, anatomic differences, methodological differences) may account for all of the observed gender differences in schizophrenia. Ultimate resolution of etiological heterogeneity in schizophrenia will come with the elucidation of disease pathophysiology or the identification of susceptibility genes. Until such resolution occurs, given the likelihood of multiple explanations (including methodological ones) for reported results, continued research that focuses exclusively on gender differences is unlikely to provide definitive answers about pathophysiology or etiology. However, the interpretation of robust gender differences in schizophrenia will continue to be of value in clinical situations (e.g., in predicting early symptomatology and social outcome).

Summary

Research on the neurobiology of schizophrenia requires continued exploration of gender differences, and future sample selection and study design must take potential gender differences into account. Explanations for gender differences in schizophrenia may reflect a variety of sources that include biological (genetic, anatomic, physiological, cognitive) and nonbiological (interpersonal, cultural) ones. Ultimately, satisfactory resolution of etiological heterogeneity within and between the genders will require elucidation of pathophysiology and identification of primary etiological factors (e.g., genes). The identification of robust gender differences in schizophrenia will yield valuable information for clinical practice.

References

Addington D, Addington J, Patten S: Gender and affect in schizophrenia. Can J Psychiatry 41:265–268, 1996

Andreasen NC, Erhardt JC, Swayze VW II, et al: Magnetic resonance imaging of the brain in schizophrenia. the pathopsychologic significance of structural abnormalities. Arch Gen Psychiatry 47:35–44, 1990

Angermeyer MC: Gender differences in schizophrenia: rehospitalization and community survival. Psychol Med 19:365–382, 1989

Angermeyer MC, Kühn L: Gender differences in age at onset of schizophrenia: an overview. Eur Arch Psychiatry Neurol Sci 237:351–364, 1988

Angermeyer MC, Kühn L, Goldstein JM: Gender and the course of schizophrenia: differences in treated outcomes. Schizophr Bull 16:293–307, 1990

Bardenstein KK, McGlashan TH: Gender differences in affective, schizoaffective, and schizophrenic disorders. Schizophr Res 3:159–172, 1990

Bellodi L, Bussoleni C, Scorza-Smeraldi R, et al: Family study of schizophrenia: exploratory analysis for relevant factors. Schizophr Bull 12:120–128, 1986

Bleuler M: The Schizophrenic Disorders. New Haven, CT, Yale University Press, 1978

Bogerts B, Ashtari M, Degreef G, et al: Reduced temporal limbic structure volumes on magnetic resonance images in first episode schizophrenia. Psychiatry Res 35:1–13, 1990

Bradbury TN, Miller GA: Season of birth in schizophrenia: a review of evidence, methodology and etiology. Psychol Bull 98:569–594, 1985

Castle DJ, Murray RM: Editorial: The neurodevelopmental basis of sex differences in schizophrenia. Psychol Med 21:565–575, 1991

Castle DJ, Sham PC, Wessely S, et al: The subtyping of schizophrenia in men and women: a latent class analysis. Psychol Med 24:41–51, 1994

Castle DJ, Abel K, Takei N, et al: Gender differences in schizophrenia: hormonal effect or subtypes? Schizophr Bull 21:1–12, 1995

Chen WJ, Yeh LL, Chang CJ, et al: Month of birth and schizophrenia in Taiwan: effect of gender, family history and age at onset. Schizophr Res 20: 133–143, 1996

Crow TJ, Done DJ: Prenatal exposure to influenza does not cause schizophrenia. Br J Psychiatry 161:390–393, 1992

Dassa D, Azorin JM, Ledoray V, et al: Season of birth and schizophrenia: sex difference. Prog Neuropsychopharmacol Biol Psychiatry 20:243–251, 1996

Done DJ, Johnstone EC, Frith CD, et al: Complications of pregnancy and delivery in relation to psychosis in adult life: data from the British perinatal mortality survey sample. BMJ 302:1576–1580, 1991

Eagles JM, Hunter D, Geddes JR: Gender-specific changes since 1900 in the season-of-birth effect in schizophrenia. Br J Psychiatry 167:469–472, 1995

Falconer DS: The inheritance of liability to certain diseases, estimated from the incidence among relatives. Ann Hum Genet 29:51–76, 1965

Falconer DS: The inheritance of liability to certain diseases with variable age of onset, with particular reference to diabetes mellitus. Ann Hum Genet 31:1–20, 1967

Faraone SV, Chen WJ, Goldstein JM, et al: Gender differences in age at onset of schizophrenia. Br J Psychiatry 164:625–629, 1994

Fennig S, Putnam K, Bromet EJ, et al: Gender, premorbid characteristics and negative symptoms in schizophrenia. Acta Psychiatr Scand 92:173–177, 1995

Foerster A, Lewis SW, Owen M, et al: Low birth weight and a family history of schizophrenia predict poor premorbid functioning in psychosis. Schizophr Res 5:13–20, 1991

Folnegovic Z, Folnegovic-Smalc V: Schizophrenia in Croatia: age of onset differences between males and females. Schizophr Res 14:83–91, 1994

Geddes JR, Black RJ, Whalley LJ, et al: Persistence of the decline in the diagnosis of schizophrenia among first admissions to Scottish hospitals from 1969 to 1988. Br J Psychiatry 163:620–626, 1993

Goldstein JM: Gender differences in the course of schizophrenia. Am J Psychiatry 145:684–689, 1988

Goldstein JM, Link BG: Gender and the expression of schizophrenia. J Psychiatr Res 22:141–155, 1988

Goldstein JM, Faraone SV, Chen WJ, et al: Sex differences in the familial transmission of schizophrenia. Br J Psychiatry 156:819–826, 1990

Gur RE, Mozley D, Resnick SM, et al: Magnetic resonance imaging in schizophrenia, I: volumetric analysis of brain and cerebrospinal fluid. Arch Gen Psychiatry 48:407–412, 1991

Häfner H, Behrens S, de Vry J, et al: Oestradiol enhances the vulnerability threshold for schizophrenia in women by an early effect on dopaminergic neurotransmission: evidence from an epidemiological study and from animal experiments. Eur Arch Psychiatr Clin Neurosci 241:65–68, 1991

Häfner H, Riecher-Rössler A, Hambrecht M: IRAOS: an instrument for the assessment of onset and early course of schizophrenia. Schizophr Res 6:209–223, 1992

Häfner H, Maurer K, Löffler W, et al: The influence of age and sex on the onset and early course of schizophrenia. Br J Psychiatry 162:80–86, 1993

Häfner H, Maurer K, Löffler W, et al: The epidemiology of early schizophrenia: influence of age and gender on onset and early course. Br J Psychiatry Suppl 164:29–38, 1994

Hambrecht M, Häfner H: Sensitivity and specificity of relatives' reports on the early course of schizophrenia. Psychopathology 30:12–19, 1997

Hambrecht M, Maurer K, Häfner H: Evidence for a gender bias in epidemiological studies of schizophrenia. Schizophr Res 8:223–231, 1992a

Hambrecht M, Maurer K, Häfner H, et al: Transnational stability of gender differences in schizophrenia? Eur Arch Psychiatry Clin Neurosci 242:6–12, 1992b

Hambrecht M, Riecher-Rössler A, Fatkenheuer B, et al: Higher morbidity risk for schizophrenia in males: fact or fiction? Compr Psychiatry 35:39–49, 1994

Harrison G, Croudace T, Mason P, et al: Predicting the long-term outcome of schizophrenia. Psychol Med 26:697–705, 1996

Harvey I, Williams M, Toone BK, et al: The ventricular brain ratio (VBR) in functional psychoses, II: the relationship of lateral ventricular and total intracranial area. Psychol Med 20:55–62, 1991

Heimbuch RC, Matthysse SW, Kidd KK: Estimating age-of-onset distributions for disorders with variable onset. Am J Hum Genet 32:564–574, 1980

Hettema JM, Walsh D, Kendler KS: Testing the effect of season of birth on familial risk for schizophrenia and related disorders. Br J Psychiatry 168:205–209, 1996

Jablensky A, Cole SW: Is the earlier age at onset of schizophrenia in males a confounded finding? Br J Psychiatry 170:234–240, 1997

Jablensky A, Sartorius N, Ernberg G, et al: Schizophrenia: manifestations, incidence and course in different cultures. A World Health Organization ten-country study. Psychol Med Monogr Suppl 20:1–97, 1992

Jeste DV, Lindamer LA, Evans J, et al: Relationship of ethnicity and gender to schizophrenia and pharmacology of neuroleptics. Psychopharmacol Bull 32:243–251, 1996

Kallmann FJ: The Genetics of Schizophrenia. New York, Augustin, 1938

Kendell RE, Malcolm DE, Adams W: The problem of detecting changes in the incidence of schizophrenia. Br J Psychiatry 162:212–218, 1993

Kendler KS, MacLean CJ: Estimating familial effects on age at onset and liability to schizophrenia, I: results of a large sample family study. Genet Epidemiol 7:409–417, 1990

Kendler KS, Walsh D: Gender and schizophrenia: results of an epidemiologically based family study. Br J Psychiatry 167:184–192, 1995

Kendler KS, Tsuang MT, Hays P: Age at onset in schizophrenia: a familial perspective. Arch Gen Psychiatry 44:881–890, 1987

Kendler KS, Karkowski-Shuman L, Walsh D: Age at onset in schizophrenia and risk of illness in relatives: results from the Roscommon Family Study. Br J Psychiatry 169:213–218, 1996

Kirov G, Jones PB, Harvey I, et al: Do obstetric complications cause the earlier age at onset in male than female schizophrenics? Schizophr Res 20:117–124, 1996

Kraepelin E: Dementia Praecox and Paraphrenia (1919). Translated by Barclay RM; edited by Robertson GM. New York, Robert K. Krieger, 1971

Lewis MS: Age incidence and schizophrenia, part I: the season of birth controversy. Schizophr Bull 15:59–73, 1989

Lewis MS, Griffin PA: An explanation for the season of birth effect in schizophrenia and certain other diseases. Psychol Bull 89:589–596, 1981

Lewis S: Sex and schizophrenia: vive la difference. Br J Psychiatry 161:445–450, 1992

Maier W, Lichtermann D, Minges J, et al: The impact of gender and age at onset on the familial aggregation of schizophrenia. Eur Arch Psychiatry Clin Neurosci 242:279–285, 1993

Marsh L, Pearlson GD, Richards SS: Structural brain changes in schizophrenia: MRI replication of a postmortem study. Paper presented at the International Congress on Schizophrenia Research, Tucson, AZ, April 21–25, 1991

Maurer K, Häfner H: Methodologic aspects of onset assessment in schizophrenia. Schizophr Res 15:265–276, 1995

McCreadie RG, Hall DJ, Berry IJ, et al: The Nithsdale Schizophrenia Surveys, X: obstetric complications, family history and abnormal movements. Br J Psychiatry 161:799–805, 1992

McGlashan TH, Bardenstein KK: Gender differences in affective, schizoaffective, and schizophrenic disorders. Schizophr Bull 16:319–329, 1990

Munk-Jorgensen P: First-admission rates and marital status of schizophrenics. Acta Psychiatr Scand 75:62–68, 1987

Nasrallah HA, Schwarzkopf SB, Olson SC, et al: Gender differences in schizophrenia on MRI brain scans. Schizophr Bull 16:205–210, 1990

Ni Nuallain M, O'Hare A, Walsh D: Incidence of schizophrenia in Ireland. Psychol Med 17:943–948, 1987

O'Callaghan E, Gibson T, Colohan HA, et al: Risk of schizophrenia in adults born after obstetric complications and their association with early onset of illness: a controlled study. BMJ 305:1256–1259, 1992

O'Callaghan E, Sham PC, Takei N, et al: The relationship of schizophrenic births to 16 infectious diseases. Br J Psychiatry 165:353–356, 1994

Ødegaard O: Hospitalized psychosis in Norway: time trends 1926–1965. Social Psychiatry 6:53–78, 1971

Offord DR: School performance of adult schizophrenics, their siblings and age mates. Br J Psychiatry 125:12–19, 1974

Opjordsmoen S: Long-term clinical outcome of schizophrenia with special reference to gender differences. Acta Psychiatr Scand 83:307–313, 1991

Owen MJ, Lewis SW, Murray RM: Obstetric complications and schizophrenia: a computed tomographic study. Psychol Med 18:331–339, 1988

Pearlson GD, Garbacz DJ, Moberg PJ, et al: Symptomatic, familial, perinatal, and social correlates of computer axial tomography (CAT) changes in schizophrenics and bipolars. J Nerv Ment Dis 173:42–50, 1985

Pulver AE, Brown CH, Wolyniec PS, et al: Schizophrenia, age at onset, gender and familial risk. Acta Psychiatr Scand 82:344–351, 1990

Pulver AE, Liang KY, Brown CH, et al: Risk factors in schizophrenia: season of birth, gender, and familial risk. Br J Psychiatry 160:65–71, 1992

Reich T, James JW, Morris CA: The use of multiple thresholds in determining the mode of transmission of semi-continuous traits. Ann Hum Genet 36: 163–184, 1972

Riecher A, Maurer K, Löffler W, et al: Gender differences in age at onset and course of schizophrenic disorders, in Search for the Causes of Schizophrenia. Edited by Häfner H, Gattaz WF. New York, Springer-Verlag, 1991, pp 14–33

Riecher-Rössler A, Häfner H: Schizophrenia and oestrogens—is there an association? Eur Arch Psychiatry Clin Neurosci 242:323–328, 1993

Sartorius N, Jablensky A, Korten A, et al: Early manifestations and first-contact incidence of schizophrenia in different cultures. Psychol Med 16:909–928, 1986

Seeman MV: Gender differences in schizophrenia. Can J Psychiatry 27:107–111, 1982

Seeman MV: Current outcome in schizophrenia: women versus men. Acta Psychiatr Scand 73:609–617, 1986

Seeman MV, Lang M: The role of estrogens in schizophrenia gender differences. Schizophr Bull 16:185–194, 1990

Sham PC, Gottesman II, MacLean CJ, et al: Schizophrenia: sex and familial morbidity. Psychiatry Res 52:125–134, 1993

Sham PC, Jones P, Russell A, et al: Age at onset, sex, and familial psychiatric morbidity in schizophrenia: Camberwell Collaborative Psychosis Study. Br J Psychiatry 165:466–473, 1994

Shimizu A, Kurachi M, Noda M, et al: Morbidity risks of schizophrenia to parents and siblings of schizophrenic patients. Japanese Journal of Psychiatry and Neurology 41:65–70, 1987

Shimizu A, Kurachi M, Noda M, et al: Influence of sex on age at onset of schizophrenia. Japanese Journal of Psychiatry and Neurology 42:35–40, 1988

Sumner BEH, Fink G: The density of 5-hydoxytryptamine$_{2A}$ receptors in forebrain is increased at pro-oestrus in intact female rats. Neurosci Lett 234:7–10, 1997

Szymanski S, Lieberman J, Pollack S, et al: Gender differences in neuroleptic nonresponsive clozapine-treated schizophrenics. Biol Psychiatry 39:249–254, 1996

Takei N, Lewis G, Sham PC, et al: Age-period-cohort analysis of the incidence of schizophrenia in Scotland. Psychol Med 26:963–973, 1996

Waddington JL, Youssef HA: Evidence for a gender-specific decline in the rate of schizophrenia in rural Ireland over a 50-year period. Br J Psychiatry 164:171–176, 1994

Wilcox JA, Nasrallah HA: Perinatal distress and prognosis of psychotic illness. Neuropsychobiology 17:173–175, 1987

Wolyniec PS, Pulver AE, McGrath JA, et al: Schizophrenia: gender and familial risk. J Psychiatr Res 26:17–27, 1992

Woolley CS, McEwen BS: Estradiol regulates hippocampal dendritic spine density via an N-methyl-D-aspartate receptor–dependent mechanism. J Neurosci 14:7680–7687, 1994

CHAPTER 10

Gender Differences in First-Episode Schizophrenia

Heinz Häfner, M.D., Ph.D., Dres.h.c.

There have long been reports of gender differences in schizophrenia. Nearly 100 years ago, Kraepelin pointed to a several-years-higher age at first admission for women with dementia praecox (Kraepelin 1909–1915). Currently, the most important issues in the field concern 1) *diagnoses, subtypes,* and *symptoms;* 2) *antecedents, course,* and *outcome;* 3) *lifetime risk of psychosis* and *age distribution of onset;* 4) *genetic and environmental risk factors* as well as associated conditions—brain morphology in particular; 5) comorbidity, *illness behavior, social status,* and *quality of life;* and 6) aspects of care, including *treatment compliance,* responsiveness to drug and other therapies as well as rehabilitation (e.g., psychotherapy, family therapy, sociotherapy) and the need for inpatient and long-term residential care. Those issues addressed in the present chapter appear in *italics.*

This chapter was previously presented as the Zubin lecture at the annual meeting of the American Psychopathological Association, New York City, February 27–28, 1997.

Initial Symptoms, Type of Onset, and Subtypes of Psychosis

The epidemiological analyses I first present rely on a population-based sample of first-episode cases. In the ABC (Age, Beginning, Course) Schizophrenia Study, my colleagues and I (Häfner et al. 1993) identified, over a 2-year period (1987–1989), 276 successive first-admission patients (ages 12–59 years) from 10 psychiatric units and hospitals serving a semi-urban, semi-rural German population of 1.5 million (Heidelberg, Mannheim, and the surrounding regions). All patients had received a broad diagnosis of schizophrenia (International Classification of Diseases, 9th Revision [ICD-9; World Health Organization 1978a] codes 295, 297, 298.3/4). A more detailed description of sample recruitment and characteristics and the methodology applied to assess the design variables has been presented by Häfner et al. (1993).

All of the patients were rated with the Present State Examination (PSE; Wing et al. 1974), the Scale for the Assessment of Negative Symptoms (SANS; Andreasen 1983), the Psychological Impairments Rating Schedule (PIRS; Biehl et al. 1989), the Disability Assessment Schedule (DAS; World Health Organization 1988; Jung et al. 1989), and other instruments by trained psychiatrists and psychologists immediately upon hospitalization. To assess the onset and early course of the disorder before first contact, we developed a semistructured Interview for the Retrospective Assessment of the Onset of Schizophrenia (IRAOS; Häfner et al. 1992) on the basis of internationally well-known and widely used instruments (Table 10–1). A prospective population study, the ideal design for determining onset, was not practical, because the onset of schizophrenia is a rare event, and three-fourths of cases begin with nonspecific symptoms. The IRAOS elicits information on prodromal signs, symptoms, social development, and social disability as well as on their time of appearance. To reduce recall deficits, the IRAOS was administered independently to two different sources: the patient within 3–5 weeks of first admission, and a close relative of the patient. In addition, available documents, such as family doctors' case notes and school records, were reviewed. The patients were interviewed with the IRAOS only after their psychotic symptoms had disappeared or considerably diminished. A time grid based on anchor events, such as birthdays, holidays, and so forth, was

TABLE 10–1.
Instrument for the Retrospective Assessment of the Onset of Schizophrenia (IRAOS)

Based on	Dimension(s) measured
Premorbid Adjustment Scale (PAS; Cannon-Spoor et al. 1982)	Premorbid adjustment
Past History and Sociodemographic Description Schedule (PHSD; World Health Organization 1977)	Changes in sociodemographic variables
Psychiatric and Personal History Schedule (PPHS; World Health Organization 1978b)	Changes in sociodemographic variables and occurrence of early symptoms
Disability Assessment Schedule (DAS; World Health Organization 1988)	Social disability
Bonn Scale for the Assessment of Basic Symptoms (BSABS; Gross et al. 1987)	Prodromal signs
Present State Examination (PSE; Wing et al. 1974)	All symptoms
Scale for the Assessment of Negative Symptoms (SANS; Andreasen 1983)	Negative symptoms
and others	—

Source. Modified from Häfner H, Riecher A, Maurer K, et al.: "Ein Instrument zur retrospektiven Einschätzung des Erkrankungsbeginns bei Schizophrenie [Instrument for the Retrospective Assessment of the Onset of Schizophrenia—IRAOS]." *Zeitschrift für Klinische Psychologie* 19:230–255, 1990. Copyright © 1990, Hogrefe. Used with permission.

constructed to help patients determine and remember the dates of relevant events. Two hundred thirty-two subjects (108 men and 124 women)—84% of the first-admission sample—were first-episode patients.

Morbid Risk

The cumulative incidence rate through 59 years of age, a good indicator of lifetime risk for schizophrenia, was almost the same for both genders: 13.2 per 100,000 for men and 13.1 per 100,000 for women (based on 5-year age bands). As Figure 10–1 shows, however, men consumed their

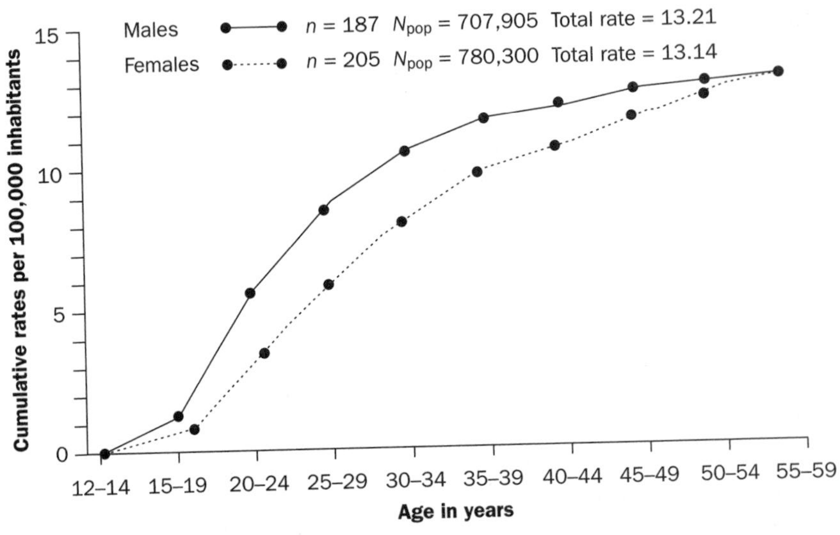

FIGURE 10–1. Cumulative incidence rates for schizophrenia—broad definition (ICD-9 codes 295, 297, 298.3, and 298.4)— in a representative first-admission sample (N = 392) from Mannheim, Heidelberg, Rhine–Neckar District, and Eastern Palatinate: ABC Schizophrenia Study, 1987–1989. *n* = number of patients in 2 years; N_{pop} = total population; ICD-9 = International Classification of Diseases, 9th Revision (World Health Organization 1978a).
Source. Reprinted from Häfner H, Behrens S, de Vry J, et al.: "Warum erkranken Frauen später an Schizophrenie?" *Nervenheilkunde* 10:154–163, 1991b. Copyright © 1991, F. K. Schattauer. Used with permission.

lifetime risk earlier, by age 30–35 years. From age 35 on, the rates for women grew increasingly closer to rates for men and finally reached the same endpoint. An early cutoff age, such as 45 years in the DSM-III (American Psychiatric Association 1980) diagnostic criteria, is bound to yield a seemingly higher morbid risk for men than for women—and, indeed, such a higher risk has been previously reported in many U.S. and Canadian studies (e.g., Lewine 1988).

A cross-sectional comparison of first psychotic episodes yielded no significant gender differences in clinical and operationalized diagnoses, subtypes, diagnostic scores, or subscores (Table 10–2). Even the six clusters we derived from the symptoms of the psychotic prephase to represent empirical subtypes did not show any significant gender differences (Table 10–3).

TABLE 10–2.

Comparison of clinical and operationalized diagnoses, CATEGO total score and syndrome subscores, and PSE index of definition: ABC Schizophrenia Study first-admission sample (N = 276[a])

	Females (n = 143), %	Males (n = 133), %	P
Diagnosis[*]			
Schizophrenia—broad definition (ICD-9: 295, 297, 298.3/4)	100	100	
Schizophrenia (ICD 295)	86.7	89.5	NS
Operationalized diagnosis[*]			
CATEGO ICD 295	79.0	72.9	NS
CATEGO class S+	74.1	66.9	NS
CATEGO affective psychosis	14.0	12.0	NS
Scores (mean values)[**]			
PSE index of definition	7.49	7.45	NS
CATEGO total score	40.73	41.36	NS
CATEGO subscores			
Delusional and hallucinatory syndromes	11.28	9.84	NS
Behavior, speech, and other syndromes	7.87	8.01	NS
Specific neurotic syndromes	6.91	7.57	NS
Nonspecific neurotic syndromes	14.67	15.94	NS

Note. [a]Of this sample, 232 (84%) were first-episode patients. CATEGO (Wing et al. 1974); PSE = Present State Examination (Wing et al. 1974); ICD-9 = International Classification of Diseases, 9th Revision (World Health Organization 1978a). NS = not significant. [*]χ^2 tests; [**]t tests.
Source. Modified from Häfner H, Maurer K, Löffler W, et al.: "The Epidemiology of Early Schizophrenia: Influence of Age and Gender on Onset and Early Course." *British Journal of Psychiatry Supplement* 164:29–38, 1994. Copyright © 1994, Royal College of Psychiatrists. Used with permission.

Age at Onset

The gender difference in age at first admission reported by Kraepelin in 1909 is a hallmark of the disorder, as Lindelius (1970), Lewine (1980),

TABLE 10–3.

Symptom clusters by gender and age at first admission: ABC Schizophrenia Study first-episode sample ($n = 232$)

Cluster	Nonspecific, negative, depressive	Delusional	Psychotic thought disorder	Auditory hallucinations, substance abuse	Disorganization/ psychotic thought disorder	Low values on all dimensions
By gender, % ($\chi^2 = 1.1$; $df = 5$; $P = .95$)						
Males	49.2	45.2	40.6	48.4	50.0	42.3
Females	50.8	54.8	59.4	51.6	50.0	57.7
By age at first admission, years ($F = 0.293$; $df = 5$; $P = .91$)	31.1	29.8	29.9	29.3	30.3	31.4

Angermeyer and Kühn (1988), and others have pointed out. In our study, mean age at emergence of the first sign, the first negative and the first positive symptom, and the climax of the first episode, was between 24 and 30 years. These milestones of the early course differed by 3–4 years between men and women (Figure 10–2). The pooled data of the World Health Organization (WHO) Determinants of Outcome Study (Jablensky et al. 1992) revealed an age difference of the same size: 3.4 years (Hambrecht et al. 1992).

The distribution of onsets over the entire age range showed an early and steep increase for men. After a pronounced peak between 15 and 25 years of age, the onset distribution for men fell monotonically. In women, the age distribution of onsets increased less steeply and reached a lower and later peak between 15 and 30 years of age. After a brief decline, new onsets again increased in the 45- to 49-year age group around menopause (Figure 10–3). A replication of these results using Danish national

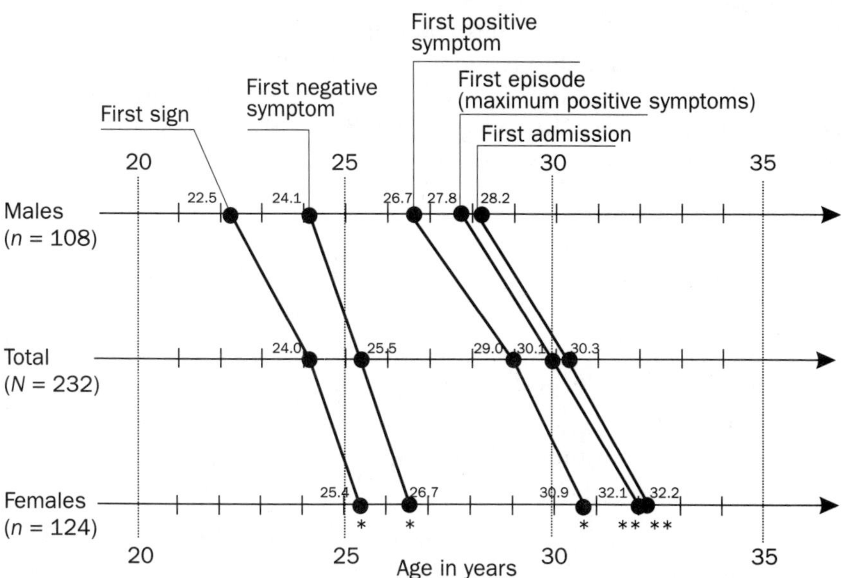

FIGURE 10–2. Mean age values by five definitions of illness onset: ABC Schizophrenia Study first-episode sample of schizophrenia (broad definition) ($n = 232$). $^{*}P \leq .05$; $^{**}P \leq .01$.

Source. Reprinted from Häfner H, Gattaz WF: "Geschlechtsunterschiede bei der Schizophrenie." *Der Gynäkologe* 28:426–433, 1995. Copyright © 1995, Springer-Verlag. Used with permission.

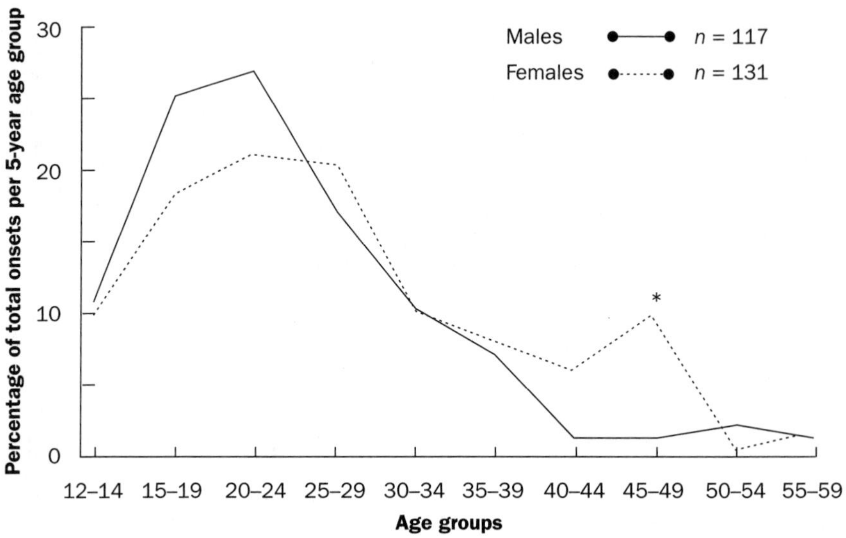

FIGURE 10–3. Distribution of age at onset of schizophrenia (first-ever sign of mental disorder), by gender (ICD-9 codes 295, 297, 298.3, and 298.4): ABC Schizophrenia Study. ICD-9 = International Classification of Diseases, 9th Revision (World Health Organization 1978a). *$P < .05$.
Source. Reprinted from Häfner H, Gattaz WF: "Geschlechtsunterschiede bei der Schizophrenie." *Der Gynäkologe* 28:426–433, 1995. Copyright © 1995, Springer-Verlag. Used with permission.

case-register data also showed a second peak of population-based female first-admission rates in the 50- to 54-year age group (Figure 10–4). Considering the fact that, on average, 4–5 years elapse between onset and first admission, the delayed peak in comparison with our true-onset data is understandable.

In explanation of these gender differences, Lewine (1980), Seeman (1982), Loranger (1984), Seeman and Lang (1990), and our group (Häfner et al. 1991a) have proposed a protective effect for estrogen. This suggestion and the distribution of onsets over the female life cycle—together with the neuroleptic-like effect of short-term estrogen applications in animals, demonstrated by Di Paolo and Falardeau (1985), Fields and Gordon (1982), and Hruska (1986)—prompted us to test the estrogen hypothesis. We studied the effects of a 4-week estrogen regimen (0.25 mg 17β-E2) versus placebo in sterilized rats compared with sham-operated rats with physiological estrogen secretion (Häfner et al. 1991a).

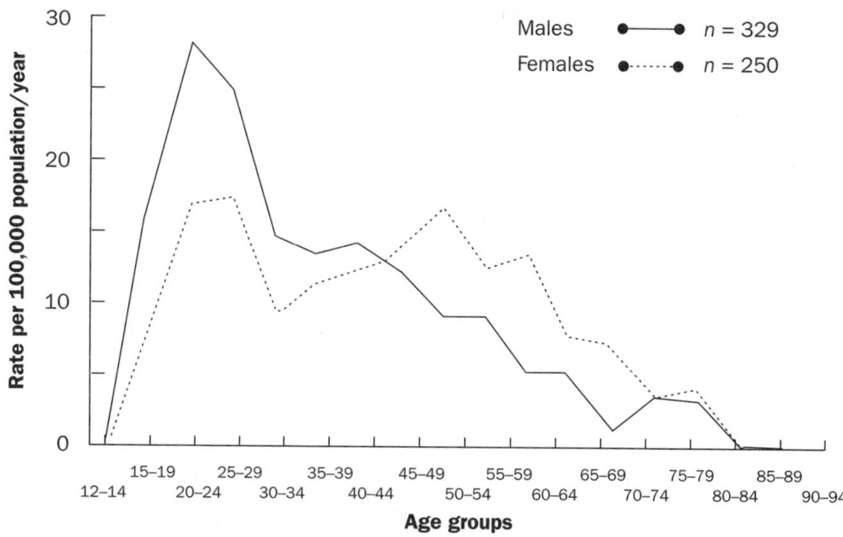

FIGURE 10–4. First-admission rates for schizophrenia (ICD-9 code 295) in Denmark, 1976. ICD-9 = International Classification of Diseases, 9th Revision (World Health Organization 1978a).
Source. Reprinted from Häfner H, Hambrecht M, Löffler W, et al.: "Is Schizophrenia a Disorder of All Ages? A Comparison of First Episodes and Early Course Across the Life-Cycle." *Psychological Medicine* 28:351–365, 1998. Copyright © 1998, Cambridge University Press. Used with permission.

Estrogen led to a significant attenuation of apomorphine-induced dopaminergic behavior (i.e., oral stereotypies, sitting and grooming) in neonatal rats and to a slightly weaker effect in adult rats. We were able to show that this effect came about via a reduced sensitivity of central D_2 dopamine receptors.

Hence, estrogen acts on dopaminergic neurotransmission both functionally and structurally. More recently, investigators have demonstrated comparable neurochemical and molecular effects of estrogen on serotonin receptors (Sumner and Fink 1995) and on glutamate receptors (Woolley and McEwen 1994).

To test the applicability of these results from animal experiments to human schizophrenia, we compared 32 women with schizophrenic and 29 women with depressive episodes, both with normal menstrual cycles, in a controlled clinical study. Increasing estrogen plasma levels showed significant correlations with schizophrenia symptom scores, but not with depressive symptom scores, in both groups of women (Table 10–4.) The only exception was the Nurses' Observation Scale for Inpatient Evaluation (NOSIE; Honigfeld et al. 1966) score, which is based on observation on the ward and measurement of behavioral disturbances and does not take diagnosis into account. We concluded that estrogen has a neuroleptic-like effect on schizophrenic symptoms in women.

However, DeLisi et al. (1994), Leboyer et al. (1992), and Albus and Maier (1996) have shown that the gender difference in age at onset disap-

TABLE 10–4.

Modulation of schizophrenic symptomatology in the menstrual cycle: comparison of women with schizophrenic and with depressive episodes

	Correlations with estrogen levels (means)	
Symptom scores	**Schizophrenic women** (n = 32)	**Depressed women** (n = 29)
BPRS—total	−0.25**	−0.03NS
BPRS—scores for		
anxiety/depression	−0.10NS	−0.00NS
anergia	−0.15**	−0.04NS
thought disorder	−0.28**	−0.13NS
activation	−0.27**	−0.06NS
hostility/suspiciousness	−0.19t	−0.13NS
NOSIE total	0.25**	0.22**
BfS total	−0.20*	−0.02NS
PDS—paranoid score	−0.17*	−0.06NS
PDS—depression score	−0.10NS	−0.01NS
HAMD total	Not assessed	−0.03NS

Note. BfS = Befindlichkeits-Skala (von Zerssen and Koeller 1976); BPRS = Brief Psychiatric Rating Scale (Overall and Gorham 1962); HAMD = Hamilton Rating Scale for Depression (Hamilton 1960); NOSIE = Nurses' Observation Scale for Inpatient Evaluation (Honigfeld et al. 1966); PDS = Paranoid-Depressivitäts-Skala (von Zerssen and Koeller 1976). Wilcoxon tests of cross-correlations: t$P < .10$; *$P < .05$; **$P < .01$; NS = not significant.

Source. Modified from Riecher-Rössler A, Häfner H, Dütsch-Strobel A, et al.: "Further Evidence for a Specific Role of Estradiol in Schizophrenia?" *Biological Psychiatry* 36:492–495, 1994. Copyright © 1994, The Society of Biological Psychiatry. Used with permission of Elsevier Science.

pears in familial schizophrenia. In contrast, the gender difference grew to 5.7 years in the definitely nonfamilial cases of Albus and Maier's sample.

In a replication study with our first-episode sample, the gender difference in familial cases (i.e., proband has at least one first-degree relative with schizophrenia) did indeed fall below the level of significance (-1.6 years), whereas in sporadic cases (i.e., proband has no relative with schizophrenia) the gender difference rose from 3.6 years in the total sample to a highly significant 4.9 years (Figure 4–5). The estrogen effect, delaying onset in women by elevating the vulnerability threshold for schizophrenia, obviously depends on the degree of genetic liability: the higher the patient's genetic load, the greater its suppression of the protective effect of estrogen.

Harrow et al. (1996), studying 18 men and 7 women with DSM-III-R (American Psychiatric Association 1987)–diagnosed schizophrenia, reported that the gender difference in age at onset was entirely attributable to a low age at onset in men who had suffered obstetric complications.

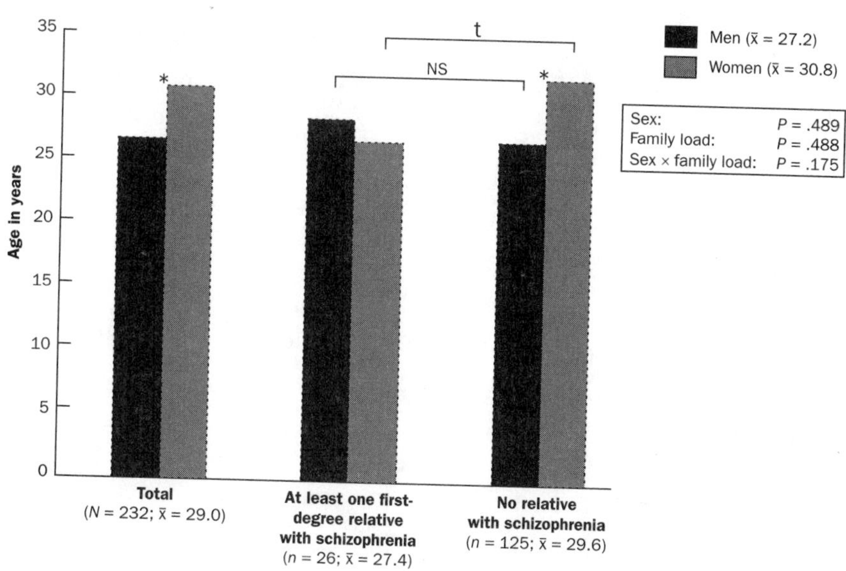

FIGURE 10–5. Age at first psychotic symptom for men and women in familial and nonfamilial schizophrenia (ICD-9 codes 295, 297, 298.3, and 298.4): ABC Schizophrenia Study first-admission sample ($n = 232$). ICD-9 = International Classification of Diseases, 9th Revision (World Health Organization 1978a). $^{t}P < .10$; $^{*}P < .01$; NS = not significant.

However, a replication using the same methodology in our large population-based first-episode sample failed to confirm this finding.

Confirmation of the estrogen effect led us to the following two hypotheses: 1) lacking a protective effect, young men should develop a majority and the most severe forms of schizophrenia, and older men should develop increasingly fewer and less severe cases; 2) women, as long as estrogen sustains their high vulnerability thresholds, might be spared in some instances, with the consequence that late-onset schizophrenias should be more frequent and more severe in women than in men.

Table 10–5 confirms what Harris and Jeste (1988) and several other authors have reported: late-onset schizophrenias are significantly more frequent in women than in men. Testing the second hypothesis, we found that men with onset at age 40 or later scored lower on all symptom dimensions as well as on disability, and in four of eight comparisons scored significantly lower, than men with early onset (Table 10–6). For late-onset women, not a single indicator was significantly reduced and one, negative symptomatology, was significantly higher. This means that first episodes of schizophrenia in late-onset women are somewhat more severe than first episodes in early-onset women and are clearly more severe than first episodes in late-onset men. This holds especially for the negative symptoms. In men, with their particularly severe early-onset schizophrenias, severity of illness decreases with increasing age at onset. These results supported our two hypotheses.

TABLE 10–5.

Schizophrenia onset by gender and age at first psychotic symptom: ABC Schizophrenia Study first-episode sample (n = 232)

Age at first psychotic symptom (years)	n	Men (%)	Women (%)	M:F ratio
12–20	49	57	43	1.33
21–35	136	48	52	0.92
36–59	47	32	68	0.47*

Note. M:F = male:female. *Odds ratio = 2.16 (sex ratio in the age group versus sex ratio in the remaining age groups); $P < .05$.

Source. Modified from Häfner H, Nowotny B: "Epidemiology of Early-Onset Schizophrenia." *European Archives of Psychiatry and Clinical Neuroscience* 245:80–92, 1995.

TABLE 10–6.

Comparison of gender differences in symptom scores at first admission, by age at first psychotic symptom (young [<21 years] versus old [≥40 years]): ABC Schizophrenia Study first-episode subjects

Symptom scores	Men			Women		
	Young (n = 28)	Versus Wilcoxon	Old (n = 9)	Young (n = 21)	Versus Wilcoxon	Old (n = 24)
CATEGO						
Delusional and hallucinatory syndromes	12.1	.02*	↓5.7	10.0	.95	10.5
Behavior, speech, and other syndromes	8.6	.29	7.3	8.9	.44	7.9
Specific neurotic syndromes	10.7	.11	7.3	8.2	.42	7.1
Nonspecific neurotic syndromes	18.9	.03	↓11.4	13.0	.58	13.8
Total score	50.3	.02*	↓31.8	40.0	.80	39.2
Scale for the Assessment of Negative Symptoms (SANS)	9.3	.29	6.6	6.7	.08ᵗ	↑ 9.5
Psychological Impairment Rating Scale (PIRS)	10.7	.26	8.4	9.8	.73	10.5
Disability Assessment Scale (DAS)	3.0	.06ᵗ	↓1.8	1.9	.61	1.8

Note. Arrows mark the direction of the age difference. *$P < .05$; ᵗ$P < .10$.
Source. Reprinted from Häfner H, an der Heiden W: "Epidemiology of Schizophrenia." *Canadian Journal of Psychiatry* 42:139–151, 1997. Copyright © 1997, Canadian Psychiatric Association. Used with permission.

Premorbid Signs (Neurodevelopmental Disorder)

Studies based on teachers' and parents' reports (Watt et al. 1984), on offspring of schizophrenic mothers (Erlenmeyer-Kimling et al. 1993; Parnas et al. 1993), and on three large-scale birth cohorts of British and North Finnish populations (Crow et al. 1995; Done et al. 1994; Jones et al. 1996; van Os 1996) as well as a retrospective sibling study (Walker et al. 1995) using family videos have shown that neuromotor and cognitive deficits and emotional and behavioral abnormalities are common in childhood and adolescence in individuals who later develop schizophrenia (Figure 10–6).

As Figure 10–7 (from Walker et al.'s [1995] study comparing siblings with and without schizophrenia) shows, premorbid signs manifest somewhat later in girls than in boys. Girls exhibit primarily internalizing ("introversive") behaviors (e.g., shyness, social withdrawal, depressive

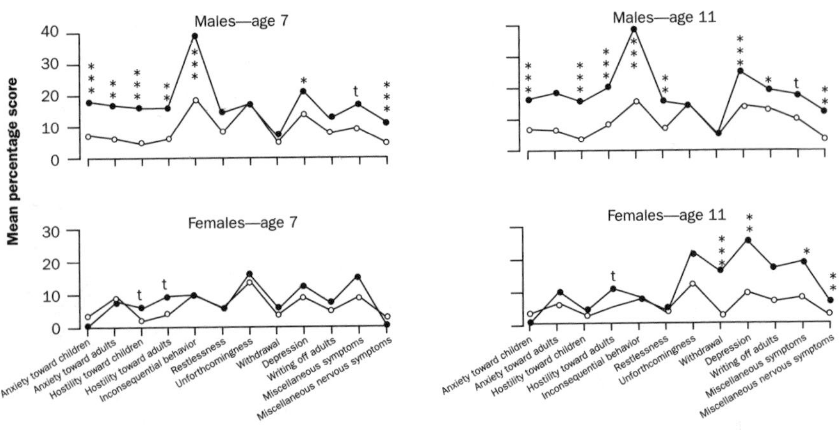

FIGURE 10–6. Antecedents of schizophrenia: social adjustment (Bristol Social Adjustment Guide; Stott 1987) of preschizophrenic boys and girls at ages 7 and 11 years: British Child Development Study. ● = preschizophrenic subjects; O = control subjects. $^{t}P < .10$; $^{*}P < .05$; $^{**}P < .01$; $^{***}P < .005$.
Source. Modified from Crow TJ, Done DJ, Sacker A: "Birth Cohort Study of the Antecedents of Psychosis: Ontogeny as Witness to Phylogenetic Origins," in *Search for the Causes of Schizophrenia,* Vol. 3. Edited by Häfner H, Gattaz WF. Berlin, Springer-Verlag, 1995, pp. 3–20. Copyright © 1995, Springer-Verlag. Used with permission.

mood, social anxiety), whereas boys manifest mainly externalizing behaviors (e.g., hyperactivity, physical and verbal aggression, failure of behavioral inhibitions). Although symptoms and dysfunctions take on a new quality with the onset of psychosis, the gender differences in the age at onset of the behavioral antecedents of schizophrenia and in the patterns of behavior will reappear in the psychosis.

Onset and Early Course

Reconstructing the early course of schizophrenia from the first sign of the disorder until first admission, we found that of the broadly defined cases of schizophrenia, only 18% had an acute onset (within 1 month of first symptoms), whereas the bulk—68%—had a chronic onset with a more than 1-year persistence of symptoms before first admission (Table 10–7). Significant gender differences were observed neither in type of onset nor in type of first symptoms; 73% of cases began with a prodromal phase of negative and/or nonspecific symptoms and only 7% with purely positive

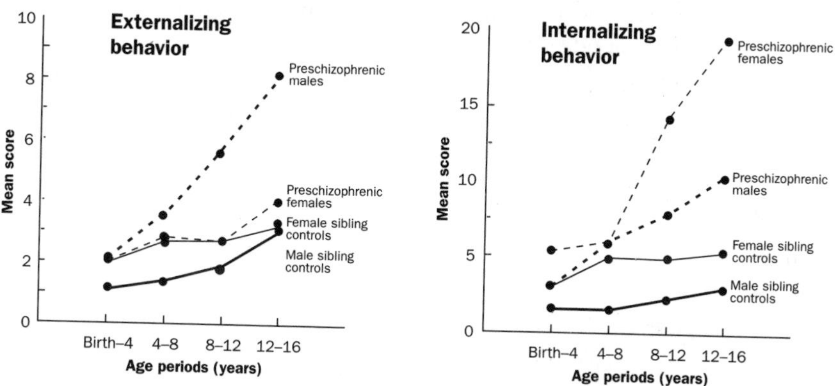

FIGURE 10–7. Antecedents of schizophrenia: comparison of preschizophrenic and control siblings—mean Achenbach Child Behavior Checklist (Achenbach 1982) externalizing/internalizing behavior problem scores (by age period and gender.

Source. Modified from Walker EF, Weinstein J, Baum K, et al.: "Antecedents of Schizophrenia: Moderating Effects of Development and Biological Sex," in *Search for the Causes of Schizophrenia*, Vol 3. Edited by Häfner H, Gattaz WF. Berlin, Springer-Verlag, 1995, pp 21–42. Copyright © 1995, Springer-Verlag. Used with permission.

symptoms. Likewise, the 10 most frequent initial symptoms did not differ between the genders, with the exception of worrying, which was slightly more frequent in women (Table 10–8). Worrying is also more frequent in women versus men in nonschizophrenic populations. In the 73% of cases that began with negative or nonspecific symptoms, the prodromal phase lasted an average of 5 years before the first positive symptom appeared, and the psychotic prephase lasted until the climax of the first episode (i.e., the maximum of positive symptoms)—about 1 year, as shown in Figure 10–8, a simplified representation of the accumulation of positive and negative symptoms.

The emergence of the milestones of the early course—first sign, first negative and first positive symptom, and climax of the first episode—was parallel in men and women, with an age difference of 3–4 years (see Figure 10–2). Symptom accumulation—based on the mean number of symptoms per year (Figure 10–9, top panel) and, for the last year preceding first admission (Figure 10–9, bottom panel), based on the mean

TABLE 10–7.

Schizophrenia onset type and type of first symptoms, by gender: ABC Schizophrenia Study first-episode sample

	Total (N = 232), %	Men (*n* = 108), %	Women (*n* = 124), %
Type of onset*			
Acute (≤1 month)	18	19	17
Subacute (>1 month to ≤1 year)	15	11	18
Insidious or chronic (>1 year)	68	70	65
Type of first symptoms*			
Negative or nonspecific	73	70	76
Positive	7	7	6
Both	20	22	19

*The variables listed showed no significant gender differences.

Source. Modified from Häfner H, Maurer K, Löffler W, et al.: "Onset and Early Course of Schizophrenia," in *Search for the Causes of Schizophrenia*, Vol. 3. Edited by Häfner H, Gattaz WF. Berlin, Springer-Verlag, 1995a, pp. 43–66. Copyright © 1995, Springer-Verlag. Used with permission.

TABLE 10–8.
Ten most frequent early signs of schizophrenia (independent of course) reported by patients: ABC Schizophrenia Study first-episode sample

	Total (N = 232), %	Men (*n* = 108), %	Women (*n* = 124), %
Restlessness	19	15	22
Depression	19	15	22
Anxiety	18	17	19
Trouble with thinking and concentration	16	19	14
Worrying	15	9	20*
Lack of self-confidence	13	10	15
Lack of energy; slowness	12	8	15
Poor work performance	11	12	10
Social withdrawal, distrust	10	8	12
Social withdrawal, lack of communication	10	8	12

Note. Based on closed questions; multiple counting possible. All items tested for gender differences; *$P \leq .05$.
Source. Modified from Häfner H, Maurer K, Löffler W, et al.: "Onset and Early Course of Schizophrenia," in *Search for the Causes of Schizophrenia*, Vol. 3. Edited by Häfner H, Gattaz WF. Berlin, Springer-Verlag, 1995a, pp. 43–66. Copyright © 1995, Springer-Verlag. Used with permission.

number of symptoms per month (because it was during this period that patients showed the most pronounced increases in symptoms)—showed that the exponential increase in negative symptoms was less steep and started several years earlier compared with the increase in positive symptoms (Figure 10–9). Just before the climax of the first episode, positive symptoms outnumbered negative symptoms. However, negative symptoms also showed an episodic course with increases and decreases, although the fluctuation was less pronounced than that of positive symptoms and no gender differences were evident.

The compelling similarity of the early course of schizophrenia, from initial symptoms to type of onset, patterns of course, and symptomatology of the first episode, in men and women raises substantial doubts about some widespread assumptions—according to which, for example, a chronic onset should be more frequent in men, an acute onset more fre-

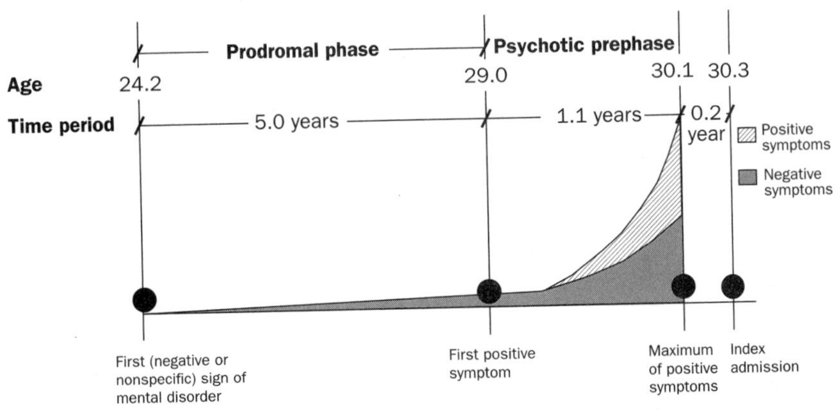

FIGURE 10–8. Schizophrenia prephases from first sign of mental disorder to first hospital admission, for both genders together: ABC Schizophrenia Study first-episode sample (*n* = 232 [108 males, 124 females]).
Source. Reprinted from Häfner H, Maurer K, Löffler W, et al.: "Onset and Early Course of Schizophrenia," in *Search for the Causes of Schizophrenia,* Vol. 3. Edited by Häfner H, Gattaz WF. Berlin, Springer-Verlag, 1995a, pp. 43–66. Copyright © 1995, Springer-Verlag. Used with permission.

quent in women, negative symptoms more frequent in men, and positive symptoms more frequent in women in the first episode (e.g., Lewis and Murray 1987). If one also considers that T. E. Goldberg et al. (1995), assessing four independent cohorts of schizophrenic men and women with a large test battery, failed to find any substantial neuropsychological differences between the genders, one cannot but agree with those authors' conclusion that "these results provide little support for the hypothesis that gender is associated with a unique pathogenesis of schizophrenia" (p. 883). This statement also holds for the proxy variables neuropsychology, symptomatology, and early course. In order to understand the influence of gender on schizophrenia, it is therefore important to analyze gender differences in variables more distant to the disease process.

Illness Behavior (Symptomatology in First Episode)

For this purpose, we compared all of the 303 single items of the instruments we used for measuring symptoms, functional impairment, and so-

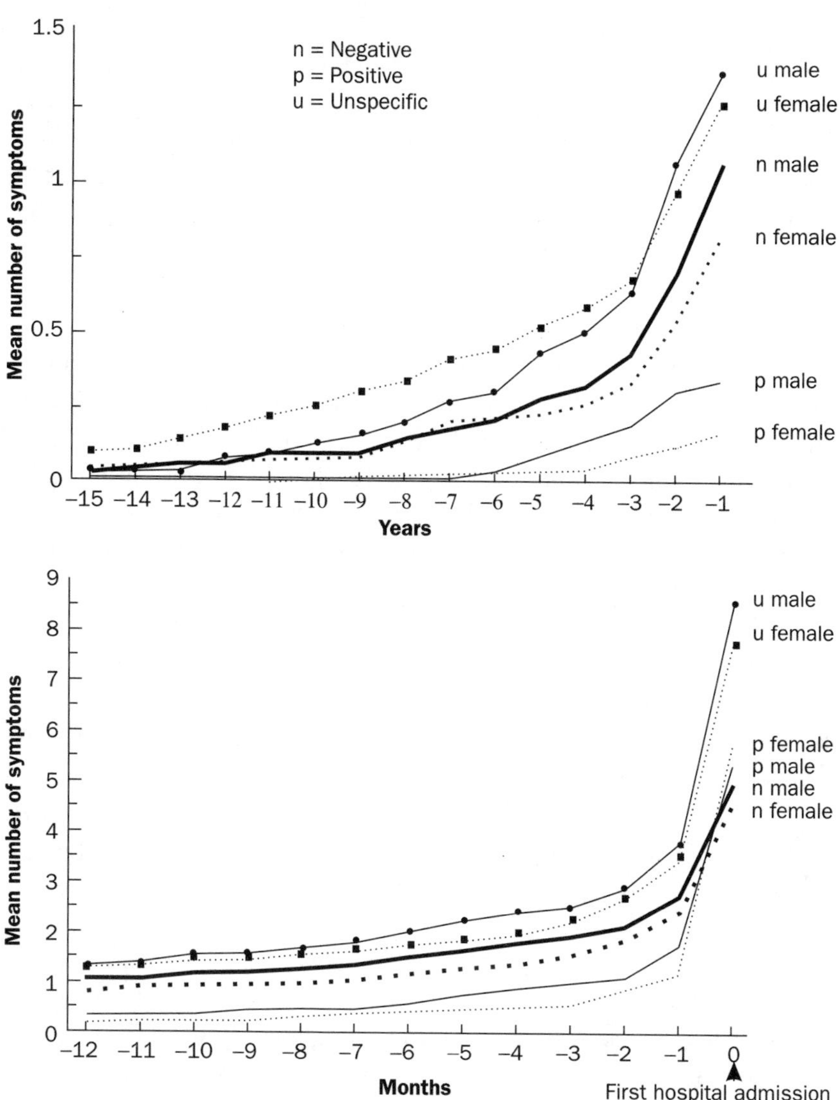

FIGURE 10–9. Cumulative numbers of positive, negative, and unspecific symptoms from symptom onset to first hospital admission, for both genders together: ABC Schizophrenia Study first-episode sample ($n = 232$ [108 males, 124 females]).

Source. Reprinted from Häfner H, Maurer K, Löffler W, et al.: "Onset and Early Course of Schizophrenia," in *Search for the Causes of Schizophrenia,* Vol. 3. Edited by Häfner H, Gattaz WF. Berlin, Springer-Verlag, 1995a, pp. 43–66. Copyright © 1995, Springer-Verlag. Used with permission.

cial disability at the climax of the first episode in our ABC Study sample. Controlling for multiple testing, we found, as expected, no significant gender differences in the positive and negative core symptoms. The few differences in the content of delusions, such as a high frequency of delusions of pregnancy in women versus zero in men, probably reflect the sense of reality schizophrenic men manage to retain in illness rather than representing an expression of the disorder.

The most pronounced gender difference was that eight socially negative behavioral items—self-neglect, reduced interest in acquiring a job, social inattentiveness, lack of free-time activities, communication deficits, overall social disability, loss of interests, and inadequate personal hygiene—assessed cross-sectionally and two items—substance and alcohol abuse—assessed cumulatively over the prephase were all considerably more frequent in men, whereas one socially positive behavioral item—overadaptiveness/conformity—was more frequent in women (Table 10–9).

This finding was not surprising, in view of the aforementioned gender differences in antecedents and the consistent reports of men's poorer premorbid social performance in schizophrenia. But this finding is not specific to schizophrenia. A series of general-population studies have consistently reported a higher frequency of conduct disorders, disruptive antisocial and also violent behavior, and substance abuse among male adolescents and young men in comparison with their female counterparts (Choquet and Ledoux 1994). Schizophrenia obviously does not abolish this gender-specific risk.

The normal psychology of behavioral gender differences, too, mentioned by Charles Darwin and reviewed, for example, by Maccoby and Jacklin (1974), has shown that boys and young men show more aggressive behavior—in particular, antisocial aggression—compared with girls and young women, who display more prosocial aggression, aggressive inhibition, and acceptance of authority.

In our first-episode sample, schizophrenic men under age 21 years scored the highest, and men over age 35 years the lowest, on the socially negative behavioral items listed in Table 10–9, thus confirming the strong age dependence of these behaviors. Obviously, with increasing age at onset—and possibly also with increasing age over the course of the disorder—men's illness behavior becomes less socially negative, indicating improved adjustment.

TABLE 10–9.

Behavioral items with significant gender differences (from a total of 303 PSE, PIRS, SANS, DAS, and IRAOS items[a]): ABC Schizophrenia Study first-episode sample (n = 232)

More frequent in women	More frequent in men
Cumulative (until first admission)	
• Restlessness	• Drug abuse
	• Alcohol abuse
Cross-sectional (at first admission)	
• Overadaptiveness/conformity	• Self-neglect
	• Reduced interest in acquiring a job
	• Social inattentiveness
	• Lack of free-time activities
	• Deficits of communication
	• Social disability (overall estimate)
	• Loss of interests
	• Inadequate personal hygiene

Note. PSE = Present State Examination (Wing et al. 1974); PIRS = Psychological Impairments Rating Schedule (Biehl et al. 1989); SANS = Scale for the Assessment of Negative Symptoms (Andreasen 1983); DAS = Disability Assessment Schedule (World Health Organization 1988); IRAOS = Instrument for the Retrospective Assessment of the Onset of Schizophrenia (Häfner et al. 1992). [a]Validated by split-half method for α-correction.

Source. Reprinted from Häfner H: "Ist es einzig die Krankheit?" in *Moderne Konzepte zu Diagnostik, Pathogenese und Therapie.* Edited by Möller H-J, Müller N. Wien, Germany, Springer, 1998, pp. 37–59. Copyright © 1998, Springer-Verlag. Used with permission.

On the other hand, this gender difference in illness behavior—that is, the greater readiness of schizophrenic women to internalize social norms and their greater cooperativeness and therapy compliance versus the higher frequency of aversive, noncooperative, and socially negative behavior of young schizophrenic men—might lead to differences in course and outcome.

Medium-Term Course

There are more reports of gender differences in the course and outcome of schizophrenia at the social than at the symptom level. Theoretically, the social consequences of the disorder depend on disease-related social disability. Studying when social disability emerges, we were surprised to find that all of the DAS items appeared, on average, as early as 2–4 years before first admission (Figure 10–10). Hence, it is as early as the prodromal phase and long before the first psychiatric contact that schizophrenic individuals exhibit deficits in social competence. Crow et al. (1986), Loebel et al. (1992), and Wiersma et al. (1996) have also shown that the length of untreated illness is a predictor of poor short-term therapy outcome.

Role of Social Environment

According to several methodologically sound epidemiological studies, for example, E. M. Goldberg and Morrison's (1963), Dohrenwend et al.'s (1992) Israel study, and the birth cohort studies mentioned, schizophrenic individuals are not born into social disadvantage. Nonetheless, the patient's stage of social development at onset might play a decisive role in determining his or her course of illness. Three-fourths of all schizophrenias manifest themselves between 15 and 30 years of age, the period of life of the steepest social ascent. To assess the level of social development at onset, we chose six key social roles characteristic of this period of life and compared their performance at the onset of schizophrenia in three age groups: ages 20 years or younger, 21–35 years, and 36 years and older.

Early Social Course

Our results illustrate the enormous impact of age on patients' social conditions at the onset of schizophrenia (Figure 10–11). Men become ill 3–4 years earlier than women, which means an earlier intrusion of the disorder into their social biographies. The figures were significantly more favorable for women, not only in terms of school education but also in terms of the roles taken up later (employment and own accommodation

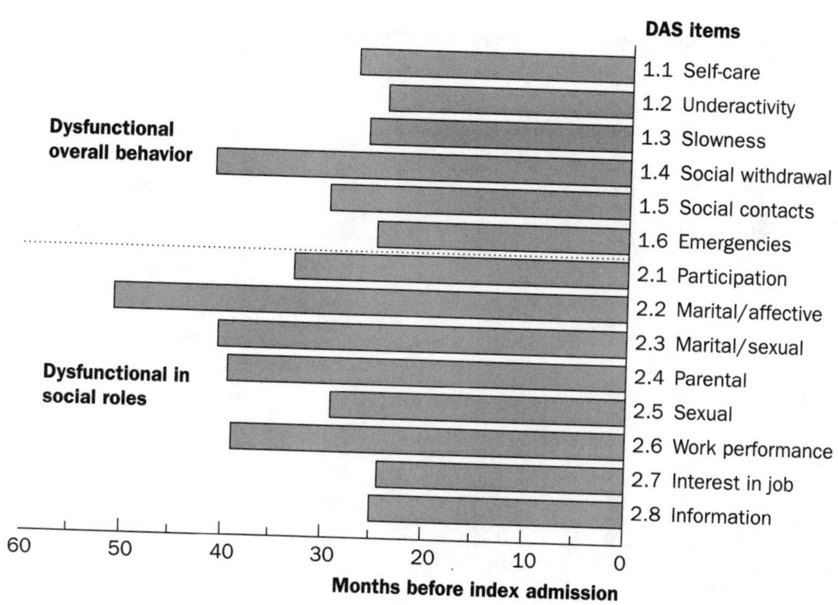

FIGURE 10–10. Onset of social disabilities (months before first admission), as assessed with the Disability Assessment Schedule (DAS; World Health Organization 1988): ABC Schizophrenia Study first-episode sample ($n = 232$).
Source. Reprinted from Häfner H, Maurer K, Löffler W, et al.: "Der Frühverlauf den Schizophrenie." *Zeitschrift für Medizinische Psychologie* 5:22–31, 1996. Copyright © 1996, Spcktrum Akademischer Verlag GmbH. Used with permission.

[i.e., versus living with parents or in a group home]). The most pronounced difference emerged with marriage or stable partnership and was attributable not only to men's lower age at onset but also to their higher age at marriage (2.5 years older) in comparison with women (Table 10–10). Hence, social conditions at the onset of schizophrenia are on average better for women than for men. For this reason, and because of the socially negative illness behavior of young men, social course and outcome would be expected to be worse for men than for women, at least for a limited period of time after onset.

To test this hypothesis, we followed a population-based cohort of 115 first-episode patients from our ABC sample at five cross sections over 5 years beginning at first admission. As an indicator of the objective social situation, we selected the patients' ability to earn their own living. Of the three age groups, it was the oldest, the group with the highest social status

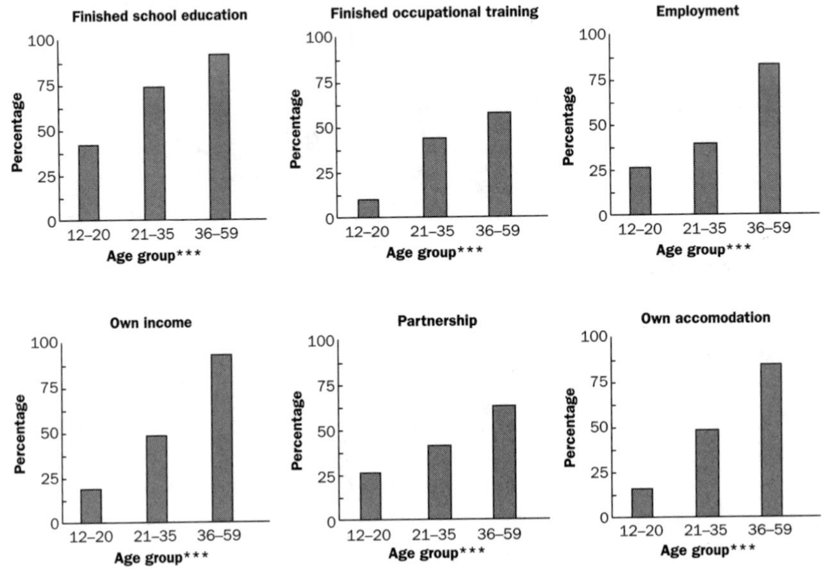

FIGURE 10–11. Stage of social development, as assessed by performance of six key roles, at the onset of schizophrenia (first sign), by age: ABC Schizophrenia Study first-episode sample ($n = 232$). ***Group differences $P < .001$ (χ^2).
Source. Modified from Häfner H, Nowotny B: "Epidemiology of Early-Onset Schizophrenia." *European Archives of Psychiatry and Clinical Neuroscience* 245:80–92, 1995. Copyright © 1995, Springer-Verlag. Used with permission.

at onset, that suffered the most pronounced social decline in the period extending from onset until 5 years after first admission—that is, a period encompassing about 11 years (Figure 10–12). In terms of social outcome, however, these patients still fared better than the younger age groups. The youngest and the intermediate age groups even experienced a slight improvement in social status during the prodromal phase, but remained at these still rather low levels in the five years following first admission.

Because of their higher age at onset, women's social conditions surpassed those of men by about the same amount at both the beginning and the end of the follow-up period (Figure 10–13). These analyses demonstrate that the gender difference persisting from onset through the medium-term course is in fact determined by patients' stages of social development at onset: the earlier the disorder intruded into their social biographies, the lower the level of social development patients had achieved at that point.

TABLE 10–10.

Social role performance at emergence of first sign of mental disorder: ABC Schizophrenia Study first-episode sample

	Men (n = 108)	Women (n = 124)	Total (N = 232)	P
Mean age, years	22.5	25.4	24.0	
Completed school education, %	70	69	70	
Occupational training, %	41	38	39	NS
Employment, %	37	52	45	*
Own income, %	44	55	50	NS
Own living accommodations, %	39	54	47	*
Marriage or stable partnership, %	28	52	41	**

Note. $^{*}P \leq .05$; $^{**}P \leq .01$; NS = not significant.
Source. Reprinted from Häfner H, Fätkenheuer B, Nowotny B, et al.: "New Perspectives in the Epidemiology of Schizophrenia." *Psychopathology* 28 (Suppl. 1):26–40, 1995b. Copyright © 1995, S. Karger. Used with permission.

To obtain objective measures of the social course of schizophrenia before first admission, we compared a representative subsample of 57 first-admission patients from Mannheim with 57 age- and gender-matched control subjects drawn from the city's population register. As an indicator of social development, performance on six key roles of the IRAOS interview was assessed for both schizophrenic patients and control subjects at the same age, determined by the patients' age at onset, age at first positive symptom, and age at first admission.

Again, at illness onset, no significant difference—and hence, no significant indication of social disadvantage before onset—was found. After onset, while the control subjects were filling a growing number of social roles, schizophrenic men and women more or less remained at their initially low stages in employment, own income, and own accommodation. Here, too, the most pronounced differences between patients and controls and between the genders was found in marriage or stable partnership. Whereas at baseline both schizophrenic and control men lagged significantly behind women as a result of their lower age at onset and

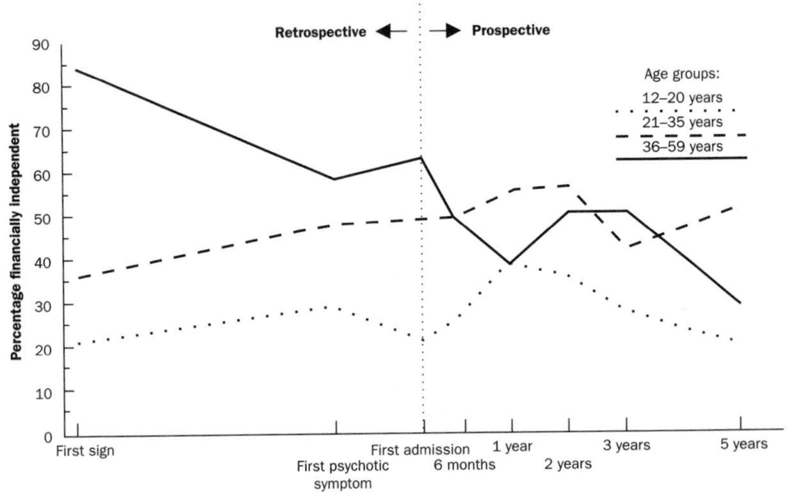

FIGURE 10–12. Social course: financial independence by age group—ABC Schizophrenia Study follow-up sample (n = 115). Autonomy = living on own or partner's income.
Source. Reprinted from Häfner H, Hambrecht M, Löffler W, et al.: "Is Schizophrenia a Disorder of All Ages? A Comparison of First Episodes and Early Course Across the Life-Cycle." *Psychological Medicine* 28:351–365, 1998. Copyright © 1998, Royal College of Psychiatrists. Used with permission.

higher age at marriage, respectively, healthy men reduced this gap, whereas schizophrenic men and women suffered a continuous decline after onset (Figure 10–14). In the particularly sensitive domain of mating behavior, the early emergence of social disability in schizophrenic individuals causes not only social stagnation but also social decline in some younger patients.

Women, however, retained their significant advantage over men: at first admission, 33% of the schizophrenic women, but only 17% of the schizophrenic men, were living with a spouse or partner (comparable figures in control subjects were 78% for women and 60% for men).

Role of Symptom-Related Early Course

As was the case in the prodomal and psychotic prephases through the climax of the first episode, the CATEGO total score (Wing et al. 1974) in the 5 years following first admission indicated no relevant gender differ-

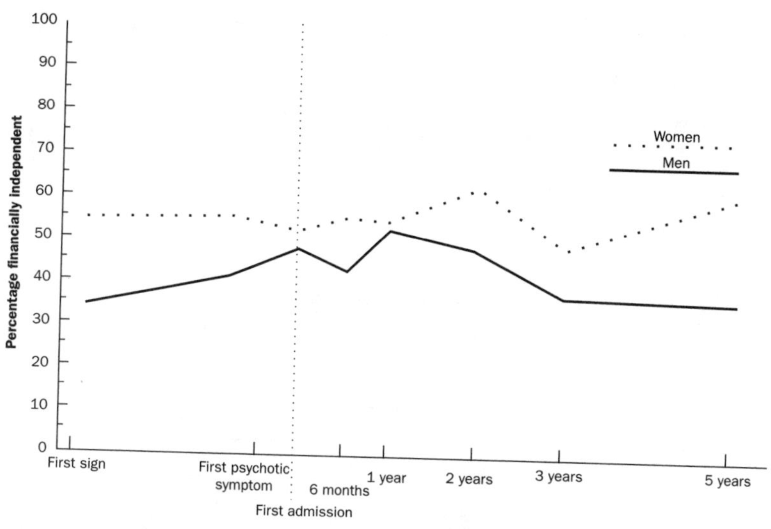

FIGURE 10–13. Social course: financial independence by gender—ABC Schizophrenia Study follow-up sample (n = 115).
Source. Reprinted from Häfner H: "Ist es einzig die Krankheit?" in *Moderne Konzepte zu Diagnostik, Pathogenese und Therapie*. Edited by Möller H-J, Müller N. Wien, Germany, Springer, 1998, pp. 37–59. Copyright © 1998, Springer-Verlag. Used with permission.

ences in symptomatology (Figure 10–15A). This finding was in agreement with results reported from the few existing epidemiological follow-up studies covering at least 5 years (Biehl et al. 1986; Salokangas et al. 1987; Shepherd et al. 1989). Unlike symptoms, however, social disability showed a significant gender difference, with lower DAS scores for women than for men (Figure 10–15B). The main reason for this difference lies in men's socially negative illness behavior. The fact that a number of socially negative behavioral items, such as self-neglect, reduced interest in acquiring a job, and substance abuse, are included in the DAS score explains, at least to some extent, why men's scores are significantly higher than women's.

Long-Term Course and Outcome

Epidemiological follow-up studies extending 10 years or more and satisfying methodological standards are rare. However, the first results of the 13-

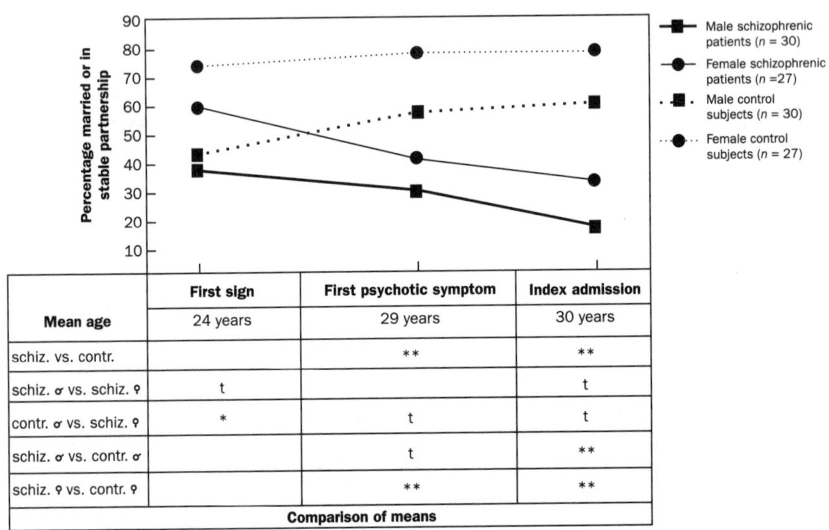

	First sign	First psychotic symptom	Index admission
Mean age	24 years	29 years	30 years
schiz. vs. contr.		**	**
schiz. ♂ vs. schiz. ♀	t		t
contr. ♂ vs. schiz. ♀	*	t	t
schiz. ♂ vs. contr. ♂		t	**
schiz. ♀ vs. contr. ♀		**	**
Comparison of means			

FIGURE 10–14. Marriage or stable partnership in schizophrenia patients and control subjects, by gender: ABC Schizophrenia Study first-episode sample ($n = 232$). schiz. = schizophrenia patients; contr. = control subjects; ♀ = women; ♂ = men. $^{t}P \leq .10$; $^{*}P \leq .05$; $^{**}P \leq .01$.
Source. Reprinted from Häfner H, Fätkenheuer B, Nowotny B, et al.: "New Perspectives in the Epidemiology of Schizophrenia." *Psychopathology* 28 (Suppl. 1):26–40, 1995b. Copyright © 1995, S. Karger. Used with permission.

to 15-year follow-ups of the Groningen, Netherlands; Nottingham, England; and Mannheim, Germany, first-admission cohorts of the WHO Disability Study, studied with standardized instruments, have appeared (an der Heiden et al. 1995, 1996; Sartorius et al. 1996). These results confirm what was indicated by our analyses of early and medium-term course and outcome. As illustrated in Figure 10–16, which depicts the Nottingham cohort studied by Mason et al. (1996), time spent with psychotic symptoms after remission of the first episode showed a plateau that began 2 years after first admission and continued for the duration of the follow-up period. The same was true for other measures of symptomatology and course in a stricter sense (an der Heiden et al. 1995, 1996). Individual courses, too, such as good versus poor outcome, proved remarkably stable over the long follow-up period. A comparison of the PSE DAH (delusions, hallucinations) scores in our Mannheim cohort (an der Heiden et al. 1995) 1, 5, and 14 years after first admission did not indicate any

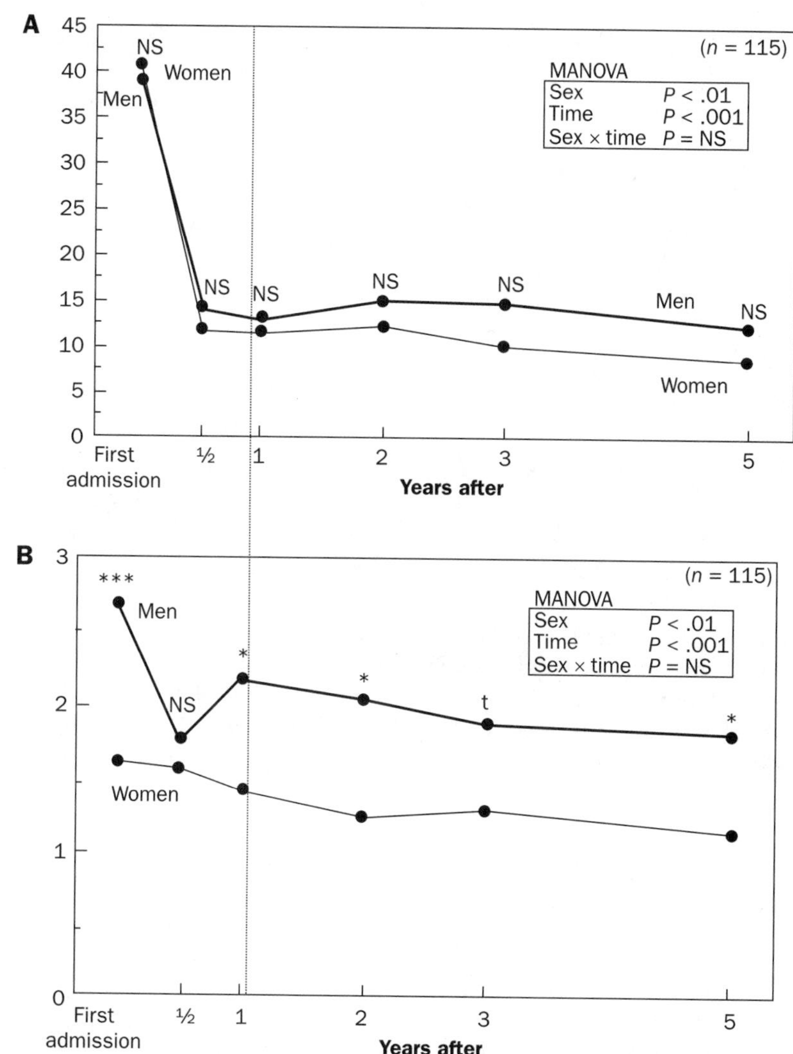

FIGURE 10–15. Five-year course of symptomatology and social disability by gender, as assessed (A) with the CATEGO (Wing et al. 1974) total score from first admission (six cross sections) and (B) with the Disability Assessment Schedule (DAS; World Health Organization 1988) total score from first admission (six cross sections): ABC Schizophrenia Study first-episode sample ($n = 232$). MANOVA = multivariate analysis of variance. $^{t}P < .10$; $^{*}P < .05$; $^{***}P < .001$; NS = not significant.

Source. Reprinted from Häfner H: "Ist es einzig die Krankheit?" in *Moderne Konzepte zu Diagnostik, Pathogenese und Therapie*. Edited by Möller H-J, Müller N. Wien, Germany, Springer, 1998, pp. 37–59. Copyright © 1998, Springer-Verlag. Used with permission.

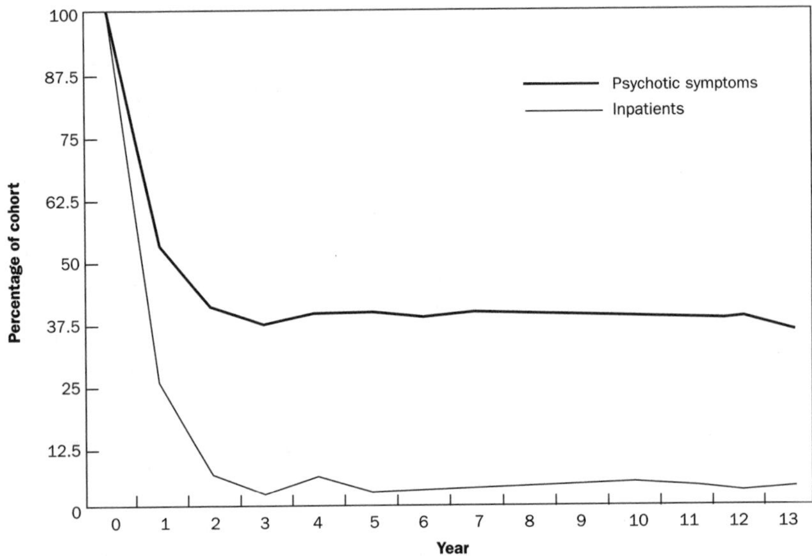

FIGURE 10–16. Proportion of time spent with psychotic symptoms and as a psychiatric inpatient: WHO Disability Study, Nottingham cohort.
Source. Reprinted from Mason P, Harrison G, Glazebrook C, et al.: "The Course of Schizophrenia Over 13 Years." *British Journal of Psychiatry* 169: 580–586, 1996. Copyright © 1996, Royal College of Psychiatrists. Used with permission.

substantial changes in symptom frequency or profiles (Figure 10– 17). Although the DAS profiles (overall behavior) showed no change from 5 to 14 years after first admission, there was a slight increase in underactivity compared with the profiles 1 year after admission.

Men and women did not differ in their symptomatologies 14 years after first admission, and the gender difference in social disability, which had still been present 5 years after first admission, had disappeared. The initial gender differences probably level out over time, possibly as a result of the age-related decrease in men's socially negative behavior.

At the 14-year follow-up, about 60% of the male and female patients showed a poor outcome, reporting having experienced positive symptoms and/or social impairment in the last year. However, an unusual gender difference was seen within the 40% of good-outcome patients (Figure 10–18): 28% of the good-outcome women, but only 3% of the good-outcome men, continued to take neuroleptic drugs. We do not know

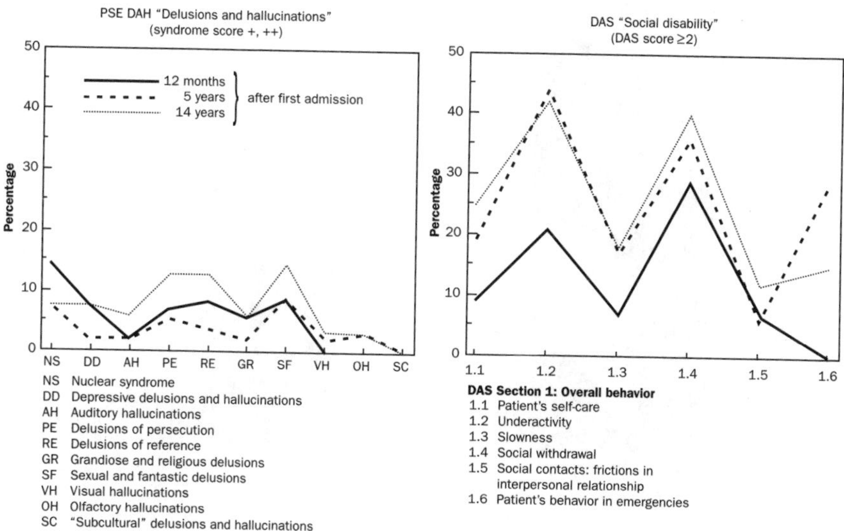

FIGURE 10–17. Positive symptoms and social disability (percentage of conspicuous cases; $n = 56$): WHO Disability Study, Mannheim cohort. + = one of the constituent symptoms clearly present; ++ = at least two symptoms present. *Source.* Reprinted from an der Heiden W, Krumm B, Müller S, et al.: "Mannheimer Langzeitstudie der Schizophrenie." *Nervenarzt* 66:820–827, 1995. Copyright © 1995, Springer-Verlag. Used with permission.

whether these women would have suffered more relapses—and, consequently, a relative increase in poor outcomes—if they discontinued the medication. But this gender difference, too, probably results from illness behavior; that is, women's generally greater cooperativeness and compliance with treatment and their greater concern for health. These factors might motivate the two-thirds of the women to keep on taking the prescribed neuroleptics despite stable remissions, whereas almost all symptom-free men cease taking them.

These relatively good long-term outcomes must be weighed against the patients' actual living situations. To obtain an objective picture, Weber (1996) assessed 48 (30 men and 18 women) of the 63 surviving patients of the Mannheim cohort 15.5 years after first admission (33–58 years of age) and compared them with age- and gender-matched control subjects from the same population of origin. Even after 15 years of perceivably nonprogressive illness, the schizophrenic patients showed

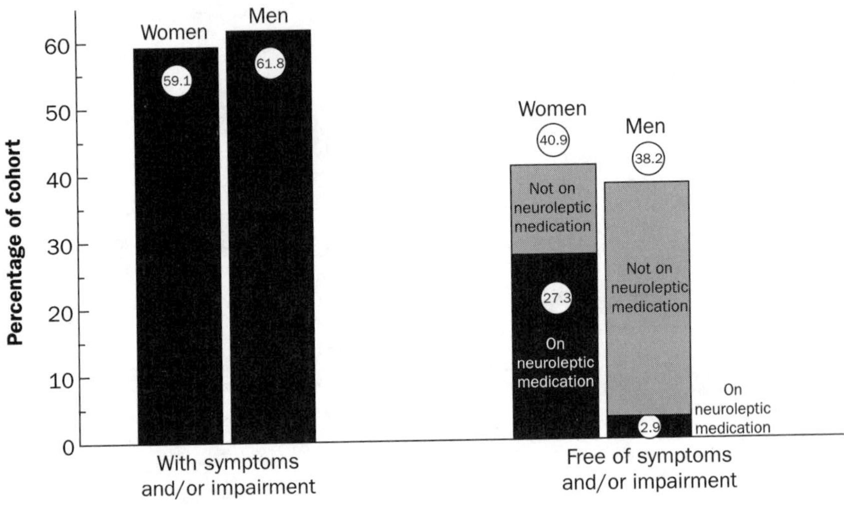

FIGURE 10–18. Symptomatology and impairment 14 years after first admission in two outcome groups, by gender (Fisher exact test: $P < .05$): WHO Disability Study, Mannheim cohort.
Source. Based on data from an der Heiden et al. 1996.

serious deficits in all main domains of life (Table 10–11). The more favorable living situation of women in comparison with men, above all in the domain of marriage or stable partnership, despite a similar symptom-related outcome, is obviously accounted for by women's age-related more favorable social conditions at illness onset and better social adjustment (Table 10–12).

Weber (1996) also assessed cognitive coping with the illness and subjective life satisfaction in this fairly homogeneous cohort by using the FLL (Der Fragebogen zu Lebenszielen und zur Lebenszufriedenheit; Kraak and Nord-Rüdiger 1989), a life goal and satisfaction questionnaire. On the basis of Lehman's (1983a, 1983b) interactional model, Weber assessed subjective importance of life goals, goal achievement, and life-domain-related satisfaction. In the patients studied, there was no correlation between symptom measures and social disability on the one hand and overall life satisfaction on the other (Figure 10–19). However, significant differences emerged between patients and controls: whereas 82% of the control men and 84% of the control women reported a high degree of overall life satisfaction, only 43% of the schizophrenic men and 58% of

TABLE 10–11.

Life-domain outcomes of 48 (30 male, 18 female) subjects with a PSE CATEGO 295 diagnosis of schizophrenia 15.5 years after first admission compared with 48 age- and gender-matched control subjects from the same population of origin: WHO Disability Study, Mannheim cohort

Domain	Schizophrenic subjects (%)	Control subjects (%)
Marital status/partnership		
Never married	52.1	14.6
Married	29.2	66.7
Lives with a spouse/partner	35.4	81.3
Lives in a home	20.8	—
Employment/financial independence		
No occupational training	29.2	10.4
Employed	23.1	83.5
Unemployed	62.5	8.4
Unable to earn own living	73.0	10.5

Note. PSE CATEGO = Present State Examination (PSE) and CATEGO (Wing et al. 1974).
Source. Based on data from Weber 1996.

the schizophrenic women did so. Schizophrenic individuals rated many life goals as only slightly less important than did the healthy controls. For example, to be loved and to maintain stable relationships and self-esteem were almost equally important to both schizophrenic and healthy individuals. However, only schizophrenic men rated sexual relationships and employment as highly as did the healthy controls. Women had significantly reduced their expectations in these life domains, obviously as a means of coping with their diminished capacities. As a consequence, despite having only modest achievements in the life domains of sexual relationships and employment, schizophrenic women were generally more satisfied than schizophrenic men, whose goal achievement and satisfaction with current status differed markedly from their high expectations, and healthy control subjects. Although schizophrenic women obviously adjust their expectations to the changed circumstances in illness, they nonetheless manage to achieve—to a greater extent than schizophrenic

TABLE 10–12.
Living situations of schizophrenic men and women 15.5 years after first admission: WHO Disability Study, Mannheim cohort

	Women (n = 18), %	Men (n = 30), %	P
Mean age, years	45	42	NS
Outcome			
Symptoms or disability present	61	60	NS
Living situation			
Never married	22	70	**
Married	44	20	**
Lives with a spouse/partner	50	23	t
Lives in a home	6	30	t
Own children	53	23	*

Note. $^{t}P \leq .10$; $^{*}P \leq .05$; $^{**}P \leq .01$; NS = not significant.
Source. Based on data from Weber 1996.

men—some highly valued goals in the domain of interpersonal relationships. These factors contribute to the more favorable living situations of schizophrenic women and to their slightly higher life satisfaction despite having illness-related outcomes similar to those of schizophrenic men.

Conclusion

Our systematic investigation of possible gender differences in the antecedents, age at onset, prodromal signs, symptoms, social consequences, and course of schizophrenia over a period of 11 years from onset through 5 years after first admission produced some surprising perspectives. The stringent methodology applied in examining a large population-based first-episode sample was probably the reason why many of the traditionally held opinions—such as a higher lifetime risk and predominance of a chronic type of onset and negative symptoms in men, in contrast with predominance of an acute type of onset and positive symptoms in women—were not supported. None of the proxy variables of the disorder

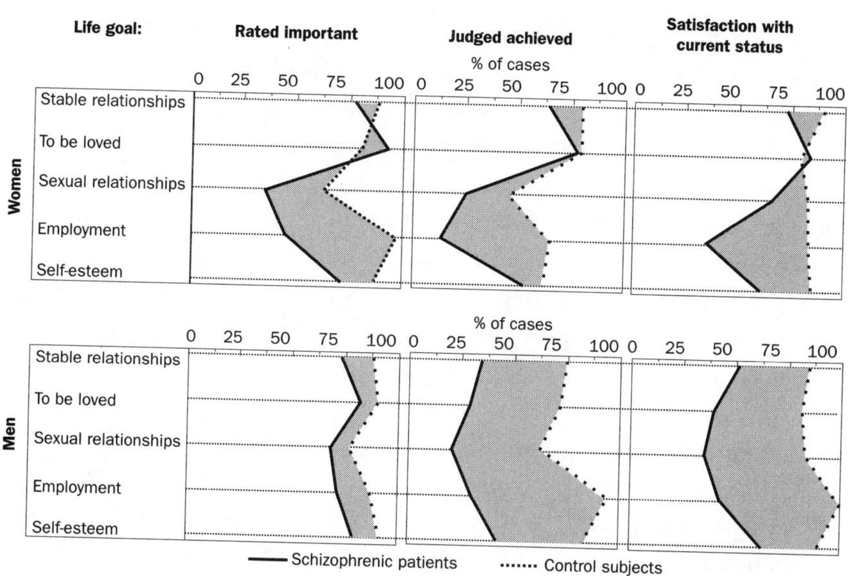

FIGURE 10–19. Life-goal importance, achievement, and satisfaction 15.5 years after first admission in schizophrenic men ($n = 30$) and women ($n = 18$) compared with age- and gender-matched control subjects: WHO Disability Study, Mannheim cohort.
Source. Based on data from Weber 1996.

studied—for example, initial symptoms, type of onset, pattern of early course—yielded significant gender differences. Moreover, a cross-sectional assessment of the first psychotic episode showed no significant gender differences in positive and negative core symptoms, syndromes, subtypes, and diagnostic categories. These findings were in line with the results of a systematic comparative study using a comprehensive neuropsychological test battery (T. E. Goldberg et al. 1995), which likewise failed to find any considerable gender differences. Analysis of the illness course after remission of the first episode yielded stable mean symptom scores without significant gender differences.

The course of schizophrenia, however, was by no means the same in men and women. In this respect, we were able to confirm some of the findings reported in the literature. Factors other than the pathophysiological process of the disorder, which is presumably the same in men and women, seem to be responsible for these gender differences in course.

In addition to the higher age at onset for women reported in many studies (e.g., Angermeyer and Kühn 1988), significant gender differences emerged, especially in social and behavioral variables more distant to the disease process. The causes underlying these gender differences are 1) women's higher age at onset, entailing a higher social status at the onset of the disorder compared with the earlier intrusion of the disorder into men's social biographies; and 2) men's socially negative illness behavior, also to be found in the general population as an expression of age- and gender-specific behavioral patterns, and probably also a reason for their poorer compliance with therapy. Both factors contribute to the less favorable social course of schizophrenia in men.

Given that the illness frequently begins, in both men and women, with signs of functional impairment, and that social disability emerges, on average, long before first admission, it is primarily in the early stages of illness that the social consequences of schizophrenia appear. As a result, there is a risk of confusing the early social course of the disorder with poor premorbid adjustment, the main predictor of course and outcome.

The impact of the gender difference in age at onset on the social course of schizophrenia via the level of social development is reduced by genetic load and eliminated altogether in familial cases (Albus and Maier 1996). Estrogen's delaying effect on the onset of schizophrenia in women depends on the degree of genetic liability: presumably, the lower the patients' genetic load, the more powerful estrogen's protective effect.

Systematic analyses of gender differences are obviously capable of contributing to a better understanding of the processes determining course and outcome in schizophrenia. We are confident that what presents itself as schizophrenia at cross-sectional assessments and over time is the product of an interplay between various causal factors, including genetic load, neurodevelopmental abnormalities (as nonspecific additional risk factors), neuromodulatory influences (e.g., reduced sensitivity of central D_2 receptors due to estrogen), effects delaying the onset of the disorder, age and level of social development at illness onset, and gender- and age-specific behavioral patterns reflected in illness behavior. With this interactional model—which includes multifarious factors—our understanding of schizophrenia has become more complex but also better grounded. It is such a model that might in the future yield interesting hints for targeted therapies and further research into the etiology of the disorder.

References

Achenbach TM: Child Behavior Checklist. Burlington, VT, University of Vermont, 1982

Albus M, Maier W: Lack of gender differences in age at onset in familial schizophrenia. Schizophr Res 18:51–59, 1996

American Psychiatric Association: Diagnostic and Statistical Manual of Mental Disorders, 3rd Edition. Washington, DC, American Psychiatric Association, 1980

American Psychiatric Association: Diagnostic and Statistical Manual of Mental Disorders, 3rd Edition, Revised. Washington, DC, American Psychiatric Association, 1987

an der Heiden W, Krumm B, Müller S, et al: Mannheimer Langzeitstudie der Schizophrenie. Nervenarzt 66:820–827, 1995

an der Heiden W, Krumm B, Müller S, et al: Eine prospektive Studie zum Langzeitverlauf schizophrener Psychosen: Ergebnisse der 14-Jahres-Katamnese. Zeitschrift für Medizinische Psychologie 5:66–75, 1996

Andreasen NC: The Scale for the Assessment of Negative Symptoms (SANS). Iowa City, University of Iowa, 1983

Angermeyer MC, Kühn L: Gender differences in age at onset of schizophrenia: an overview. European Archives of Psychiatry and Neurological Sciences 237:351–364, 1988

Biehl H, Maurer K, Schubart C, et al: Prediction of outcome and utilization of medical services in a prospective study of first onset schizophrenics—results of a prospective 5-year follow-up study. European Archives of Psychiatry and Neurological Sciences 236:139–147, 1986

Biehl H, Maurer K, Jablensky A, et al: The WHO Psychological Impairments Rating Schedule (WHO/PIRS), I: introducing a new instrument for rating observed behaviour and the rationale of the psychological impairment concept. Br J Psychiatry Suppl 155:68–70, 1989

Cannon-Spoor HE, Potkin SG, Wyatt RJ: Measurement of premorbid adjustment in chronic schizophrenia. Schizophr Bull 8:470–484, 1982

Choquet M, Ledoux S: Epidémiologie et adolescence, in Confrontations psychiatriques, vol 27 (no 35). Paris, Rhone-Poulenc rorer specia, 1994, pp 287–309

Crow TJ, MacMillan JF, Johnson AL, et al: A randomised controlled trial of prophylactic neuroleptic treatment. Br J Psychiatry 148:120–127, 1986

Crow TJ, Done DJ, Sacker A: Birth cohort study of the antecedents of psychosis: ontogeny as witness to phylogenetic origins, in Search for the Causes of Schizophrenia, Vol 3. Edited by Häfner H, Gattaz WF. Berlin, Springer-Verlag, 1995, pp 3–20

DeLisi LE, Bass N, Boccio A, et al: Age of onset in familial schizophrenia. Arch Gen Psychiatry 51:334–335, 1994

Di Paolo T, Falardeau P: Modulation of brain and pituitary dopamine receptors by estrogens and prolactin. Prog Neuropsychopharmacol Biol Psychiatry 9:473–480, 1985

Dohrenwend BP, Levav I, Shrout PE, et al: Socioeconomic status and psychiatric disorders: the causation-selection issue. Science 255:946–952, 1992

Done DJ, Crow TJ, Johnstone EC, et al: Childhood antecedents of schizophrenia and affective illness: social adjustment at ages 7 and 11. BMJ 309: 699–703, 1994

Erlenmeyer-Kimling L, Cornblatt BA, Rock D, et al: The New York High-Risk Project: anhedonia, attentional deviance, and psychopathology. Schizophr Bull 19:141–153, 1993

Fields JZ, Gordon JH: Estrogen inhibits the dopaminergic supersensitivity induced by neuroleptics. Life Sci 30:229–234, 1982

Goldberg EM, Morrison SL: Schizophrenia and social class. Br J Psychiatry 109:785–802, 1963

Goldberg TE, Gold JM, Torrey EF, et al: Lack of sex differences in the neuropsychological performance of patients with schizophrenia. Am J Psychiatry 152:883–888, 1995

Gross G, Huber G, Klosterkötter J, et al: Bonner Skala für die Beurteilung von Basissymptomen (BSABS) [Bonn Scale for the Assessment of Basic Symptoms]. Geneva, Switzerland, World Health Organization, 1987

Häfner H: Ist es einzig die Krankheit? in Moderne Konzepte zu Diagnostik, Pathogenese und Therapie. Edited by Möller H-J, Müller N. Wien, Germany, Springer, 1998, pp 37–59

Häfner H, an der Heiden W: Epidemiology of schizophrenia. Can J Psychiatry 42:139–151, 1997

Häfner H, Gattaz WF: Geschlechtsunterschiede bei der Schizophrenie. Der Gynäkologe 28:426–433, 1995

Häfner H, Nowotny B: Epidemiology of early-onset schizophrenia. Eur Arch Psychiatry Clin Neurosci 245:80–92, 1995

Häfner H, Riecher A, Maurer K, et al: Ein Instrument zur retrospektiven Einschätzung des Erkrankungsbeginns bei Schizophrenie [Instrument for the Retrospective Assessment of the Onset of Schizophrenia—IRAOS]. Zeitschrift für Klinische Psychologie 19:230–255, 1990

Häfner H, Behrens S, de Vry J, et al: Oestradiol enhances the vulnerability threshold for schizophrenia in women by an early effect on dopaminergic neurotransmission: evidence from an epidemiological study and from animal experiments. Eur Arch Psychiatry Clin Neurosci 241:65–68, 1991a

Häfner H, Behrens S, de Vry J, et al: Warum erkranken Frauen später an Schizophrenie? Nervenheilkunde 10:154–163, 1991b

Häfner H, Riecher-Rössler A, Hambrecht M, et al: IRAOS: an instrument for the assessment of onset and early course of schizophrenia. Schizophr Res 6:209–223, 1992

Häfner H, Maurer K, Löffler W, et al: The influence of age and sex on the onset and early course of schizophrenia. Br J Psychiatry 162:80–86, 1993

Häfner H, Maurer K, Löffler W, et al: The epidemiology of early schizophrenia: influence of age and gender on onset and early course. Br J Psychiatry Suppl 164:29–38, 1994

Häfner H, Maurer K, Löffler W, et al: Onset and early course of schizophrenia, in Search for the Causes of Schizophrenia, Vol 3. Edited by Häfner H, Gattaz WF. Berlin, Springer-Verlag, 1995a, pp 43–66

Häfner H, Fätkenheuer B, Nowotny B, et al: New perspectives in the epidemiology of schizophrenia. Psychopathology 28 (suppl 1):26–40, 1995b

Häfner H, Maurer K, Löffler W, et al: Der Frühverlauf den Schizophrenie. Zeitschrift für Medizinische Psychologie 5:22–31, 1996

Häfner H, Hambrecht M, Löffler W, et al: Is schizophrenia a disorder of all ages? A comparison of first episodes and early course across the life-cycle. Psychol Med 28:351–365, 1998

Hambrecht M, Maurer K, Sartorius N, et al: Transnational stability of gender differences in schizophrenia? An analysis based on the WHO Study on Determinants of Outcome of Severe Mental Disorders. Eur Arch Psychiatry Clin Neurosci 242:6–12, 1992

Hamilton M: A rating scale for depression. J Neurol Neurosurg Psychiatry 23: 56–62, 1960

Harris MJ, Jeste DV: Late-onset schizophrenia: an overview. Schizophr Bull 14: 39–55, 1988

Harrow M, MacDonald III AW, Sands JR, et al: Vulnerability to delusions over time in schizophrenia and affective disorders. Schizophr Bull 21:95–109, 1996

Honigfeld G, Roderic D, Klett JC: NOSIE-30: a treatment-sensitive ward behavior scale. Psychol Rep 19:180–182, 1966

Hruska RE: Elevation of striatal dopamine receptors by estrogen: dose and time studies. J Neurochem 47:1908–1915, 1986

Jablensky A, Sartorius N, Ernberg G, et al: Schizophrenia: manifestations, incidence and course in different cultures. A World Health Organization ten-country study. Psychol Med Monogr Suppl 20:1–97, 1992

Jones P, Rantakallio P, Hartikainen A-L: Does schizophrenia result from pregnancy delivery and perinatal complications? A 28-year study in the 1966 North Finland birth cohort (abstract). European Psychiatry 11 (suppl 4): 242, 1996

Jung E, Krumm B, Biehl H, et al: DAS-M: Mannheimer Skala zur Einschätzung Sozialer Behinderung. Weinheim, Beltz, 1989

Kraak B, Nord-Rüdiger D: Der Fragebogen zu Lebenszielen und zur Lebenszufriedenheit (FLL). Göttingen, Germany, Hogrefe, 1989

Kraepelin E: Psychiatrie, 8th Edition, Vols 1–4. Leipzig, Barth, 1909–1915

Leboyer M, Filteau M-J, Jay M, et al: No gender effect on age of onset in familial schizophrenia? (letter). Am J Psychiatry 149:1409, 1992

Lehman AF: The well-being of chronic mental patients. Arch Gen Psychiatry 40:369–375, 1983a

Lehman AF: The effects of psychiatric symptoms on quality of life assessments among the chronic mentally ill. Evaluation and Program Planning 6:143–151, 1983b

Lewine RJ: Sex differences in age of symptom onset and first hospitalization in schizophrenia. Am J Orthopsychiatry 50:316–322, 1980

Lewine RRJ: Gender and schizophrenia, in Handbook of Schizophrenia, Vol 3. Edited by Nasrallah HA. Amsterdam, Elsevier, 1988, pp 379–397

Lewis SW, Murray RM: Obstetric complication, neurodevelopmental deviance and schizophrenia. J Psychiatr Res 21:413–421, 1987

Lindelius R: A study of schizophrenia: a clinical, prognostic and family investigation. Acta Psychiatr Scand Suppl 216:1–125, 1970

Loebel AD, Lieberman JA, Alvir JMJ, et al: Duration of psychosis and outcome in first-episode schizophrenia. Am J Psychiatry 149:1183–1188, 1992

Loranger AW: Sex differences in age of onset of schizophrenia. Arch Gen Psychiatry 41:157–161, 1984

Maccoby EE, Jacklin CN: The Psychology of Sex Differences. Stanford, CA, Stanford University Press, 1974

Mason P, Harrison G, Glazebrook C, et al: The course of schizophrenia over 13 years. Br J Psychiatry 169:580–586, 1996

Overall JE, Gorham DR: The Brief Psychiatric Rating Scale. Psychol Rep 10: 799–812, 1962

Parnas J, Cannon TD, Jacobsen B, et al: Lifetime DSM-III-R diagnostic outcomes in offspring of schizophrenic mothers: results from the Copenhagen High-Risk Study. Arch Gen Psychiatry 50:707–714, 1993

Riecher-Rössler A, Häfner H, Dütsch-Strobel A, et al: Further evidence for a specific role of estradiol in schizophrenia? Biol Psychiatry 36:492–495, 1994

Salokangas RKR, Stengard E, Räkköläinen V, et al: New schizophrenic patients and their families (English summary), in Reports of Psychiatria Fennica, No 78. Helsinki, Finland, Foundation for Psychiatric Research in Finland, 1987, pp 119–216

Sartorius N, Gulbinat W, Harrison G, et al: Long-term follow-up of schizophrenia in 16 countries. Soc Psychiatry Psychiatr Epidemiol 31:249–258, 1996

Seeman MV: Gender differences in schizophrenia. Can J Psychiatry 27:107–112, 1982

Seeman MV, Lang M: The role of estrogens in schizophrenia gender differences. Schizophr Bull 16:185–194, 1990

Shepherd M, Watt D, Falloon I, et al: The natural history of schizophrenia: a five-year follow-up study of outcome and prediction in a representative sample of schizophrenics. Psychol Med Monogr Suppl 15:1–46, 1989

Stott DH: The Social Adjustment of Children: Manual to the Bristol Social Adjustment Guide. London, Holder & Stoughton, 1987

Sumner BEH, Fink G: Oestradiol-17β in its positive feedback mode significantly increases 5-HT_{2A} receptor density in the frontal, cingulate and piriform cortex of the female rat. J Physiol (Lond) 483:52, 1995

van Os JJ: Evidence for similar developmental precursors of chronic affective illness and schizophrenia in a general population birth cohort. Poster presented at the 8th Congress of the Association of European Psychiatrists ("European Psychiatry—A Force for the Future"), London, July 7–12, 1996

von Zerssen D, Koeller DM: Klinische Selbstbeurteilungs-Skalen (KSb-Si) aus dem Münchener Psychiatrischen Informations-System (PSYCHIS München) (Manual). Weinheim, Germany, Belz, 1976

Walker EF, Weinstein J, Baum K, et al: Antecedents of schizophrenia: moderating effects of development and biological sex, in Search for the Causes of Schizophrenia, Vol 3. Edited by Häfner H, Gattaz WF. Berlin, Springer-Verlag, 1995, pp 21–42

Watt NF, Grubb TW, Erlenmeyer-Kimling L: Social, emotional, and intellectual behavior at school among children at high risk for schizophrenia, in Children at High Risk for Schizophrenia. Edited by Watt NF, Anthony J, Wynne LC, et al. London, Cambridge University Press, 1984, pp 212–226

Weber J: Die Lebenszufriedenheit einer Kohorte Schizophrener 15,5 Jahre nach stationärer Erstaufnahme (doctoral thesis). Mannheim, Germany, Faculty of Clinical Medicine, University of Heidelberg, 1996

Wiersma D, Nienhuis FJ, Giel R, et al: Assessment of the need for care 15 years after onset of a Dutch cohort of patients with schizophrenia, and an international comparison. Soc Psychiatry Psychiatr Epidemiol 31:114–121, 1996

Wing JK, Cooper JE, Sartorius N: Measurement and Classification of Psychiatric Symptoms: An Instruction Manual for the PSE and CATEGO Program. London, Cambridge University Press, 1974

Woolley CS, McEwen BS: Estradiol regulates hippocampal dendritic spine density via an N-methyl-D-aspartate receptor–dependent mechanism. J Neurosci 14:7680–7687, 1994

World Health Organization: Past History and Sociodemographic Description Schedule (PHSD), 3rd Draft. Geneva, Switzerland, World Health Organization, June 1977

World Health Organization: Mental Disorders: Glossary and Guide to Their Classification in Accordance With the Ninth Revision of the International Classification of Diseases. Geneva, Switzerland, World Health Organization, 1978a

World Health Organization: Psychiatric and Personal History Schedule (PPHS). WHO 5365 MNH (70/78). Geneva, Switzerland, World Health Organization, 1978b

World Health Organization: Psychiatric Disability Assessment Schedule (WHO/DAS). Geneva, Switzerland, World Health Organization, 1988

SECTION IV

Substance Abuse and Dependence

CHAPTER 11

Gender Differences in the Epidemiology of Substance Dependence in the United States

Denise B. Kandel, Ph.D.

The epidemiology of drug use in the general population includes two distinct streams of research. The much more common stream measures consumption patterns in the population by asking individuals whether they have ever used drugs, and, if so, how frequently they have used them. The second stream, and one implemented much more rarely, measures the extent of problematic drug use by asking individuals about behaviors and symptoms that meet criteria for a substance use disorder. Progress in our understanding of the development of substance use and dependence and of problems related to substance use will come about only when these different research traditions are brought more closely together. These two perspectives are rarely combined in the same study.

This chapter is based on data from Kandel et al. (1997) and from Chen et al. (1997). The material in this chapter was previously presented at the Symposium on Patterns of Prevalence, Symptom Presentation, and Course, American Psychopathological Association, February 27, 1997.

This research is supported by research grant DA09110 and by a Research Scientist Award (DA00081) from the National Institute on Drug Abuse.

The author wishes to acknowledge the contributions of Kevin Chen, Mark Davies, Bridget Grant, Ronald Kessler, Lynn Warner, and Christine Schaffran to the research.

Important exceptions include the work of Ronald Kessler (Kessler et al. 1994; Warner et al. 1995) and Naomi Breslau (Breslau et al. 1994).

To date, the most extensive national data on substance use disorders are provided by three surveys: the Epidemiological Catchment Area (ECA) Study (Robins and Regier 1991) carried out in the early 1980s, the National Comorbidity Survey (NCS) implemented in 1990–1992 (Kessler et al. 1994; Warner et al. 1995), and the National Longitudinal Alcohol Epidemiologic Survey (NLAES) conducted in 1992 (Grant et al. 1994).

From a comparative and life-span perspective, existing epidemiological surveys of substance use disorders have two important limitations. No data are available for adolescents in comparison with older age groups, because most existing surveys have sampled persons 18 years of age and older. Although the NCS participants ranged in age from 15 to 54 years, findings have been reported for those aged 15–24 years as a group; there were too few respondents 15–17 years old to provide reliable estimates for those ages. In addition, in existing surveys, limited data are provided for nicotine dependence, the most common substance use disorder. In the ECA Study, questions about nicotine dependence were included in only two sites, and only very limited epidemiological results have been reported (Covey et al. 1994; Robins et al. 1986). In the NCS, supplemental funding from the National Institute of Mental Health (NIMH) allowed questions on tobacco use and nicotine dependence to be added to the interview. Although the questions were added after the survey had already been initiated and were not as detailed as those for the other substances, nationally representative estimates of cigarette use and dependence could be generated from the reported findings (Anthony et al. 1994). Nicotine dependence was not assessed in the NLAES.

In this chapter I present data from ongoing research on the epidemiology and phenomenology of substance use disorders from comparative and life-span perspectives. This research is based on data from the National Household Survey on Drug Abuse (NHSDA; National Institute on Drug Abuse 1991; Substance Abuse and Mental Health Services Administration 1993, 1994). Although this data set has many limitations, it also has certain advantages not provided by any other study.

I will deal with four issues:

- What is the prevalence of dependence on the following four substances: 1) nicotine or cigarettes, 2) alcohol, 3) marijuana, and

4) cocaine? (I use the terms *nicotine* and *cigarettes* interchangeably here.)

- How does the prevalence of dependence on these four substances vary by age and by gender?
- What is the relationship between intensity of substance use, indexed by quantity/frequency measures, and diagnostic criteria of dependence?
- What aspects of substance consumption account for gender- and age-specific differences in rates of dependence?

The National Household Survey on Drug Abuse: Marijuana Dependence

The NHSDA is a national annual survey of drug use patterns in the general population aged 12 years and over. It constitutes an important, and mostly unused, source of data for assessing the epidemiology of drug dependence in the United States among adolescents and adults.

Sample

The present analyses are based on three aggregated surveys (1991, 1992, and 1993) totaling 87,915 respondents, including more than 22,000 adolescents. The universe for the NHSDA sample is the civilian noninstitutionalized U.S. population, which represents more than 98% of the country's total population. Persons living in noninstitutional group quarters, such as homeless shelters, rooming houses, and college dormitories, are included as well. Young persons (12–34 years old) and minorities are oversampled. Completion rates in 1991 through 1993 were 79% or above. For more details about these surveys, see National Institute on Drug Abuse (1991) and Substance Abuse and Mental Health Services Administration (1993, 1994).

Methods of Data Collection

The data were collected through anonymous personal structured household interviews, each approximately 1 hour long. The schedule included separate self-administered modules about patterns of use (e.g., lifetime, last-year, and last-month frequency of use; quantities used) for 12 classes of drugs, including cigarettes. A separate module asked whether respondents had experienced each of six symptoms of dependence in the last year with respect to each drug class. Another module asked about having experienced problems related to the use of specific drugs in the last year. No information on lifetime symptoms of dependence or drug-related problems was available.

Definition of Substance Dependence

The questions on drug-related symptoms of dependence and drug-related problems experienced within the last year were used to develop approximate measures of DSM-IV (American Psychiatric Association 1994) diagnostic criteria for substance use disorders involving nicotine, alcohol, marijuana, or cocaine. The analyses focused mainly on dependence, because that concept is more clearly conceptualized in the DSM nosology and is better measured than abuse.

DSM-IV defines seven diagnostic criteria and associated symptoms related to substance dependence. An individual must have met three of these seven criteria at any time in the last 12 months in order to be diagnosed with a current psychoactive substance dependence disorder. NHSDA items that approximated the seven DSM-IV criteria were identified. Table 11–1 lists the DSM-IV criteria and the corresponding NHSDA measures. An individual was defined as being dependent on cigarettes, alcohol, marijuana, or cocaine within the last year if he or she met three of the seven approximate indicators for DSM-IV diagnostic criteria from the items listed in Table 11–1. The identification of dependence (and abuse) allowed by the NHSDA cannot be as systematic as that based on structured schedules developed specifically to measure psychiatric disorders—for example, the Diagnostic Interview Schedule (DIS; Robins et al. 1981), the Composite International Diagnostic Interview (CIDI; World Health Organization 1990), or the Alcohol Use Disorder and Associated Disabilities Interview Schedule (AUDADIS; Grant et al. 1995). The NHSDA measure is a proxy measure of dependence. However, the NHSDA makes possible certain assessments and comparisons not possible in other data sets. These include the assessment of dependence (and abuse) on nicotine and other substances as well as the assessment of dependence among different demographic groups in the

TABLE 11–1.

Comparison of DSM-IV criteria for substance dependence and corresponding questions in the National Household Survey on Drug Abuse (NHSDA)

DSM-IV criteria	NHSDA questions
(1) tolerance, as defined by either of the following: (a) a need for markedly increased amount of the substance to achieve intoxication or desired effect (b) markedly diminished effect with continued use of the same amount of the substance	DR-3. *During the past 12 months,* for which drugs have you *needed larger amounts to get the same effect;* that is, for which drugs could you no longer get high on the same amount you used to use?
(2) withdrawal, as defined by either of the following: (a) the characteristic withdrawal syndrome for the substance (b) the same (or a closely related) substance is taken to relieve or avoid withdrawal symptoms	DR-6. For which drugs have you had withdrawal symptoms; that is, you *felt sick because you stopped or cut down* on your use of them *during the past 12 months?*
(3) the substance is often taken in larger amounts or over a longer period than was intended	DR-5. Which drugs have you *felt that you needed* or were dependent on *in the past 12 months?*
(4) there is a persistent desire or unsuccessful efforts to cut down or control substance use	DR-1. *During the past 12 months,* for which drugs have you consciously *tried to cut down* on your use?
	DR-2. *During the past 12 months,* for which drugs have you *been unable to cut down* on your use, even though you tried?

(continued)

TABLE 11–1. *(continued)*

Comparison of DSM-IV criteria for substance dependence and corresponding questions in the National Household Survey on Drug Abuse (NHSDA)

DSM-IV criteria	NHSDA questions
(5) a great deal of time is spent in activities necessary to obtain the substance (e.g., visiting multiple doctors or driving long distances), use the substance (e.g., chain smoking), or recover from its effects	Drug-specific pattern of heavy use as follows: • Tobacco: smoking 2+ packs daily in the past 30 days • Alcohol: drinking 5+ drinks a day for 15+ days in the past 30 days; or "gotten very high or drunk" near daily (3+ days a week) in the past 12 months • Marijuana: used 3+ joints near daily (3+ times a week) in the past 30 days; or 2+ ounces (86+ joints or 43+ grams) in the past 30 days; or traded services for marijuana • Cocaine: about 2+ grams (37+ big lines of powder) used in the past 30 days, or traded services for cocaine/crack
(6) important social, occupational, or recreational activities are given up or reduced because of substance use	DP-1. As a result of drug use at any time in your life, did you, in the past 12 months . . . (h) get less work done than usual at school or on the job?

(continued)

TABLE 11–1. *(continued)*

Comparison of DSM-IV criteria for substance dependence and corresponding questions in the National Household Survey on Drug Abuse (NHSDA)

DSM-IV criteria	NHSDA questions
(7) the substance use is continued despite knowledge of having a persistent or recurrent physical or psychological problem that is likely to have been caused or exacerbated by the substance (e.g., current cocaine use despite recognition of cocaine-induced depression, or continued drinking despite recognition that an ulcer was made worse by alcohol consumption)	DP-1. As a result of drug use at any time in your life, did you, in the past 12 months . . . (a) Become depressed or lose interest in things? (b) Have arguments/fights with family and friends? (c) Feel completely alone and isolated? (d) Feel very nervous and anxious? (e) Have health problems? (f) Find it difficult to think clearly? (g) Feel irritable and upset? (i) Feel suspicious and distrustful of people? (j) Find it harder to handle your problems? (k) Have to get emergency medical help? (l) Have someone suggest you seek treatment?[a] Respondent had any one of the 11 problems listed.

Note. DSM-IV = Diagnostic and Statistical Manual of Mental Disorders, 4th Edition (American Psychiatric Association 1994); NHSDA = National Household Survey on Drug Abuse. [a]Not asked in 1991 NHSDA. An additional problem in the NHSDA (1992–1993) list, "Drive unsafely," is a DSM-IV abuse but not a dependence criterion.

population—in particular, age, gender, and ethnic groups. These subgroup assessments are possible because of the sample characteristics—namely, its large size and the oversampling of minorities and of individuals aged 12–34 years (i.e., the populations at highest risk for drug use)—and because the same methodology has been used to assess substance use dependence and abuse at all ages and for all substances. Thus, adolescents can be compared with adults. Although age, gender, and ethnic differences in rates of drug use in the population 12 years old and over, and in rates of substance use disorders among adults, have been well described, corresponding rates for dependence on nicotine and other drugs based on identical criteria and for these three demographic correlates concurrently remain to be documented.

Rates of Substance Dependence in Adolescence and Adulthood

Prevalence rates of last-year dependence were examined both for the total sample and as a function of age and gender. The rates were examined *conditional on use* rather than in the total population in order to avoid confounding drug-specific liability for dependence with baseline rates of experimentation with each specific drug.

To provide a broad overview of the relative rates of dependence on different drug classes, I first present the rates for the total sample for the four drug classes, without differentiation as to demographic characteristics (Figure 11–1). The right panel of Figure 11–1 displays the conditional rates of dependence on each drug among users of each drug class in the total population 12 years of age and older; the left panel displays the overall rates of use of each drug class in the last 12 months in the same historical period in the total population.

Two trends are readily apparent. First, of the four drugs, cigarettes are associated with the highest rate of dependence, and alcohol with the lowest. Of the individuals who have smoked in the past year, 28% meet criteria for dependence on nicotine. The next highest percentages are observed for marijuana and for cocaine. More than twice as many last-year users are dependent on nicotine (28%) as on cocaine (12%); 5% are dependent on alcohol. Second, the rank order of prevalence of current dependence among the users of each drug class does not follow the rank order of prevalence of the use of these drugs. Although the highest rates of use within the last year are observed for alcohol, the highest rates of dependence given use are observed for cigarettes. Nicotine is clearly the most addictive of the psychoactive substances with which people experiment.

There are important gender- and age-specific differences in these trends.

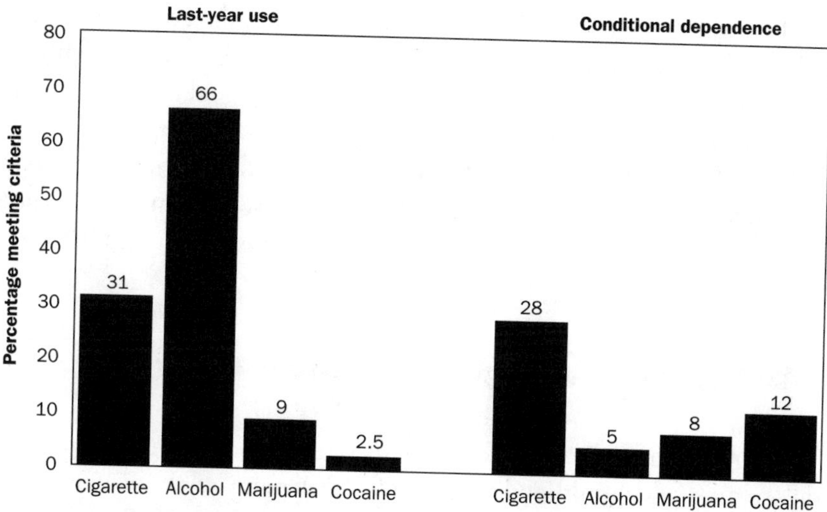

FIGURE 11–1. Prevalence of last-year use and conditional dependence of cigarettes, alcohol, marijuana, and cocaine among last-year users ages 12 years and older: National Household Survey on Drug Abuse (NHSDA), 1991–1993 (N = 9,284).

Differences by Gender

Overall, more male than female last-year users are dependent on alcohol and marijuana, whereas slightly more female than male last-year users are dependent on nicotine and cocaine, the two stimulant drugs (Table 11–2). With the exception of cocaine, all of the gender differences are statistically significant.

Among males, the conditional rate of last-year dependence for nicotine is four times higher than that for alcohol, three times higher than that for marijuana, and more than twice as high as that for cocaine. Among females, the rate of last-year dependence for nicotine is eight times higher than that for alcohol, more than four times higher than that for marijuana, and two times higher than that for cocaine.

Differences by Age

There are striking age differences in the rates of dependence for different drug classes (Table 11–2). In adulthood, a higher proportion of users are dependent on cocaine than on marijuana; in adolescence, there is a slight trend in the opposite direction. For cigarettes, the conditional rates of dependence are higher in adulthood than in adolescence. In contrast, for alcohol and especially for marijuana, the conditional rates of dependence are higher in adolescence than in adulthood. There are no age-related differences for cocaine. The differences across drug categories are accentuated among adults compared with adolescents. In adolescence the ratio between the lowest and the highest rate is 4, whereas in adulthood it is 6.

Differences by Age and Gender

Important gender-related differences in rates of dependence appear in adolescence and adulthood (Table 11–2). Among adolescent users, a somewhat higher proportion of females than of males are dependent on marijuana, although this difference is not statistically significant. More than three times as many adolescent females as adolescent males are dependent on cocaine, a highly statistically significant difference. Among adult users, the rates of dependence are higher in males than in females for alcohol and especially for marijuana but are only very slightly higher in females versus males for cigarettes and cocaine. Almost twice as many male as female adult marijuana users meet criteria for last-year dependence; this difference is highly statistically significant.

Given use of certain drug classes, males and females appear to be differentially susceptible to dependence. Furthermore, with the exception of cigarettes, the pattern of gender differences varies with age. Here I focus on one drug, marijuana, because it provides a particularly vivid illustration of age and gender differences in rates of dependence.

Relationship Between Intensity of Use and Dependence

The question of interest is why different gender and age groups experience differential liability to drug dependence. For instance, why do adolescents, and especially females, become more dependent on marijuana than do adults? Why do adult males become more dependent than adult females? Differences in extensiveness of use and in the relationships be-

TABLE 11–2.

Conditional prevalence of proxy measure of last-year dependence on alcohol, cigarette, marijuana, and cocaine in the United States among last-year users, by gender and age: National Household Survey on Drug Abuse (NHSDA), 1991–1993***[a]

	Alcohol, *n* (%) [SE]			Cigarettes, *n* (%) [SE]			Marijuana, *n* (%) [SE]			Cocaine, *n* (%) [SE]		
	Total	Male	Female	Total	Male	Female	Total	Male	Female	Total	Male	Female
Total sample	54,998 (5.2) [0.2]	26,226 (6.7) [0.3]	28,772 (3.6) [0.2]***[b]	28,392 (28.0) [0.7]	13,894 (26.5) [0.9]	14,498 (29.5) [1.0]*[b]	11,273 (8.2) [0.5]	6,408 (9.3) [0.6]	4,865 (6.4) [0.6]***[b]	3,410 (11.6) [1.0]	2,042 (10.6) [1.2]	1,368 (13.6) [1.5]
Ages 12–17 years	7,510 (8.1) [0.6]	3,879 (7.5) [0.7]	3,631 (8.7) [0.8]	3,509 (19.9) [1.1]	1,801 (20.8) [1.6]	1,708 (18.9) [1.5]	2,092 (14.4) [1.4]	1,154 (13.3) [1.8]	938 (15.8) [2.1]	321 (11.3) [3.0]	161 (4.7) [1.8]	160 (17.5) [5.1]*[b]
Ages 18+ years	47,488 (5.0) [0.2]	22,347 (6.6) [0.3]	25,141 (3.3) [0.2]***[b]	24,883 (28.5) [0.7]	12,093 (26.9) [0.9]	12,790 (30.2) [1.0]**[b]	9,181 (7.4) [0.5]	5,254 (8.9) [0.7]	3,927 (5.1) [0.6]***[b]	3,089 (11.6) [1.0]	1,881 (10.8) [1.3]	1,208 (13.3) [1.6]
χ^2 age difference[c]	***	NS	***	***	***	***	***	*	***	NS	**	NS

[a]Prevalence and standard errors were estimated on weighted sample, with correction of sampling design effects by SUDAAN (Shah et al. 1997).
[b]Gender differences were tested by chi-square; [c]Age differences were tested by chi-square.
*$P < .05$; **$P < .01$; ***$P < .001$; NS = not significant.

tween frequency and quantity of use and dependence may explain the different rates of dependence observed among subgroups of users of different drug classes.

With the exception of alcohol, there is very little epidemiological research in the field that integrates information on patterns of drug use (e.g., frequency and quantity) with information on substance use disorders. My colleagues and I (Chen et al. 1997) conducted analyses to examine the relationship between marijuana use and dependence at different levels of frequency and quantity of use by gender and by age. Adolescent males (but not females) use marijuana at a lower frequency than do adult males and females. In adolescence, males and females use the drug at similar frequency levels; in adulthood, men consistently use marijuana more frequently and more extensively than do women (Table 11–3). The gender difference in rates of marijuana use among adolescents, which is not statistically significant at the univariate level, becomes significant when intensity of use is controlled.

As expected, there is a strong relationship between extent of marijuana use and dependence. Figure 11–2 displays the relationship between frequency of use and 12-month dependence by gender separately for adolescents and adults. With few exceptions, the results for quantity used are similar to those obtained for frequency (Figure 11–3). In these analyses, we excluded extensiveness of use from the definition of dependence so as not to confound the two variables being correlated. The definition for dependence was changed from three of seven criteria to three of six criteria. The higher the frequency and quantity of use, the higher the rates of dependence. The association is stronger for adolescents than for adults and for adolescent females than for adolescent males, although a slight reversal of this pattern occurs in adulthood.

As an explanation for group-specific rates of dependence, intensity of marijuana use (indexed by frequency and/or quantity of use) could be important in several ways.

Groups that have *higher* rates of dependence . . .

1. may be using marijuana more heavily, or
2. may be more sensitive to the effects of marijuana at the same intensity of use, or
3. may be using marijuana more heavily *and* be more sensitive to the effects of marijuana at the same intensity of use.

TABLE 11–3.

Distribution of frequency and quantity of marijuana use in last year and quantity of use in last 30 days among last-year users by gender and age: National Household Survey on Drug Abuse (NHSDA), 1991–1993 (N = 9,284[a])

	Adolescents (12–17 years), %			Adults (18+ years), %		
	Total (N = 1,779)	Males (*n* = 990)	Females (*n* = 789)	Total (N = 7,505)	Males (*n* = 4,369)	Females (*n* = 3,136)
Frequency of use last year						
1–2 times	27.9	26.5	29.7	21.8	19.0	26.6
3–5 times	13.6	13.0	14.4	14.7	13.1	17.4
6–11 times	9.1	8.9	9.4	10.8	9.4	13.0
1–2 times per month	13.1	14.4	11.4	12.3	13.4	10.5
Several times per month	9.2	8.1	10.7	9.3	9.8	8.4
1–2 times a week	10.9	10.8	11.0	11.9	13.4	9.5
Almost daily	7.9	8.8	6.7	10.7	12.8	7.2
Daily	8.3	9.6	6.6	8.5	9.1	7.4
χ^2 (gender difference) (*df* = 7)		9.2			198.7***	
χ^2 (age difference) (*df* = 7)		Total = 26.1***		Male = 26.4***		Female = 11.5

(continued)

TABLE 11–3. *(continued)*

Distribution of frequency and quantity of marijuana use in last year and quantity of use in last 30 days among last-year users by gender and age: National Household Survey on Drug Abuse (NHSDA), 1991–1993 (N = 9,284[a])

	Adolescents (12–17 years), %			Adults (18+ years), %		
	Total (N = 1,779)	Males (*n* = 990)	Females (*n* = 789)	Total (N = 7,505)	Males (*n* = 4,369)	Females (*n* = 3,136)
Average amount used per day in last 30 days						
No use	54.6	53.8	55.6	46.3	42.5	52.6
Up to 1 joint	20.8	20.9	20.8	29.1	29.7	28.1
2 joints	10.7	10.4	11.1	12.0	14.0	8.8
3 joints	5.0	4.5	5.8	5.8	6.3	5.1
4+ joints	8.8	10.4	6.7	6.7	7.4	5.5
χ^2 (gender difference) ($df = 4$)		4.7			94.1^{***}	
χ^2 (age difference) ($df = 4$)		Total = 39.7^{***}		Male = 39.2^{***}		Female = 11.1^{*}

[a]Unweighted N, excluding those missing last-year frequency of use; weighted rates.
$^{*}P < .05$; $^{**}P < .01$; $^{***}P < .001$.

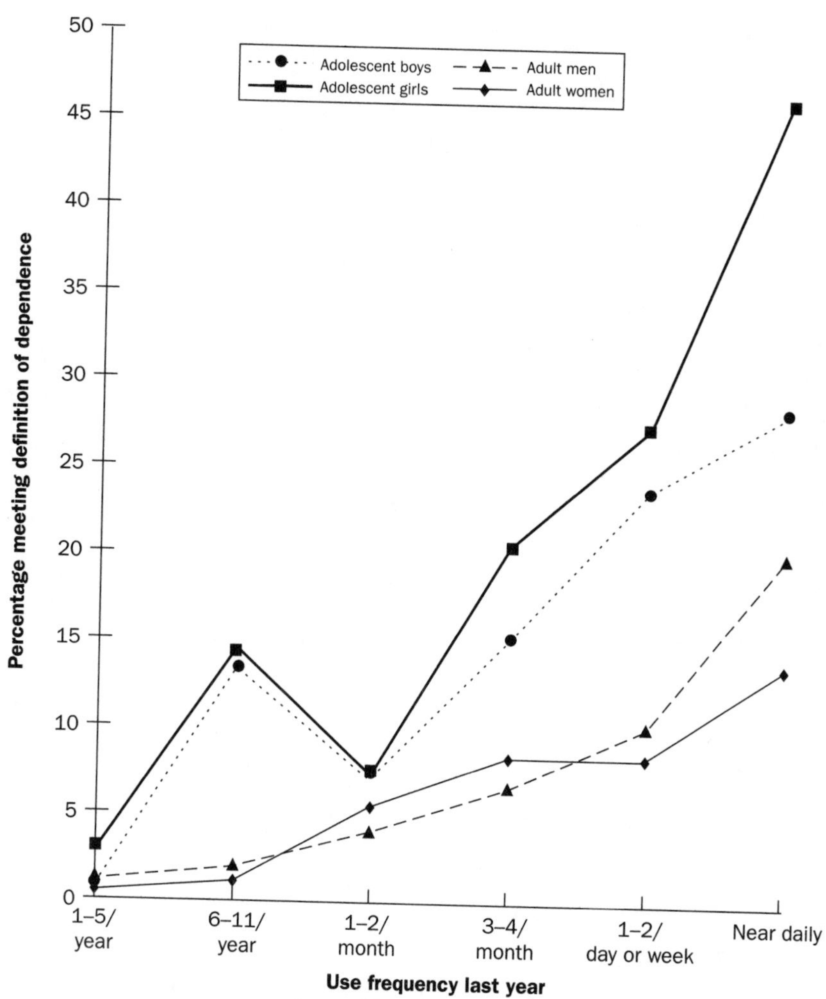

FIGURE 11–2. Relationship between last-year frequency of marijuana use and 12-month dependence among adolescent and adult last-year users, by gender: National Household Survey on Drug Abuse (NHSDA), 1991–1993 ($N = 9{,}284$).

Groups that have *similar* rates of dependence . . .

4. may be using marijuana at different levels of intensity but be differentially responsive to similar doses (different groups may experience different liability to dependence at the same levels of use).

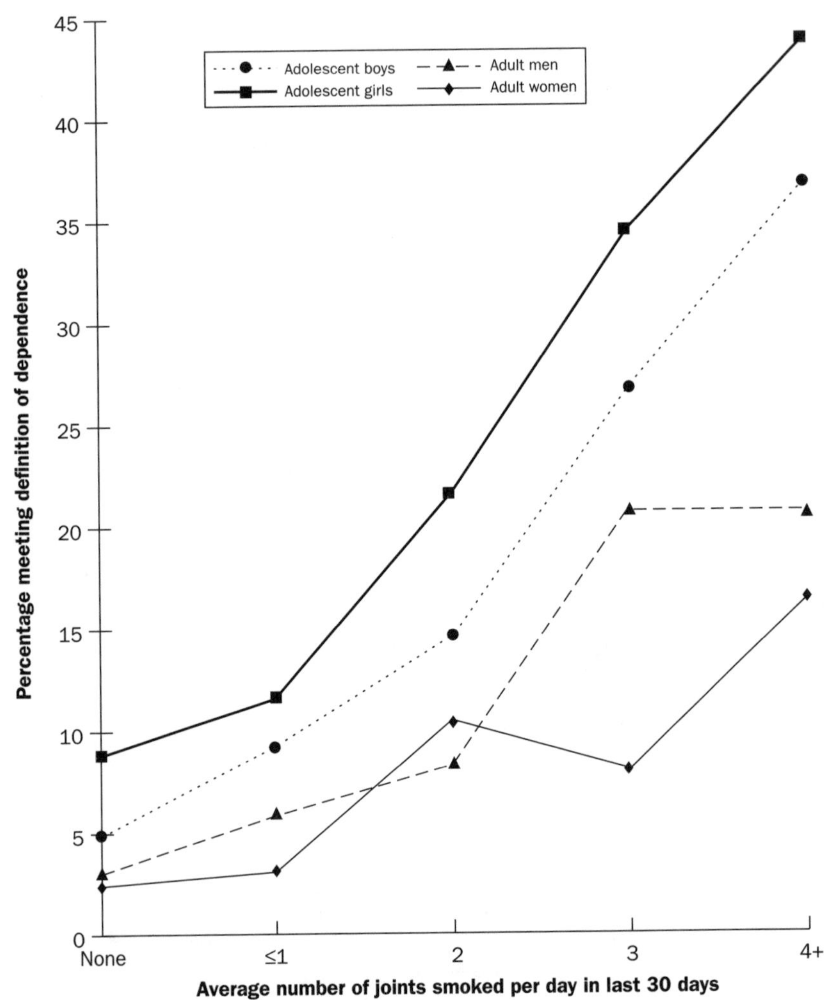

FIGURE 11–3. Relationship between quantity of marijuana used per day in last 30 days and last-year dependence among adolescent and adult last-year users, by gender: National Household Survey on Drug Abuse (NHSDA), 1991–1993 (N = 9,284).

We conducted a formal test of these hypotheses to explain the gender- and age-related differences observed in conditional rates of marijuana dependence. As previously noted, adolescents have higher rates of dependence than do adults; among adolescent marijuana users, females are slightly more likely than males to be dependent; among adult users, males are significantly more likely than females to be dependent. We estimated separate hierarchical logistic regressions predicting dependence from frequency of marijuana use (or quantity used) for adolescents and adults together to permit a systematic test of the age and gender effects of frequency (and quantity) of marijuana use on dependence. The models included gender, age, and all two-way and three-way interactions between age, gender, and frequency (or quantity) of use. The only significant interaction was the age-by-gender interaction. Results for frequency of use are presented in Table 11–4.

These regressions provide two parameters of interest for our purposes: a slope and an intercept for each group. The slope indexes the rate of response (i.e., dependence) to increasing levels of use. The intercept indexes (in part) the response threshold to the drug. A high intercept reflects a low threshold—that is, a high proportion of persons dependent at low doses. By contrast, a low intercept reflects a high threshold—that is, a low proportion of persons dependent at low doses. We used statistical tests (i.e., *z* tests of the differences) to compare the regression coefficients from these logit models across groups to determine whether variations in

TABLE 11–4.

Logistic regressions of last-year marijuana dependence on frequency and quantity of use among last-year users, by gender and age[a]: National Household Survey on Drug Abuse (NHSDA), 1991–1993

	Use level indexed by frequency of use[a]		Use level indexed by quantity of use	
	Beta	SE	Beta	SE
Level of use	.64***	(.05)	.55***	(.05)
Gender (male vs. female)	–.49[t]	(.26)	–.43[t]	(.26)
Age (adults vs. adolescents)	–1.44***	(.23)	–1.35***	(.24)
Gender × Age	.78*	(.31)	.81**	(.23)
(Intercept)	–3.82***	(.24)	–2.41***	(.21)

Note. Coefficients and standard errors were estimated on weighted sample with correction of complex sample design effects by SUDAAN (Shah et al. 1997). [a]Frequency of use is coded as the log of the midpoint in terms of numbers of days used in last year. [t]$P < .10$; *$P < .05$; **$P < .01$; ***$P < .001$.

rates between any two groups were due to differences in thresholds of response to the drug (indexed by the intercept), differences in the rate of response to increasing levels of use (indexed by the slope), or both. Different intercepts would indicate that groups have different threshold responses to marijuana and that the levels at which dependence develops are different. A *high* intercept would indicate that a group has a *low* threshold, because a higher proportion of individuals become dependent at a low dose of marijuana. A *low* intercept would indicate a *high* threshold. Different slopes would indicate that the associations between frequency (or quantity) of use and marijuana dependence differ.

Four pairs of groups were compared: 1) among females, adolescents versus adults; 2) among males, adolescents versus adults; 3) among adolescents, males versus females; 4) among adults, males versus females. Similar processes hold for frequency and quantity of use.

We found that frequency (and quantity) of marijuana use was linearly associated with the probability of becoming dependent on marijuana in every group. As reflected in the slopes, the associations did not vary significantly by age or by gender in adolescents or adults. However, as reflected in the higher intercepts for adolescents compared with adults, adolescents of both genders become dependent at a lower threshold of frequency than do adults. At low intensity of use, a higher proportion of adolescents than of adults become dependent. Similarly, adult males become dependent at a lower threshold than do adult females. An opposite gender difference obtains in adolescence: adolescent males become dependent at a higher threshold than do females—that is, they have a lower rate of dependence than do females at low frequency of use.

These results provide insight into the processes underlying the age and gender differentials observed in the prevalence of marijuana dependence. Once having used marijuana, adolescents—and especially female adolescents—appear to experience higher rates of dependence than do adults, although not because they use marijuana more frequently than adults. In fact, adolescent males use marijuana less frequently than do adult males. Adolescents experience higher rates of dependence than adults because they appear to be more sensitive than adults to the effects of marijuana: at low intensity of use, adolescents become more dependent than adults. Given increasing intensity of use, the relative rate of increase is the same irrespective of age. However, at the same levels of frequency (or quantity) of use, adolescents experience higher rates of dependence than do adults because the threshold at which they first become dependent is lower than that for adults.

Adolescent males experience lower rates of dependence than do adolescent females because they appear to be less sensitive to the drug and become dependent at a higher frequency of use. Adolescent males and females use marijuana at the same frequency. However, in addition to a difference in threshold, frequency of use becomes important in accounting for gender differences in adulthood. Adult males experience higher rates of dependence than do adult females because they are more likely than adult females to become dependent at low levels of marijuana use, and also because they use marijuana more frequently than do females.

Conclusion

In this chapter I have highlighted several issues related to gender and age differences in the epidemiology of substance use disorders. In adolescence, the rates of dependence in females are the same as, or even slightly higher than, those in males, although this difference is statistically significant only with respect to cocaine. In adulthood, the rates are higher for males than for females for alcohol and marijuana but are essentially the same for the other two drug classes. A particularly intriguing difference is a greater liability to selected substance dependence disorders among adolescent females than among adolescent males.

A better understanding of gender and age differences in substance use and addictive behavior can only come from a multidisciplinary approach in which biological, physiological, and sociological factors are taken into account. Comprehensive studies of this kind must include the collection of longitudinal epidemiological data. Such data not only generate insights that can be applied to clinical settings but also advance our research agenda by suggesting hypotheses regarding the connection between drug use patterns and their proximal and distal etiologies and consequences.

The results of our analyses provide some understanding of the specific patterns of drug use that underlie problematic use and the need for treatment in the general population. These findings also shed some light on the factors that account for differences in rates of drug dependence observed among different demographic groups—in particular, between adolescents and adults and between males and females in adolescence and adulthood.

It is important to keep in mind that the conclusions of the study are affected by limitations in the measurement of marijuana dependence. Furthermore, the DSM criteria were developed for adults and, to the best of my knowledge, have not been validated for adolescents. The finding that adolescents are more likely than adults to be dependent on marijuana may be due to differential validity of the assessment of dependence symptoms in adolescents versus adults. Adolescents may be more likely than adults to assess their symptoms incorrectly or to attribute social and psychological problems to their drug use. However, the proxy measure used in this study showed internal validity. Indeed, compared with users who do not meet dependence criteria, a much higher proportion of those who do meet such criteria report having been in treatment for a drug problem within the last year (3.6% versus 15.8%). This proportion is even slightly higher among adolescents than among adults, although the difference is not statistically significant. Thus, the measure of dependence appears to identify individuals with drug-related problems among both adolescents and adults. The relationship between dependence and treatment experience obtains irrespective of the frequency of use, although at low frequency it is weaker. These findings need to be replicated with better measurement of the dependence criteria.

Besides their implications for policy, the results underscore the mutual relevance of epidemiology and biology for understanding addiction. In particular, the research illustrates how epidemiological studies generate hypotheses to be tested in the laboratory. The findings on gender and age differences in the relationships between extent of marijuana use and dependence illustrate how epidemiological data provide new insights and may frame new questions for research into the biological bases of drug dependence and addiction. At present, epidemiological and biological investigations are, by and large, carried out independently of each other. Yet much is to be gained by a closer interchange and collaboration between the two disciplines, as has been shown to be the case for lung cancer, the slow viruses of the nervous system, and coronary heart disease. The relevance of biology to the epidemiology of substance use disorders is obvious. Biological factors, and not only social and psychological factors, underlie the natural history of drug use and the causes and consequences of using drugs. What are less obvious are the contributions that epidemiology can make in providing novel insights into the biology of addiction and in suggesting new hypotheses to be pursued and tested in the laboratory.

References

American Psychiatric Association: Diagnostic and Statistical Manual of Mental Disorders, 4th Edition. Washington, DC, American Psychiatric Association, 1994

Anthony JC, Warner LA, Kessler RC: Comparative epidemiology of dependence on tobacco, alcohol, controlled substances and inhalants: basic findings from the National Comorbidity Survey. Exp Clin Psychopharmacol 2:244–268, 1994

Breslau N, Kilby M, Andreski P: DSM-III-R nicotine dependence in young adults: prevalence, correlates and associated psychiatric disorders. Addiction 89:743–754, 1994

Chen K, Kandel DB, Davies M: Relationships between frequency and quantity of marijuana use and last year proxy dependence among adolescents and adults in the United States. Drug Alcohol Depend 46:53–67, 1997

Covey LS, Hughes DC, Glassman AH, et al: Ever-smoking, quitting, and psychiatric disorders: evidence from the Durham, North Carolina, Epidemiologic Catchment Area. Tob Control 3:222–227, 1994

Grant BF, Harford TC, Dawson DA, et al: Prevalence of DSM-IV alcohol abuse and dependence: U.S. 1992. Alcohol Health Res World 18:243–248, 1994

Grant BF, Harford TC, Dawson DA, et al: The Alcohol Use Disorder and Associated Disabilities Interview Schedule (AUDADIS): reliability of alcohol and drug modules in a general population sample. Drug Alcohol Depend 39:37–44, 1995

Kandel DB, Chen K, Warner L, et al: Prevalence and demographic correlates of symptoms of dependence on cigarettes, alcohol, marijuana and cocaine in the U.S. population. Drug Alcohol Depend 44:11–29, 1997

Kessler RC, McGonagle KA, Zhao S, et al: Lifetime and 12-month prevalence of DSM-III-R psychiatric disorders in the United States: results from the National Comorbidity Study. Arch Gen Psychiatry 51:8–19, 1994

National Institute on Drug Abuse: National Household Survey on Drug Abuse: Population Estimates 1991. Rockville, MD, National Institute on Drug Abuse, 1991

Robins LN, Regier DA: Psychiatric Disorders in America: The Epidemiologic Catchment Area Study. New York, Free Press, 1991

Robins LN, Helzer JE, Croughan J, et al: National Institute of Mental Health Diagnostic Interview Schedule: its history, characteristics, and validity. Arch Gen Psychiatry 38:381–389, 1981

Robins LN, Helzer JE, Przybeck T: Substance abuse in the general population, in Mental Disorders in the Community: Progress and Challenge. Proceedings of the American Psychopathological Association, Vol 42. Edited by Barrett J, Rose RM. New York, Guilford, 1986, pp 9–31

Shah BV, Barnwell BG, Bieler GS: SUDAAN User's Manual, Release 7.5. Research Triangle Park, NC, Research Triangle Institute, 1997

Substance Abuse and Mental Health Services Administration (SAMHSA): National Household Survey on Drug Abuse: Population Estimates 1992. Rockville, MD, SAMHSA Office of Applied Studies, 1993

Substance Abuse and Mental Health Services Administration (SAMHSA): National Household Survey on Drug Abuse: Population Estimates 1993. Rockville, MD, SAMHSA Office of Applied Studies, 1994

Warner LA, Kessler RC, Hughes M, et al: Prevalence and correlates of drug use and dependence in the United States: results from the National Comorbidity Survey. Arch Gen Psychiatry 52:219–229, 1995

World Health Organization: Composite International Diagnostic Interview (CIDI), Version 1.0. Geneva, Switzerland, WHO, 1990

CHAPTER 12

Gender Effects in Gene–Environment Interactions in Substance Abuse

Remi J. Cadoret, M.D.
Kristin Riggins-Caspers, Ph.D.
William R. Yates, M.D.
Edward P. Troughton, B.A.
Mark A. Stewart, M.D.[†]

In this chapter we present the results of adoption studies conducted at the University of Iowa that are relevant to gender differences in gene–environment interactions associated with adult substance abuse. Various relationships between gene and environment—such as gene–environment correlation and interaction—have assumed importance in recent years with the discovery of specific examples in human behavior (Plomin et al. 1994). *Gene–environment interaction* refers to the dependence of a phenotypic trait's expression on a particular environment.

The adoption paradigm is the most direct and effective way to detect and measure specific gene–environment interactions. For example, in the Colorado Adoption Project, children with a genetic background of sociopathy were more likely than those without such a background to exhibit delinquent behavior when adopted into families with low scores on a family system maintenance subscale derived from the Moos Family En-

[†]Deceased.

vironment Scale (DeFries et al. 1994) but not when adopted into families with a high system maintenance score. The most recent Iowa adoption study (Cadoret et al. 1995b) found significant evidence that an antisocial biological background is expressed differently in adoptees with psychiatrically or behaviorally disturbed adoptive parents than it is in adoptees without such parents. It is this relationship that the present chapter will address.

The Iowa adoption studies are based on examination of adult adoptees who, as infants, were separated from their birth parents and placed with nonrelatives for adoption. Over the years, a variety of methods have been applied to obtain information about the birth parents and about the adoptees and the environment in which they were brought up in the adoptive home. The experimental paradigm used in these studies is shown in Figure 12–1. Index adoptees are those who have some psychopathology in a biological relative (usually the birth parents). In earlier Iowa adoption studies, this information was gathered from adoption agency records. However, in the most recent study (Cadoret et al. 1995a, 1995b), hospital and prison records were examined for birth par-

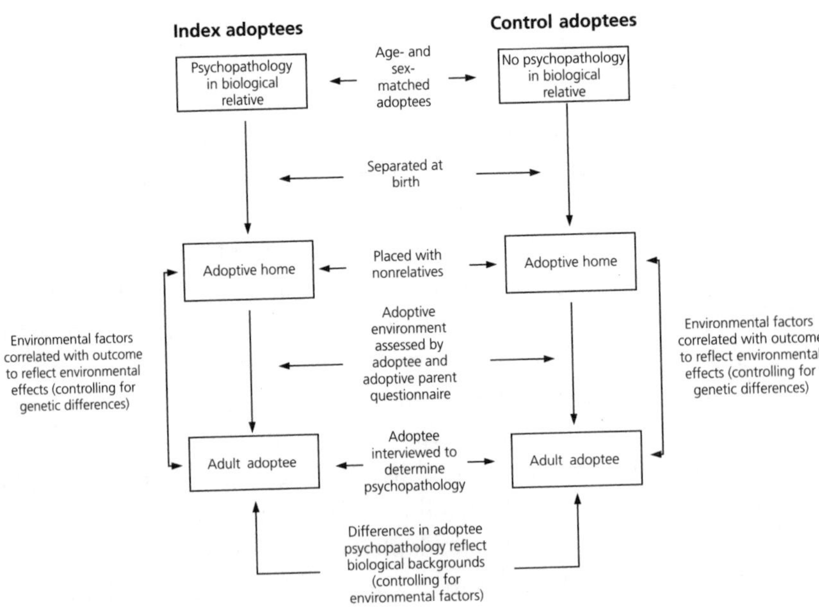

FIGURE 12–1. Paradigm used in Iowa adoption studies.

ents' psychopathology, and diagnoses were made on the basis of these more complete sources of information. Control adoptees were selected from adoptees placed in the same year by the same agency as the index adoptees and matched for age, gender, and age of biological mother at the time of birth. All adoptees had been separated at birth from their birth parents and placed with nonrelatives.

The adoptive environment has been assessed by a variety of measures obtained from interviews of the adult adoptee and of the adoptive parents. The adoptive parent interview (Cadoret et al. 1995a) contains a number of questions dealing with early development; preschool, grade school, and high school adjustment; and adult adjustment of the adoptee, allowing for the evaluation of behaviors such as attention-deficit disorder (Cadoret and Gath 1980; Cadoret and Stewart 1991), childhood temperament (Maurer et al. 1980), and other conditions (e.g., antisocial personality) (Cadoret et al. 1987). Over the years, adoptive parents have come under greater scrutiny; in our most recent studies (Cadoret et al. 1995a) we are administering the Diagnostic Interview Schedule (DIS; Robins et al. 1989) to each adoptive parent in addition to gathering information about family environment and marital problems from interviews and additional questionnaires. The adult adoptee is also interviewed in person and administered the DIS to determine psychopathology.

As can be seen from Figure 12–1, the adoption paradigm can be analyzed as a factorial design that assesses main effects for biological background by testing differences in adult adoptee psychopathology between the index adoptees and the control adoptees. The factorial design also allows for evaluation of environmental factors by correlating environmental factors with adoptee outcomes. As shown in the figure, there are two possible correlations between environment and adoptee outcome. One correlation involves adoptees with psychopathology in their biological backgrounds (index adoptees), and the other involves control adoptees without such backgrounds. The main effect for an environmental factor is the average of these two correlations. However, if the correlation between adoptive home environment and adult adoptee outcome in the index adoptees is different from the same correlation in the control adoptees, then evidence exists for a gene–environment interaction. In the factorial analysis, the direction of the effect may not be clear from the correlation itself; other arguments must be adduced to determine the possible direction of effect.

In earlier Iowa adoption studies, we found evidence of several pathways from genetic background to substance abuse (Cadoret et al. 1985, 1986, 1987). Figure 12–2 presents the best-fitting log-linear analysis for a study done with Lutheran Social Services of Iowa (Cadoret et al. 1985) in which adoptee outcomes—DSM-III (American Psychiatric Association 1980) diagnoses of adoptee alcoholism or antisocial personality disorder—were correlated with alcohol abuse and antisocial personality disorder in birth parents. Odds ratios for male adoptees appear outside parentheses; ratios for female adoptees appear inside parentheses. Figure 12–2 demonstrates one pathway leading to alcohol abuse, in which alcohol abuse or dependency in a birth parent is highly predictive of alcohol abuse or dependency in the adult adoptee. This relationship is indicated by the odds ratios of 6.0 (males) and 7.1 (females) positioned along the arrow connecting the alcohol abuse/dependency factor with adult adoptee

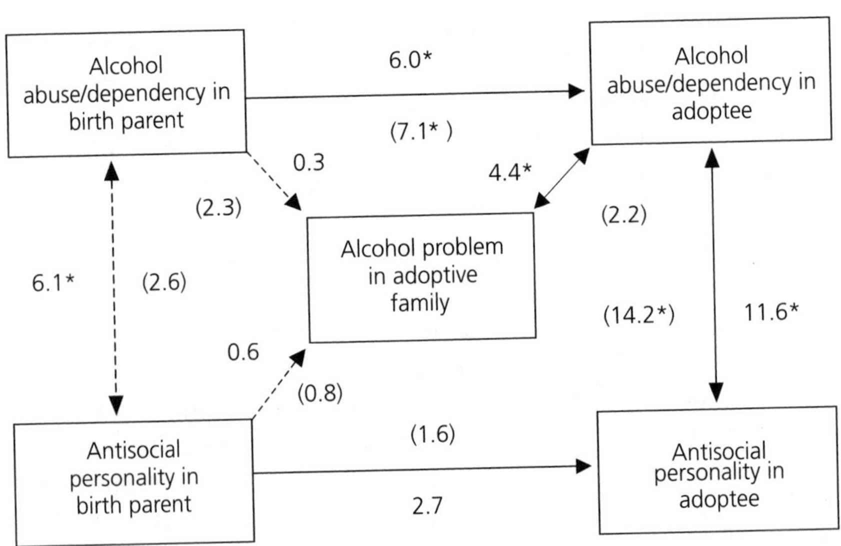

FIGURE 12–2. Interaction diagram for the best-fitting log-linear model for the Iowa Lutheran Social Services adoption study. Numbers represent odds ratios between items; asterisks indicate significant correlation. Arrows represent direction of relationship. When direction of effect cannot be determined, the arrow is bidirectional. Solid arrows represent the relationship found in the data; broken arrows represent the relationship forced into the model to control for genetic effects. Numbers in parentheses represent the values for female adoptees.
Source. Cadoret et al. 1985.

alcohol abuse. Also depicted in this model is a second pathway wherein antisocial birth parents are more likely to have antisocial offspring, and antisocial offspring are more likely to have alcohol use problems, as shown by the large odds ratio between adoptee antisocial personality disorder and adoptee alcohol abuse/dependency. This antisocial pathway was previously described by Cloninger et al. (1981) as type II alcoholism and was further delineated by Cadoret et al. (1985, 1987).

The special importance of the antisocial pathway lies in its strong association with the development of drug abuse/dependency, as illustrated in Figure 12–3. The interaction diagram in this figure shows the best-fitting log-linear model predicting substance abuse (drug abuse/dependency and alcohol abuse/dependency) in an independent adoption study

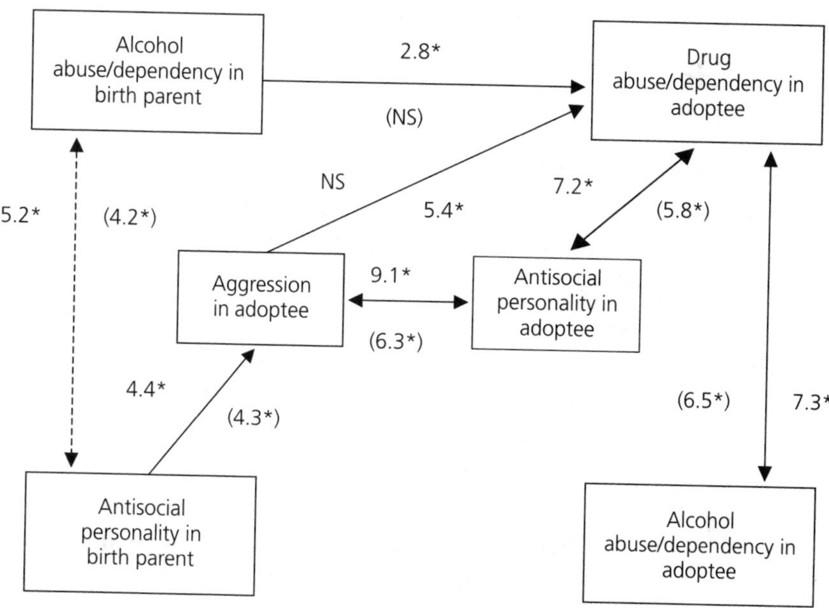

FIGURE 12–3. Interaction diagram for the best-fitting log-linear model for the National Institute on Drug Abuse adoption study, with aggression as intervening variable. Numbers represent odds ratios between items; asterisks indicate significant correlation. Arrows represent direction of relationship. When direction of effect cannot be determined, the arrow is bidirectional. Solid arrows represent the relationship found in the data; broken arrows represent the relationship forced into the model to control for genetic effects. Numbers in parentheses represent the values for female adoptees.
Source. Adapted from Cadoret et al. 1995a, 1995b, 1996.

involving 197 adoptee subjects (Cadoret et al. 1995a, 1996). As can be seen in the diagram, there is a robust relationship between adolescent aggressivity and later adult antisocial personality and drug abuse/dependency.

Our focus in this chapter is the developmental pathway between birth parents with antisocial personality and aggressivity and antisocial behavior in the offspring. Our adoption paradigm (see Figure 12–1) has allowed us to estimate how environmental influences interact with genetic antisocial background to produce intervening variables that precede substance abuse: aggressivity and conduct disorder (Cadoret et al. 1995b). We use a structured equation modeling approach here to assess the effect of adoptees' gender on this gene–environment interactive process.

Methods

In this chapter we use data from a study most recently done under the auspices of the National Institute on Drug Abuse (Cadoret et al. 1995a, 1995b, 1996). One hundred ninety-seven adult adoptees—and, wherever possible, their adoptive parents—were interviewed in person. The index adoptees in this sample were selected on the basis of having a birth parent with a history (documented from hospital or prison records) of antisocial behavior or substance abuse. Details of how this record search was accomplished were reported in previously cited studies (Cadoret et al. 1995a, 1995b, 1996). Adoptive parents were evaluated with the DIS, as were the adoptees.

In order to concentrate on the antisocial pathway to substance abuse in adoptees, additional information was gathered from the adoptive parents and from other sources, including treatment records. This information was used to identify possible intervening variables in the pathway between antisocial personality disorder in the biological background and eventual drug and alcohol abuse in the adoptee. The two intervening variables assessed were conduct disorder and aggressivity. Conduct disorder was evaluated by asking adoptive parents and the adoptee about a set of behaviors occurring before the age of 15 years (Table 12–1; Robins 1966). Aggressivity symptoms during adolescence were evaluated mostly from adoptive parent interviews; the questions used were adapted from

TABLE 12–1.
Symptoms of conduct disorder, aggressivity, and adverse adoptive home

Child conduct disorder (symptoms occurring before age 15 years)	
Alcohol or drug use	Sex
Arrest	Starts fights
Expelled, suspended	Stealing
Lying	Trouble at school
Poor grades	Truant
Run away from home	Vandalism
Aggression symptoms	
Bully	Overreacts
Cruel	Physically attacks others
Defiant	Quarrelsome
Destructive	Rebellious
Difficult to control	Resentful
Disturbs others	Sets fires
Easily upset	Steals
Excitable	Sullen
Explosive	Swears
Fights	Tantrums
Hard to manage	Teases
Insolent	Threatens others
Irritable	Touchy
Lies	Uncooperative
Loses temper	Verbally abuses others
Low frustration tolerance	Won't mind
Mean	
Adverse adoptive parent factors	
Alcohol abuse/dependency	Drug abuse/dependency
Anxiety	Legal problems
Depression	Marital problems
Divorced	Other psychiatric problems

Source. Loney et al. 1980; Robins 1966.

the aggressivity evaluation developed by Loney et al. (1980; see Table 12–1). The adoptive parent interview covered a number of health and environmental issues, such as sibling behaviors, marital difficulties, and family problems (see Table 12–1).

For analyses of the antisocial pathway from genetic background through aggressivity and conduct disorder to substance abuse, we used two measures of drug and alcohol use derived from the DIS. For alcohol, DIS items detailing abuse/dependency symptoms were totaled to derive an alcohol symptom measure. For drugs, DIS items detailing abuse/dependency symptoms for cannabis, amphetamines, sedative-hypnotics, opioids, cocaine, and hallucinogens were added to obtain a drug symptom measure.

Results

The results of the log-linear analysis of these data confirmed the presence of a pathway between antisocial personality in a birth parent and drug abuse/dependency and alcohol abuse/dependency in the adult adoptee. These results are shown in Figure 12–3 (adapted from Cadoret et al. 1995a, 1995b, 1996), where it can be seen that aggressivity or conduct disorder in the adoptee acted as an intervening variable between antisocial personality in the birth parent and drug abuse in the adoptee. For male adoptees (see Figure 12–3), conduct disorder could be substituted for antisocial personality disorder in the adoptee with no significant change in the model.

In this chapter we investigate the effect on adoptee aggressivity and conduct disorder of environmental conditions in the home as they interact with the antisocial personality background of the adoptee. To evaluate gene–environment interaction, we follow the approach suggested by Plomin et al. (1977), which uses factorial analysis of variance (as described earlier in this chapter) to assess main effects (genetic and environmental) and their interaction. In this model, aggressivity or conduct disorder will be predicted by independent variables that include a genetic effect (such as alcoholism or antisocial personality disorder in a birth parent), an environmental effect (such as conditions in the adoptive family), and an interaction term.

The environmental effect involves factors reported by adoptive parents and adoptees; it is referred to here as the "adverse adoptive parent" factor. A similar factor had been reported to influence substance abuse in earlier work with Iowa adoptees, and the current adverse adoptive parent factor reflects this previous finding (Cadoret et al. 1986). Adverse adoptive parent factors include psychopathology in the parents as well as marital problems such as divorce and separation (see Table 12–1).

The results of the multiple regression analyses for aggressivity with the subjects separated by gender are shown in Figure 12–4. Three different models are presented in the figure. In the first model (see first pair of bars on left), only the environmental factor (adverse adoptive parent) is used as a predictor. The percentage of the variance in aggressivity predicted by this and subsequent models can be read off the ordinate at the extreme left. By itself, the adverse adoptive parent factor does not predict a significant amount of variation. However, when the genetic factor of antisocial birth parent is added (see middle pair of bars), both male and female equations significantly predict aggressivity. When the interaction term is added to the model, only females show a significant improvement in R^2 (bar pair, extreme right). Figure 12–5 shows that for males the environmental factor of adverse adoptive parent accounts for practically all of

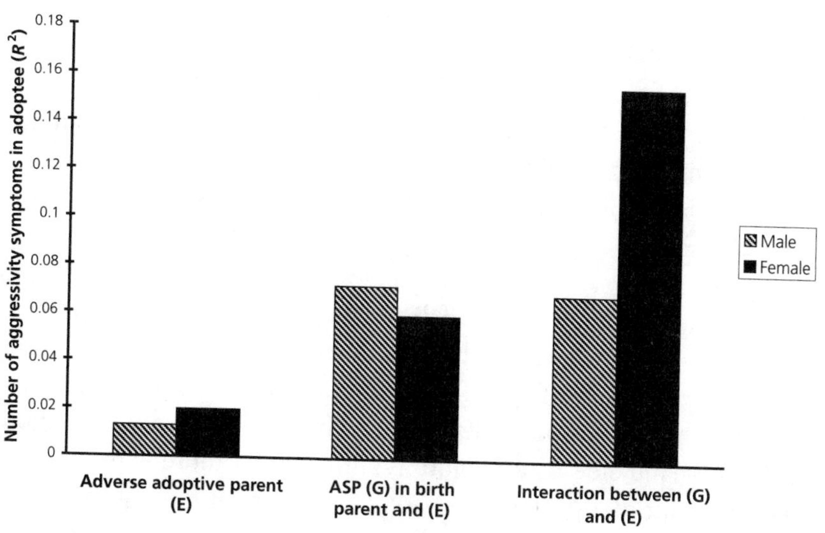

FIGURE 12–4. Gender differences and gene (G) × environment (E) interaction in adoptee aggressivity symptoms. ASP = antisocial personality.

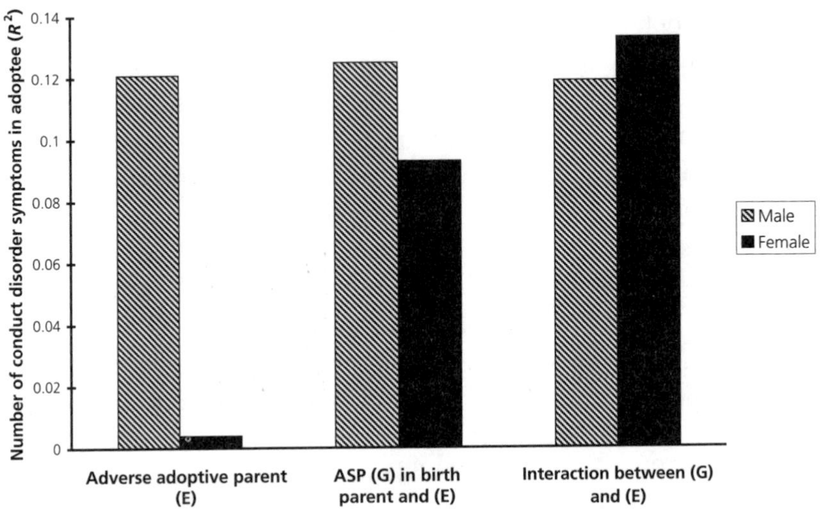

FIGURE 12–5. Gender differences and gene (G) × environment (E) interaction in adoptee conduct disorder symptoms. ASP = antisocial personality.

the variance predicted in conduct disorder, whereas for females the genetic factor and the interaction factor were stronger predictors.

The interactions between genes and the environment for adoptees are shown for males in Figure 12–6 and for females in Figure 12–7. In these figures, the aggressivity scores for individual adoptees are plotted against the total of the adverse adoptive parent factor in each adoptee's home. The results are plotted separately for adoptees from antisocial backgrounds (on the right) and for control adoptees (on the left).

As can be seen in Figure 12–6, there is little evidence that the slopes differ between males with no antisocial personality in the birth parent and those with antisocial personality in the birth parent. In contrast, a significant difference in the slope of the relationship between the number of adverse factors in the adoptive home and the number of aggression symptoms in the adoptee is found for females (see Figure 12–7) when separated into those with no antisocial personality background, as shown on the left-hand side of the figure (controls), and those with antisocial personality disorder in the birth parent, as shown on the right-hand side of the figure (index cases). Results for conduct disorder in males and females were similar to those found for aggressivity, showing greater evidence of gene–environment interaction for females. The other differ-

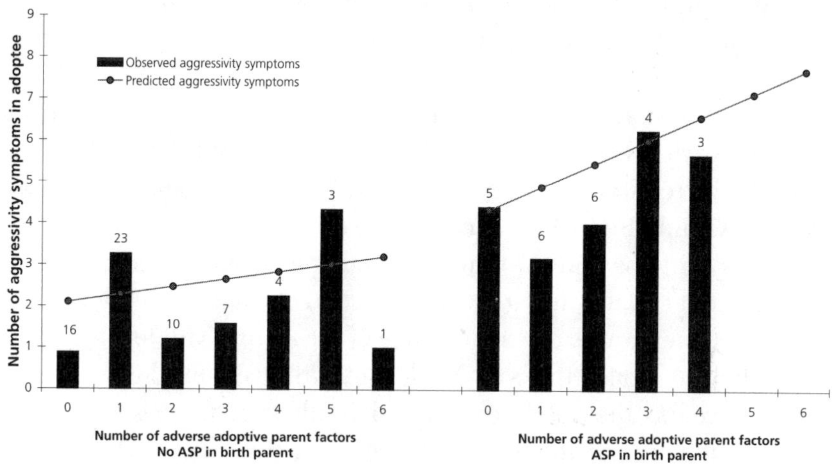

FIGURE 12–6. Aggressivity symptoms by adverse adoptive home in male adoptees. Numbers on tops of bars indicate number of observations. ASP = antisocial personality.

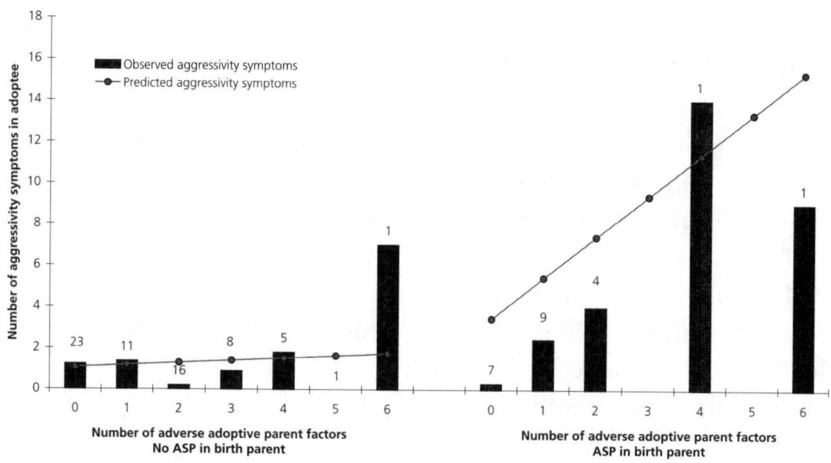

FIGURE 12–7. Aggressivity symptoms by adverse adoptive home in female adoptees. Numbers on tops of bars indicate number of observations. ASP = antisocial personality.

ence demonstrated in these figures is the general finding that both aggressivity and conduct disorder are significantly higher in males than in females.

To demonstrate the gender differences just described and to show how aggressivity and conduct disorder relate to adult substance abuse, we have fitted structural equation models to these data. Path analysis was used to examine the potential mechanisms contributing to alcohol and drug use symptoms. A series of nested models were compared, separately for males and females, using the difference in chi-square and normed fit index test to determine the significance of the change (Bollen 1989).

In the first model, the Null Model, all paths were fixed to zero. This model served as the baseline with which all other models were compared. In the second model of the sequence, the Genetic Model, the paths from birth parent alcoholism and birth parent antisocial personality were identified as predictors of adoptee alcohol use symptoms and adoptee aggression and child conduct disorder symptoms, respectively. The third model in the sequence, the Gene plus Environment Model, included environmental effects by adding the adverse adoptive parent factor as a predictor of adoptee aggression and child conduct disorder symptoms. In the final model, the Fully Recursive Model (or the Gene plus Environment and Interactive Model), the gene–environment interaction terms were added. The interaction between adverse adoptive parent and birth parent alcoholism was added as a predictor of adoptee alcohol or drug use symptoms, whereas the interaction between adverse adoptive parent and birth parent antisocial personality disorder was added as a predictor of adoptee aggression and child conduct disorder symptoms. Polyserial correlations were analyzed with LISREL-VII using the generalized least squares estimation procedure (Jöreskog and Sörbom 1989).

The findings for male adoptees' alcohol use showed significant improvement in fit for both the Genetic Model and the Gene plus Environment Model (see Table 12–2, top half). Adding the interaction terms did not result in a significant improvement in fit. The significant paths predicting male adoptees' alcohol symptoms are shown in Figure 12–8. No direct effects were found in predicting alcohol use symptoms; however, birth parent antisocial personality disorder and the adverse adoptive parent factor were found to indirectly affect male adoptee alcohol use in two different ways. Antisocial personality disorder in the birth parent indi-

TABLE 12–2.

Fit indices for nested sequence for path model of alcohol use for male and female adoptees

	df	χ^2	GFI	AGFI	$\Delta\chi^2$	NFI	ΔNFI
				Male adoptees			
Null Model	18	42.85	.67	.24			
Genetic Model	12	14.98	.94	.82	27.60*	.64	
Gene plus Environment Model	9	7.49	.97	.88	7.49*	.83	.19
Gene plus Environment and Interactive Model	6	4.64	.98	.89	2.85	.89	.06
				Female adoptees			
Null Model	18	40.59	.87	.73			
Genetic Model	12	19.91	.93	.80	20.68*	.51	
Gene plus Environment Model	9	18.48	.94	.75	1.43	.54	.03
Gene plus Environment and Interactive Model	6	1.69	.99	.97	16.79*	.96	.42

Note. GFI = goodness-of-fit index; NFI = normed fit index; AGFI = adjusted goodness-of-fit index; $\Delta\chi^2$ = change in chi-square; ΔNFI = change in NFI. The NFI is a ratio between the baseline model and a model of comparison and uses the following formula: $(\Delta 0 - \Delta k)/\Delta 0$, where 0 = Null Model and k = Theoretical Model. *$P < .05$.

rectly influenced alcohol symptoms by increasing aggression symptoms (see Figure 12–8). Higher aggression was, in turn, positively related to a greater number of child conduct disorder symptoms, which positively predicted alcohol use. The adverse adoptive parent factor indirectly influenced alcohol use by increasing child conduct disorder symptoms (see Figure 12–8).

For female adoptee alcohol use, the Genetic Model showed a significant increase in fit (see Table 12–2, bottom half). The Gene plus Environment Model did not show any improvement; however, addition of the interaction terms resulted in a significant improvement in fit for female adoptees for that model. Despite the significance discussed above, no direct or indirect path was found to predict alcohol use symptoms in female adoptees. The significance emerged from genetic and interactive predictions of female adoptee aggression and child conduct disorder symptoms. The final model predicting female adoptee alcohol symptoms is shown in Figure 12–9.

The results for the models predicting male (upper half) and female adoptee drug use (lower half) are presented in Table 12–3. As previously

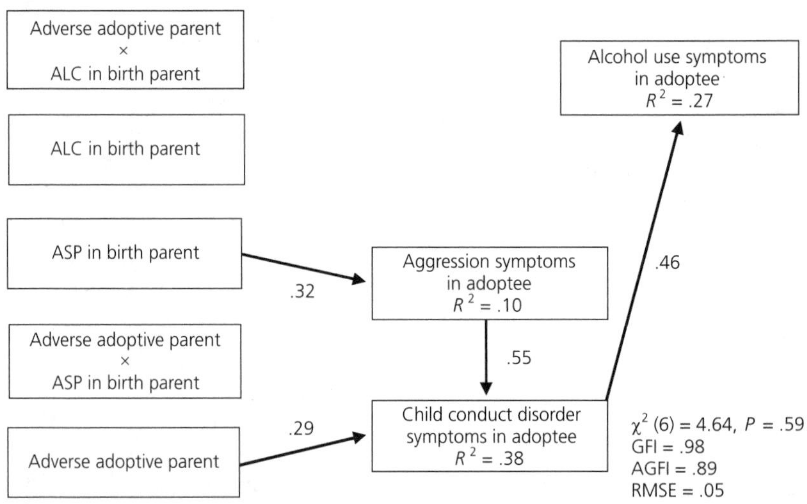

FIGURE 12–8. Main effect and interaction effect model for male adoptee alcohol use (significant paths only). Numbers on lines represent significant partial betas. ALC = alcoholism; ASP = antisocial personality; GFI = goodness-of-fit index; AGFI = adjusted goodness-of-fit index; RMSE = root-mean-square error.

found for male alcohol use, the Genetic Model and the Gene plus Environment Model showed significant improvements in fit. The path model predicting drug use symptoms showed findings identical to those previously shown for male adoptee alcohol symptoms and is therefore not replicated here.

For female adoptee drug use symptoms, the Genetic Model and the Gene plus Environment and Interactive Model showed significant improvement in fit (see Table 12–3, bottom half). As with the model predicting alcohol use, the total effects of antisocial personality disorder in the birth parent, the adverse adoptive parent factor, and the interaction terms on drug use were indirect and influenced both aggression and child conduct disorder symptoms. Unlike the model predicting female adoptee alcohol use, however, the model predicting drug use showed a significant path between child conduct disorder symptoms and adult adoptee drug use symptoms (β = .41). Again, because of the similarities in the models predicting female adoptee substance abuse, the figures for drug use are not replicated here.

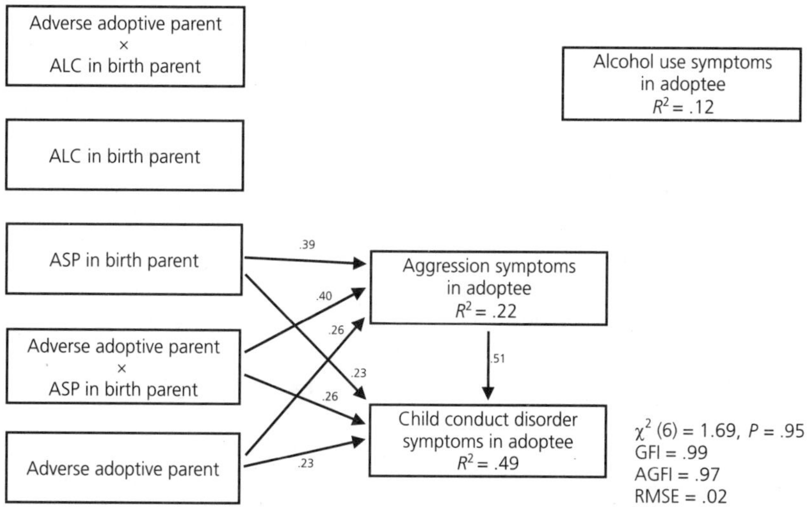

FIGURE 12–9. Main effect and interaction effect model for female adoptee alcohol use (significant paths only). Numbers on arrows represent significant partial betas. ALC = alcoholism; ASP = antisocial personality; GFI = goodness-of-fit index; AGFI = adjusted goodness-of-fit index; RMSE = root-mean-square error.

TABLE 12–3.

Fit indices for nested sequence for path model of drug use for male and female adoptees

	df	χ^2	GFI	AGFI	$\Delta\chi^2$	NFI	ΔNFI
				Male adoptees			
Null Model	18	45.38	.82	.65			
Genetic Model	12	16.82	.93	.80	28.56*	.64	
Gene plus Environment Model	9	9.10	.96	.86	7.72*	.80	.16
Gene plus Environment and Interactive Model	6	5.98	.98	.86	3.12	.87	.07
				Female adoptees			
Null Model	18	57.55	.81	.61			
Genetic Model	12	28.58	.90	.71	28.97*	.50	
Gene plus Environment Model	9	27.03	.91	.64	1.55	.53	.03
Gene plus Environment and Interactive Model	6	6.79	.98	.86	20.24*	.88	.35

Note. GFI = goodness-of-fit index; NFI = normed fit index; AGFI = adjusted goodness-of-fit index; $\Delta\chi^2$ = change in chi-square; ΔNFI = change in NFI. The NFI is a ratio between the baseline model and a model of comparison and uses the following formula: $(\Delta 0 - \Delta k)/\Delta 0$, where 0 = Null Model and k = Theoretical Model. *$P < .05$.

Multisample comparison analyses were used to test for gender differences in the genetic contributions to alcohol and drug use symptoms, as well as the interactions among adoptee gender, adverse adoptive parent factors, and genetic effects (Jöreskog and Sörbom 1989). With this analytical technique, a series of nested comparisons were made. The first model (i.e., the nonrestrictive model) allows the paths of the model to be predicted separately for each group. Once this model is estimated, paths can be forced to be equal across groups, and a change in chi-square between the subsequent models and the first nonrestrictive model is computed. If the change in chi-square is significant, then those paths forced to be equal are judged to differ across the groups being compared. Complete invariance means that all components of the model have been restricted.

For this chapter, two series of multisample comparisons were conducted, with the goal of the analyses being identification of significant gender differences in the presence of interaction effects. For purposes of these analyses, the adverse adoptive parent factor was defined as absent if 0 or 1 adverse factor was present and as present if 2–6 adverse factors were present. The first series of analyses compared males and females separately at each level of the adverse adoptive parent factor. The second series compared the effects of the adverse adoptive parent factor separately for males and females. If differences in results are found across each of the four groups (i.e., male—no adverse adoptive parent, male—adverse adoptive parent, female—no adverse adoptive parent, female—adverse adoptive parent), gender differences can be argued to exist.

For the multisample comparisons across levels of the adverse adoptive parent factor, main exogenous genetic effects were included (see Figure 12–10), but not main exogenous environmental effects, since the effect of adverse adoptive parent is taken into account by conducting the analyses separately for absence/presence of adverse adoptive parent factors. *Gammas* refer to the paths from the exogenous variables (i.e., birth parent alcoholism or antisocial personality disorder; birth parent alcohol or drug symptoms). *Betas* refer to the paths between endogenous variables only.

Alcohol Use

The results of the analyses comparing paths across levels of the adverse adoptive parent factor for male adoptees' alcohol use showed a significant

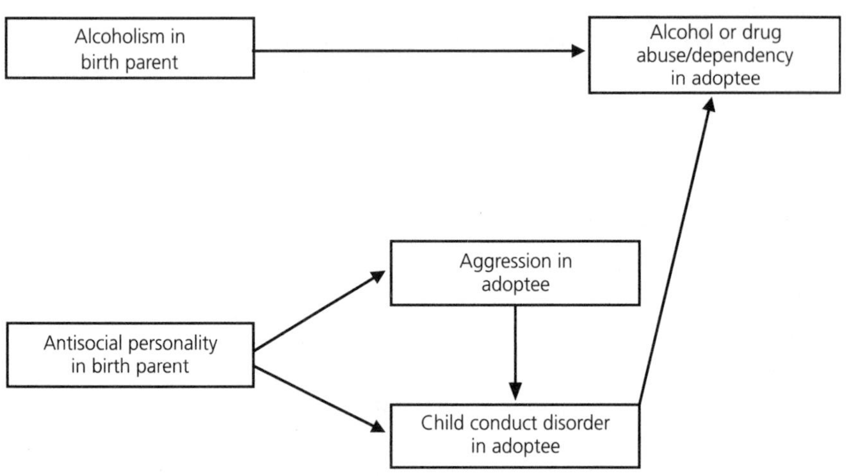

FIGURE 12–10. Model tested in multisample comparisons for adoptee gender differences in effect of adverse adoptive home.

decrease in fit after the gammas were fixed to be equal (see Table 12–4, top half). This means that the genetic main effect predicting male adoptee aggression or child conduct disorder was not the same across levels of the adverse adoptive parent factor.

For female adoptees' alcohol use, a significant decrease in fit was found both for the model equating the gammas and for the completely invariant model (see Table 12–4, bottom half). Again, the genetic paths predicting female adoptee child aggression and child conduct disorder symptoms differed according to the level of the adverse adoptive parent factor.

The results of the analyses comparing the alcohol use models for male and female adoptees at each level of the adverse adoptive parent factor are presented in Table 12–5. In the absence of the adverse adoptive parent factor, no significant reductions in fit were found after the model parameters were fixed to be equal across male and female adoptees. However, when the adverse adoptive parent factor *was* present, fixing the gammas to be equal resulted in a significant decrease in fit (see Table 12–5). By combining the findings from both analyses, it can be concluded that the genetic predictors of alcohol use, aggression, and child conduct disorder symptoms differed across males and females.

TABLE 12–4.
Multisample comparisons for level of adverse adoptive parent conducted separately for male and female adoptee alcohol use

	df	χ^2	GFI	RMSE	$\Delta\chi^2$
			Male adoptees		
Nonrestrictive model	12	16.10	.78	.13	
Gammas equal	15	25.64	.69	.12	9.54*
Gammas and betas equal	18	29.44	.68	.18	3.80
Complete invariance	21	33.65	.68	.15	4.21
			Female adoptees		
Nonrestrictive model	12	3.22	.97	.08	
Gammas equal	15	13.15	.93	.16	9.93*
Gammas and betas equal	18	16.87	.88	.25	3.72
Complete invariance	21	23.34	.94	.16	6.47*

Note. GFI = goodness-of-fit index; RMSE = root-mean-square error; $\Delta\chi^2$ = change in chi-square. *$P < .05$.

Substance Use

The same approaches described above were used to examine gender differences in predictors of substance use. No significant reduction in fit was found for male adoptees when restrictions across the adverse adoptive parent factor were made (see Table 12–6, upper half). In contrast, significance *was* found for female adoptees after the gammas and the error terms were fixed to be equal across levels of adverse adoptive parent (see Table 12–6, lower half).

When analyzed separately at each level of the adverse adoptive parent factor, significant reductions in fit were found only when the adverse adoptive parent factor was present (see Table 12–7). Fixing the gammas to be equal across males and females in this group resulted in a signifi-

TABLE 12–5.
Multisample comparisons for adoptee gender conducted separately for level of adverse adoptive parent in predicting alcohol use

	df	χ^2	GFI	RMSE	$\Delta\chi^2$
		No adverse adoptive parent			
Nonrestrictive model	12	7.57	.94	.11	
Gammas equal	15	12.58	.92	.12	5.01
Gammas and betas equal	18	13.87	.91	.14	1.29
Complete invariance	21	14.97	.91	.13	1.10
		Adverse adoptive parent			
Nonrestrictive model	12	8.72	.86	.11	
Gammas equal	15	16.19	.75	.19	7.47*
Gammas and betas equal	18	20.85	.76	.16	4.66
Complete invariance	21	21.16	.74	.17	.31

Note. GFI = goodness-of-fit index; RMSE = root-mean-square error; $\Delta\chi^2$ = change in chi-square. *$P < .05$.

cant decrease in fit. As before, this means that the genetic effect differed across males and females only when the adverse adoptive parent factor was present.

Spearman rho correlations among all study variables at each level of the adverse adoptive parent factor are presented in Table 12–8 for female and male adoptees. Correlations between birth parent alcoholism and adoptee alcohol/drug use symptoms or between birth parent antisocial personality disorder and aggression and adoptee child conduct disorder symptoms represent the paths designated as gammas in the previous analyses. The findings for the multisample comparisons involving the adverse adoptive parent factor and adoptee gender were confirmed by the presence of significant correlations between birth parent antisocial personality disorder and adoptee aggression and child conduct disorder symptoms for female adoptees with adverse adoptive parents only. These same associations were not present for male adoptees with adverse adoptive parents (see Table 12–8). No differences in significance were found between males and females within the no-adverse-adoptive-parent group.

TABLE 12–6.
Multisample comparisons for level of adverse adoptive parent conducted separately for male and female adoptee drug use

	df	χ^2	GFI	RMSE	$\Delta\chi^2$
			Male adoptees		
Nonrestrictive model	12	15.61	.79	.10	
Gammas equal	15	19.17	.76	.10	3.56
Gammas and betas equal	18	23.69	.72	.18	4.52
Complete invariance	21	27.60	.72	.14	3.91
			Female adoptees		
Nonrestrictive model	12	8.97	.90	.14	
Gammas equal	15	20.80	.77	.42	11.83*
Gammas and betas equal	18	26.17	.80	.28	5.37
Complete invariance	21	36.68	.81	.16	10.51*

Note. GFI = goodness-of-fit index; RMSE = root-mean-square error; $\Delta\chi^2$ = change in chi-square. *$P < .05$.

Discussion

The results described in this chapter confirm the important role of adolescent aggressivity and conduct disorder in adult substance abuse, a role reflected in the nosologies of Cloninger and colleagues (i.e., type II alcoholism; Cloninger et al. 1981) and Babor and associates (i.e., type B alcoholism; Babor et al. 1992). The antisocial path to substance abuse continues to be reported in more recent studies (Zucker et al. 1996). At the same time, important gender differences are present in this pathway: 1) the development of conduct disorder and aggressivity in females appears to depend on significant gene–environment interaction, and 2) aggressivity and conduct disorder are less predictive of adult alcohol abuse symptoms in females than in males. However, the conduct disorder–aggressivity pathway to drug abuse disorders appears to be important in both genders. These findings are important in that they focus attention on possible mechanisms by which a genetic propensity to substance

TABLE 12–7.
Multisample comparisons for adoptee gender conducted separately for level of adverse adoptive parent in predicting drug use

	df	χ^2	GFI	RMSE	$\Delta\chi^2$
		No adverse adoptive parent			
Nonrestrictive model	12	6.34	.93	.11	
Gammas equal	15	10.85	.91	.13	4.24
Gammas and betas equal	18	11.18	.90	.13	.93
Complete invariance	21	8.91	.90	.11	2.27
		Adverse adoptive parent			
Nonrestrictive model	12	18.35	.88	.07	
Gammas equal	15	27.99	.86	.12	9.64*
Gammas and betas equal	18	31.99	.78	.20	4.00
Complete invariance	21	27.17	.70	.22	4.82

Note. GFI = goodness-of-fit index; RMSE = root-mean-square error; $\Delta\chi^2$ = change in chi-square. *$P < .05$.

abuse is manifested. Gene–environment interaction further highlights the importance of environmental factors in the development of risk behaviors for substance abuse.

One of the unresolved issues in this gene–environment interactive factor is the causal direction of the effect. Put crudely but simply, do disturbed parents "cause" aggression and conduct disorder in children, or do aggression and conduct disorder in children "cause" psychiatric or other significant behavior changes such as marital discord in parents? A partial answer to this question is available by considering the consequences of one of these directions of effect—say, from children to parent. In such a scenario, one might expect that parents of children with a greater number of aggressive or conduct disorder symptoms would demonstrate greater psychopathology. Examination of the proportions of parents with different numbers of problems in families with and without adoptees from antisocial backgrounds (e.g., aggressivity, as shown in Figures 12–6 and 10–7) reveals that adoptees with an antisocial personality

TABLE 12–8.

Spearman rho correlations between biological parent characteristics and adoptee aggression, child conduct disorder, alcohol use, and drug use symptoms

Variables	1	2	3	4	5	6
			Female adoptees			
Biological parent alcoholism		.41*	.25	.26	.24	.02
Biological parent ASP	.59***		.58***	.70***	.33	.06
Aggression	.06	.02		.67***	.67***	.21
Child conduct disorder	.15	.07	.48***		.58***	.12
Drug use	.21	.20	.35*	.55***		.28
Alcohol use	.02	-.03	.11	.25	.33*	
			Male adoptees			
Biological parent alcoholism		.58**	.05	.12	.02	.10
Biological parent ASP	.20		.38	.20	−.07	.16
Aggression	.30	.22		.73***	.24	.31
Child conduct disorder	.13	.05	.33*		.46*	.56**
Drug use	.28	.22	.39*	.62***		.21
Alcohol use	.29	.17	.38*	.53***	.79***	

Note. Numbers below the diagonal represent correlations for the absent adverse-factor group, and numbers above the diagonal represent correlations for the present adverse-factor group. ASP = antisocial personality.
*$P < .05$; **$P < .01$; ***$P < .001$.

disorder background, although more aggressive than those without such a background, do not "produce" an excess of parents with higher numbers of problems. This lack of correlation is shown in Table 12–9, which indicates that proportions of parents with different numbers of psychiatric or behavior problems are the same in families with an aggressive child from an antisocial personality disorder background as they are in families of control children. Further indirect evidence bearing on the question of direction of effect lies in the 0 slope found in the aggressivity and conduct

TABLE 12–9.

Observed distribution of the proportion of parents having children with and without an antisocial personality (ASP) genetic diathesis, by number of adverse factors in the adoptive home

Number of adverse factors in home	Family type: Adoptee without ASP parent	Family type: Adoptee with ASP parent	Totals
0–1	73[a]	27	100
	73.71[b]	26.29	
2–3	41	14	55
	40.54	14.45	
4–6	15	5	20
	14.74	5.26	
Totals	129	46	175

Note. [a] Observed values. [b] Expected values to test hypothesis that distributions are not different.

disorder graphs for the control groups (see Figures 12–6 and 12–7). In these control group correlations, there is little evidence of any effects in the direction of aggressive adoptees to parents.

The question of direction of effect is also linked to the mechanism of gene–environment interaction. Psychiatrically disturbed parents have been shown to have impaired parenting skills (K. J. Conger and R. D. Conger 1994; R. D. Conger et al. 1992), which in turn could affect parental response to provocative antisocial behavior in a child, resulting in reinforcement of the child's antisocial stance. A possible mechanism through parent–child interaction has been suggested by Ge and associates (1996), who studied the origin of gene–environment correlation in adolescent adoptees. They found that behavioral observations of social interactions between adolescents and adoptive parents demonstrated qualities of aggressive antisocial behaviors when the adoptee's biological background contained an antisocial or alcoholic parent. Structural equation modeling of the parent–child interaction suggested a mutual-influence effect whereby the adolescent's behavior elicited a hostile response from the parents, which in turn affected the quality of the adoptee's response. This mutual-influence model is shown in Figure 12–11. If parenting factors are important, as suggested by the evidence reviewed above, then such factors could be the focus of a prospective study to elucidate the social mechanism of gene–environment interaction, which seems to be important in the genesis of conduct disorder, as shown by several independent adoption studies (Cadoret et al. 1983, 1995a).

The findings discussed in this chapter further suggest that one focal point for prevention efforts aimed at conduct disorder or aggressivity should be the interacting environmental factors, which are alterable by specific interventions. That gender differences are likely important should serve to further focus intervention protocols. This conclusion is supported by the path models presented, in which adverse adoptive parent factors moderated the relationship between birth parent characteristics and conduct disorder/aggressive behavior for female adoptees but not

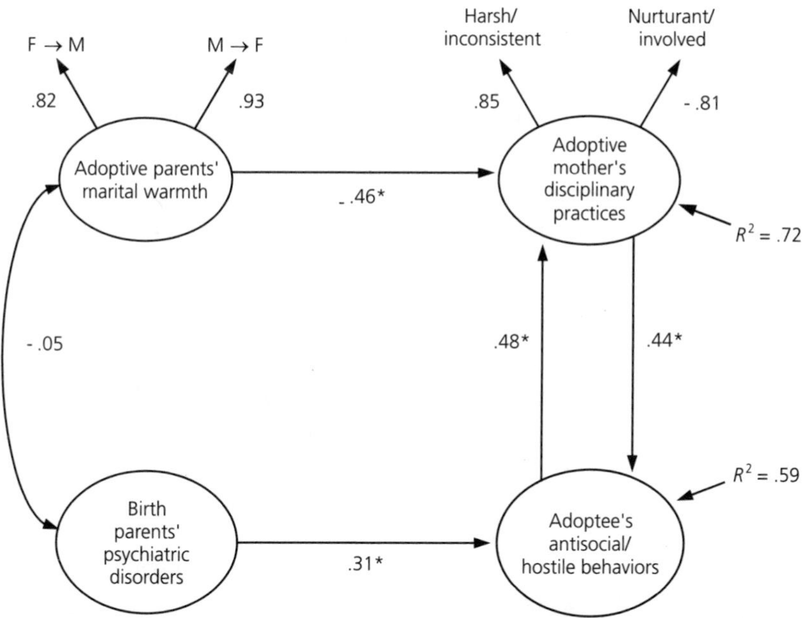

FIGURE 12–11. Evocative gene–environment correlation predicting adoptee antisocial/hostile behaviors. Standardized maximum likelihood estimates of a model of mutual influences between adoptive mothers' parenting and adopted children's antisocial/hostile behaviors ($^{*}P < .05$). Error terms are omitted. M = mother; F = father. χ^2 (6, n = 41) = 8.27, P = .219, goodness of fit = .94.
Source. Adapted from Ge et al. 1996.

for males. Consequently, interventions focused solely on altering environmental factors would be most effective for females.

These findings also suggest that interventions should be specifically tailored to the behaviors they are intended to alter and that gender differences are important to consider as well. For example, interventions designed to lower aggressive behavior or conduct disorder in both males and females might reduce drug abuse but not alcohol problems in females. For males, however, reductions in early problem behaviors could result in a lower prevalence of drug and alcohol use. Finally, the gender differences in concordance rates between alcohol and drug abuse suggest different biological or environmental precursors for males and females and, consequently, different intervention strategies.

References

American Psychiatric Association: Diagnostic and Statistical Manual of Mental Disorders, 3rd Edition. Washington, DC, American Psychiatric Association, 1980

Babor TF, Hofmann M, Del Boca FK, et al: Types of alcoholics, I: evidence for an empirically derived typology based on indicators of vulnerability and severity. Arch Gen Psychiatry 49:599–608, 1992

Bollen KA: Structural Equations With Latent Variables. New York, Wiley, 1989

Cadoret RJ, Gath A: Biologic correlates of hyperactivity: evidence for a genetic factor, in Human Functioning in Longitudinal Perspective. Edited by Sells SB, Crandall R, Roff M. Baltimore, MD, Williams & Wilkins, 1980, pp 103–114

Cadoret RJ, Stewart MA: An adoption study of attention deficit/hyperactivity/aggression and their relationship to adult antisocial personality. Compr Psychiatry 32:73–82, 1991

Cadoret RJ, Cain C, Crowe RR: Evidence for gene–environment interaction in the development of adolescent antisocial behavior. Behav Genet 13:301–310, 1983

Cadoret RJ, O'Gorman TW, Troughton E, et al: Alcoholism and antisocial personality: interrelationships, genetic and environmental factors. Arch Gen Psychiatry 42:161–167, 1985

Cadoret RJ, Troughton E, O'Gorman TW, et al: An adoption study of genetic and environmental factors in drug abuse. Arch Gen Psychiatry 43:1131–1136, 1986

Cadoret RJ, Troughton E, O'Gorman TW: Genetic and environmental factors in alcohol abuse and antisocial personality. J Stud Alcohol 48:1–8, 1987

Cadoret RJ, Yates WR, Troughton E, et al: An adoption study demonstrating two genetic pathways to drug abuse. Arch Gen Psychiatry 52:42–52, 1995a

Cadoret RJ, Yates WR, Troughton E, et al: Genetic–environmental interaction in the genesis of aggressivity and conduct disorders. Arch Gen Psychiatry 52: 916–924, 1995b

Cadoret RJ, Yates WR, Troughton E, et al: An adoption study of drug abuse/dependency in females. Compr Psychiatry 37:88–94, 1996

Cloninger CR, Bohman M, Sigvardsson S: Inheritance of alcohol abuse: cross fostering analysis of adopted men. Arch Gen Psychiatry 38:861–868, 1981

Conger KJ, Conger RD: Differential parenting and change in sibling differences in delinquency. J Fam Psychol 8:287–382, 1994

Conger RD, Conger KG, Elder GH, et al: A family process model of economic hardship and adjustment of early adolescent boys. Child Dev 63:526–541, 1992

DeFries JC, Plomin R, Fulker DW (eds): Nature and Nurture in Middle Childhood. Cambridge, MA, Blackwell, 1994

Ge X, Conger RD, Cadoret RJ, et al: The developmental interface between nature and nurture: a mutual influence model of child antisocial behavior and parent behaviors. Developmental Psychology 32:574–589, 1996

Jöreskog KG, Sörbom D: LISREL-VII: A Guide to the Program and Applications. Chicago, IL, SPSS, Inc., 1989

Loney J, Langhorne JE, Paternite CE, et al: The Iowa habit: hyperkinetic/aggressive boys in treatment, in Human Functioning in Longitudinal Perspective. Edited by Sells SB, Crandall R, Roff M, et al. Baltimore, MD, Williams & Wilkins, 1980, pp 119–140

Maurer R, Cadoret RJ, Cain C: Cluster analysis of childhood temperament data on adoptees. Am J Orthopsychiatry 50:522–534, 1980

Plomin R, DeFries JD, Loehlin JC: Genotype–environment interaction and correlation in the analysis of human behavior. Psychol Bull 54:309–322, 1977

Plomin R, Reiss D, Hetherington M, et al: Nature and nurture: genetic contributions to measures of the family environment. Dev Psychol 30:32–43, 1994

Robins L: Deviant Children Grown Up. Baltimore, MD, Williams & Wilkins, 1966

Robins LN, Helzer JE, Cottler L, et al: NIMH Diagnostic Interview Schedule, Version III, Revised. St Louis, MO, Washington University, 1989,5,10

Zucker RA, Ellis DA, Fitzgerald HE, et al: Other evidence for at least two alcoholisms, II: life course variation in antisociality and heterogeneity of alcoholic outcome. Dev Psychopathol 8:831–848, 1996

CHAPTER 13

Gender Differences in the Effects of Opiates and Cocaine

Treatment Implications

Mary Jeanne Kreek, M.D.

The National Household Surveys on Drug Abuse and the data collected by the Drug Abuse Warning Network (DAWN), as well as other studies conducted by the National Institutes of Health–National Institute on Drug Abuse (NIH–NIDA), the Substance Abuse and Mental Health Services Administration (SAMHSA), and other governmental resources, have informed us about the magnitude of the drug abuse problem in the United States. At least 11% of the U.S. population over 12 years of age have used an illicit drug at some time, according to findings from the 1998 National

This chapter is based on material previously presented at the American Psychopathological Association Annual Meeting on March 1, 1997.

This work was supported in part by the New York State Division of Substance Abuse Services; and by a Department of Health and Human Services–National Institutes of Health–National Institute on Drug Abuse (HHS-NIH-NIDA) Specialized Research Center Grant (HHS-NIH-NIDA-P50-DA05130); by a Department of Health and Human Services–National Institutes of Health–National Center for Research Resources (HHS-NIH-NCRR) General Clinical Research Center Grant (HHS-NIH-NIDA-MO1-RR00102); and by an HHS–NIH–NIDA Research Scientist Award (KO5-DA-00049) to Dr. Kreek.

Household Survey on Drug Abuse (SAMHSA 1999). It has been estimated that more than 2.7 million individuals have used heroin at some time during their lives and that 800,000 to 1 million meet the U.S. federal government criteria for entry into long-term opioid agonist treatment for heroin addiction (methadone or L-α-acetyl-methadol [LAAM] maintenance treatment). These criteria are defined as 1 year or more of daily multiple-dose self-administration of an illicitly obtained opiate, usually heroin, with development of tolerance, physical dependence, drug-seeking behavior, and harm to self, family, and/or society (Rettig and Yarmolinsky 1995). U.S. population surveys have estimated that between 22 and 24 million persons over the age of 12 years in the United States have used cocaine at some time and that between 500,000 and 1 million are regular cocaine users or cocaine addicts. Also, it is estimated that 15–20 million persons in the United States are alcohol abusers or alcoholics.

In this chapter I discuss gender differences and similarities with respect to the prevalence of drug abuse, the presence of comorbid medical and psychiatric problems, and, in particular, the impact on normal physiology of the illicit opiate heroin in women compared with men. I also present findings regarding gender differences in response to pharmacotherapy with the long-acting opioid methadone, as well as the findings of normalization of critical physiological functions during such treatment.

Prevalence of Drug and Alcohol Abuse in Women

Several recent surveys have yielded the information that women account for 35%–60% of the drug abusers or drug addicts in each of the different categories with respect to specific drugs of abuse. Survey data reported in a 1994 NIDA Capsule indicated that 8.8 million women in the United States had used illicit drugs at least during their lifetimes and that 4.3 million women had used illicit drugs at least once in the past month. It also was estimated that 1.3 million women illicitly used prescription drugs for nonmedical purposes in the past month. Of great importance from this information, it was further estimated in the report that one in two women of childbearing age (i.e., 15–44 years) had used illicit drugs at least once during their lifetimes. These surveys have also found that many women, whether addicted or not, continue to use illicit drugs of abuse throughout pregnancy. Findings from a NIDA survey of a national sample of 2,613 women who delivered at 52 different hospitals during 1992–1993 indicated that very large numbers of women used drugs of abuse during pregnancy; thus, large numbers of infants were exposed in utero to these drugs. This exposure included more than 800,000 exposures to tobacco through cigarette smoking; more than 700,000 exposures to ethanol; and more than 160,000 exposures to illicit drugs, of which marijuana, cocaine, methamphetamine, and heroin were the most common. Thus, the exposure both of women and of infants in the prenatal to perinatal period to drugs of abuse is enormous.

There is not very much literature on gender differences with respect to neurobiological, physiological, and behavioral responses to drugs of abuse.

Comorbidity of Drug Abuse and Human Immunodeficiency Virus 1 Infection

In 1983–1984, by unbanking sera that my colleagues and I had prospectively collected from 1969 onward as part of our basic clinical research on the neurobiological and molecular basis of addictions and our related treatment research efforts, removing all identifiers, and then analyzing these specimens with the first available, reliable test for human immunodeficiency virus type 1 (HIV-1) infection (studies conducted in collaboration with the Centers for Disease Control and Prevention [CDC]), we were able to determine that HIV-1 infection entered the parenteral (or "injecting") drug–abusing population in New York City in 1978 (Des Jarlais et al. 1984, 1989; Kreek et al. 1990; Novick et al. 1986a, 1986b, 1989). We also found that the prevalence of HIV-1 infection had risen rapidly, with the result that by 1982, more than 50% of the untreated injecting drug users in New York City were HIV seropositive.

A variety of studies conducted both by the New York State Health Department and by the CDC have determined that over the ensuing years, HIV-1 infection (acquired immunodeficiency syndrome [AIDS]) has become extremely common in injecting drug users (i.e., primarily users of heroin and cocaine) as well as in other types of noninjecting drug users, such as "crack" cocaine abusers and alcoholics, and that injecting drug users have represented the second-largest risk group for HIV-1 infection throughout the United States for almost a decade. Also, it has become obvious that the majority of women infected with HIV-1 are either drug abusers or partners of drug abusers and that babies born to HIV-1–infected mothers are at substantial risk (20%–35%) for developing HIV-1 infection and AIDS if expectant mothers are not receiving treatment directed at HIV-1 infection. By December 31, 1995, more than 500,000 cases of AIDS had been reported to the CDC in the United States, and of these, 184,359, or 36% of all cases, were directly or indirectly related to parenteral drug use. Also, 18,710 cases reported were in heterosexual partners of injecting drug users and 3,758 were in children of injecting drug users or their partners. Thus, it is very important to address the special problems of women who abuse or are addicted to alcohol or drugs. A related need is to consider the unique needs of women receiving long-term treatment for an addiction, as well as to develop strategies for prevention and early intervention.

Primary Sites of Action of Drugs of Abuse

Heroin, cocaine, and alcohol, three major drugs of abuse, each alter both the dopaminergic system and the endogenous opioid system, as has been shown by numerous studies from our laboratory and many others (reviewed in Kreek 1996c, 1996d, 1996e). Heroin acts primarily by binding at specific mu opioid receptors, leading toward a cascade of events following activation of those receptors. However, it has also been shown that heroin and its major metabolite morphine cause enhancement of extracellular fluid levels of dopamine in critical regions of the brain, with respect to the effects of drugs of abuse and their reinforcing properties as well as their locomotor effects, including regions of the mesolimbic-mesocortical dopaminergic system, especially the nucleus accumbens, and of the nigrostriatal dopaminergic system. The action of heroin, morphine, and other opiates in causing such a change in dopamine levels is thought to be effected in a specific brain region, the ventral tegmental area, where many dopaminergic neurons are located, which then project to the mesolimbic-mesocortical dopaminergic system. Opioids, by binding at the mu opioid receptors, inhibit the release of gamma-aminobutyric acid (GABA), the major tonic inhibitor of release of dopamine from the dopaminergic neurons. The inhibition of GABAergic neurons causes release of dopamine above basal levels.

Cocaine, in contrast, acts primarily at the specific dopamine transporter sites to prevent presynaptic reuptake of dopamine (Maisonneuve and Kreek 1994; Maisonneuve et al. 1995). This results in an increased dopaminergic tone in brain regions that have abundant dopaminergic terminals, including the nucleus accumbens and related regions of the mesolimbic-mesocortical dopaminergic system, the site of nerve terminals from neurons in the ventral tegmental area, as well as in the caudate putamen, the site of dopaminergic terminals from neurons in the substantia nigra. The binding of cocaine to the dopamine transporter, therefore, causes a significant and abrupt increase in synaptic and perisynaptic extracellular fluid concentrations of dopamine in these critical brain regions. It has been shown that alcohol also acts to enhance dopaminergic tone in these regions. These actions appear to be similar in males and females, both in animal models and, to the extent possible to be studied, in humans. However, some recent studies (e.g., Quiñones-Jenab et al. 1999) suggest possible resultant behavioral differences in these effects, a finding that needs to be further investigated.

Studies from our laboratories and others have shown that whereas heroin has obvious action at opioid receptors and thus impacts the endogenous opioid system, cocaine administration also causes significant alterations in specific components of the endogenous opioid system by enhancing activation of specific dopaminergic receptors, triggering a cascade of events that in turn alters dynorphin opioid peptide gene expression and kappa and mu receptor gene expression and release and causes subsequent changes in the density of mu and kappa opioid receptors (Spangler et al. 1993a, 1993b, 1996, 1997; Unterwald et al. 1992, 1993, 1994a, 1994b, 1999; Yuferov et al. 1999). Alcohol self-administration in animal models and alcohol consumption by alcoholic individuals has been shown to be attenuated by use of specific opioid antagonists, including naloxone, naltrexone, and nalmefene, implicating a role for the endogenous opioid system in the effects of alcohol (Mason et al. 1994; O'Malley et al. 1992; Volpicelli et al. 1992, 1995).

Pharmacotherapy of Opiate Addiction

Early Studies of Methadone Treatment

In our earliest research related to attempts to develop a pharmacotherapy for long-term treatment of heroin addiction, work conducted under the leadership of Professor Vincent P. Dole, we first evaluated both the stages of opiate addiction and the impact of heroin addiction on the individual (Cooper et al. 1983; Dole et al. 1966; Kreek 1973a, 1978, 1996a, 1996b, 1996c; Kreek et al. 1972, 1976). In late 1963, the conceptualization of the studies was initiated in 1964 by Professor Dole, who recruited the late Dr. Marie Nyswander, a psychiatrist with years of involvement in the management of heroin addiction, as well as myself as a young physician–scientist. Initial studies were conducted in 1964 at The Rockefeller Institute for Medical Research (now the Rockefeller University) and in its hospital. It had been well documented by numerous groups over many years that chronic, illicit self-administration of short-acting opiates, such as heroin, could lead to addiction. First, tolerance develops to the effects of the short-acting opiate, with needs for increasing amounts of opiate—first to get the desired euphoria ("high") or, alternatively, a sense of well-being, and later simply to prevent the onset of the signs and symptoms of opiate withdrawal (i.e., the abstinence syndrome, a physiological syndrome demonstrable both in animal models of opiate addiction and in humans, but the mechanisms for which have not been fully elucidated in molecular, biochemical, or neurobiological terms). The short-acting properties of illicit opiates, primarily heroin, lead to self-administration of the drug three to six times each day. The potential impact of very frequent use of unsterile needles (often with direct sharing of needles) on the spread of infectious diseases, such as hepatitis B and C and HIV-1, is obvious; the average heroin addict self-administers the drug 1,000 to 2,000 times each year.

The initial goals in developing a pharmacotherapeutic treatment were 1) to prevent opiate abstinence symptoms, 2) to reduce or prevent drug "hunger", and 3) to allow normalization of physiological abnormalities caused by chronic use of short-acting illicit opiates (Kreek 1992). An ideal medication was conceptualized as one that would be orally effective and have a very slow onset of action (to prevent any reinforcing effects), a long duration of action, and a slow offset of action—and thus would provide a steady state of action with no resultant opiate or euphoric effects and no withdrawal effects. The medication identified and selected for our first studies in 1964 was methadone, a synthetic opiate agonist that had been used on a very limited basis for the management of pain and in a few medical centers for short-term detoxification treatment of addiction. Although in both of those clinical settings it was thought that methadone had a short duration of action, similar to that of morphine or heroin, some findings from the early studies suggested that it might have a longer duration of action (reviewed in Kreek 1996a, 1996c, 1996d).

We learned in our early research studies that methadone could be effectively administered orally and that it had a very slow onset of action, with no effects until about 30 minutes after oral administration, a modest peak effect 2–4 hours after oral administration, and a sustained effect for a 24-hour dosing interval (Dole et al. 1966; Kreek 1978, 1992; Kreek et al. 1976). Thus, we found in our early studies that methadone, administered once per day orally, allowed a former heroin addict to have no abstinence symptoms or signs and symptoms of narcotic withdrawal over a 24-hour dosing interval, and had no opiate or narcotic-like effect, even at times of peak action of methadone (Dole et al. 1966; Kreek 1991, 1992). We also found that drug "craving" or "hunger" was markedly reduced or eliminated and that the thoughts of each patient subsequently turned to finishing education, getting a job, or returning to a more stable family life.

Although the initial studies of methadone maintenance were conducted in men, when in 1965 the treatment research was extended to various urban sites that had previously been used for detoxification treatment, women were also allowed into the treatment research (Cooper et al. 1983; Finnegan et al. 1982; Kreek 1978, 1979; Pond et al. 1985). It was found that methadone was just as effective in the long-term treatment of female heroin addicts as it was in males.

Pharmacokinetics of Effective Opiate-Addiction Treatment

Although analytical technologies were not available in the initial 1964 studies to determine the pharmacokinetics of methadone (or of morphine, heroin, or any other opiate in humans), when such techniques were developed several years later in the early 1970s by our group and by Dr. C. Inturrisi at Cornell Medical Center, it was found that the plasma concentrations of methadone did indeed parallel those of the function status that we had observed and reported in the 1960s (Kreek 1973b; Hachey et al. 1982; Inturrisi and Verebey 1972a, 1972b). In those studies and studies subsequently conducted with stable isotope technology, it was found the half-life of the racemic methadone used in the treatment of opiate addiction was 24 hours in humans; later studies using stable isotope technology showed that the half-life of the active enantiomer was more than 36–48 hours (Hachey et al. 1977; Kreek et al. 1979; Nakamura et al. 1982). The metabolism and pharmacokinetics of methadone are very similar in women and men, requiring an N-demethylation pathway to form inactive metabolites. In contrast, the half-life of heroin in humans is 2–3 minutes and the half-life of the major morphine metabolite around 4–6 hours (Inturrisi et al. 1984). Thus, long-acting properties of methadone, and the even longer-acting properties of its congener LAAM, more recently approved for the treatment of heroin addiction, allow steady-state perfusion at specific opiate receptors and thus permit normalization of both physiological and behavioral indices disrupted by chronic use of short-acting opiates (Dole and Kreek 1973; Inturrisi and Verebey 1972a, 1972b; Kaiko and Inturrisi 1973; Kreek 1973b, 1978, 1992; Kreek et al. 1976).

Effects of Pregnancy on Methadone Disposition

However, in two separate studies, it has been found that biotransformation and disposition of methadone is profoundly altered during pregnancy (Kreek 1979; Pond et al. 1985). In both of these studies, women who had been maintained on methadone during pregnancy were studied. In each case, women who had no ongoing problems with polydrug or alcohol abuse were studied. Also, none of the women studied required other medications that might alter the biotransformation of methadone. In each subject it was found that the plasma levels of methadone following oral doses were significantly lowered at each time point studied during the third trimester of pregnancy compared with when the same subject was studied both earlier in pregnancy and also restudied after delivery in the postpartum period. Also, it was found that the relative amounts of biotransformation products excreted in urine gave evidence for a more rapid biotransformation of methadone during pregnancy. It is hypothesized that the accelerated biotransformation that occurs during the third trimester of pregnancy is probably due to the very high levels of progesterone and progesterone metabolites present in late pregnancy, which have been shown to accelerate the biotransformation of several medications requiring metabolism by the P450-related hepatic enzyme systems. The observed progressive lowering of methadone plasma levels—and thus the lowering of the area under the plasma concentration–time curve in late pregnancy—was often accompanied by mild to moderate symptoms of opiate withdrawal.

Unfortunately, in many clinics in diverse geographic locations within the United States, it has been the policy to treat pregnant women with very low doses of methadone, and, if they are already in treatment before pregnancy, to begin to lower their doses of methadone, all with an assumption (or even bias) that lower doses of methadone will be better for both the mother and the neonate. However, numerous studies have shown that higher methadone doses cause no problems in infants born to methadone-maintained women other than very mild to moderate withdrawal symptoms for a limited number of days in the early neonatal period. Some, but certainly not all, infants born to mothers maintained on methadone display signs and symptoms of opiate withdrawal; however, these signs and symptoms have never been found to be related to the doses of methadone that the mother was receiving. In fact, in studies in which the mothers have been well rehabilitated with no ongoing polydrug or alcohol abuse, the signs and symptoms of opiate withdrawal in neonates have been limited, with only mild to modest abstinence symptoms evident in the early neonatal period. Conversely, many studies, as well as assessments of treatment programs, have found that pregnant women maintained on low doses of methadone have a strong likelihood of using other drugs, including not only agents such as alcohol and benzodiazepines but also illicit drugs, and have a very high rate of relapse to use of illicit opiates, all resulting from attempts to self-medicate their signs and symptoms of opiate withdrawal and their feelings of drug craving or drug hunger. Although for many years it has been recommended that pregnant women be maintained on adequate doses of methadone, findings from the pharmacokinetic studies have made it clear that the plasma concentrations in a woman in the third trimester of pregnancy are lower for the dose of methadone administered than in the same woman (or any patient) when not pregnant; thus, either no change in methadone dose or only a modest elevation in dose may be needed in some patients at this time of late pregnancy. These studies also have found that methadone metabolism promptly returns to normal in the early postpartum period, with patients once again achieving higher plasma levels of methadone and a greater area under the plasma concentration–time curve for dose of methadone administered (Kreek 1979; Pond et al. 1985).

Characteristics of Heroin-Addicted Individuals Entering and Enrolled in Treatment

Special Problems of Women

In general, women entering treatment for heroin addiction—including methadone, LAAM, or buprenorphine maintenance treatment, and treatment research—have special problems. Also entering into these problems are their life on the street (many of these women have had to engage in prostitution to earn money to support their heroin addiction) and their resultant exposure to and infection with multiple infectious diseases. It has been found that reproductive biological-related functioning in heroin-addicted women is profoundly abnormal, with irregular menses, amenorrhea, or secondary amenorrhea, due to direct opiate effects in the brain leading to reduced levels of pulsatile release of luteinizing hormone (LH) and resultant reduced or absent ovulation, a problem that is reversed during steady-dose methadone treatment (Kreek 1978). Women with children or with drug-abusing partners have special additional problems that many studies have attempted to address by developing various types of peer support groups and special services.

Currently, in the United States, a total of approximately 179,000 individuals are in methadone maintenance treatment; 30%–50% of these individuals are women. In programs that provide adequate doses of methadone (i.e., 60–120 mg/day, or even higher doses in the recent setting of increased purity of heroin in the northeastern region of the United States) and adequate onsite counseling as well as access to medical and psychiatric care and other types of support services as needed, the voluntary 1-year retention in treatment exceeds 60% (Kreek 1991, 1996a, 1996b, 1996c, 1996d; Rettig and Yarmolinsky 1995), as it has done since the 1960s. In high-quality programs, heroin use drops from 100% to less than 20% within 12 months of treatment. The numbers of methadone-maintained patients with a cocaine codependence—approximately 80%–90% of heroin addicts seeking treatment in the Northeast—drops to around 30% after 12 months or more of treatment. Women have the same problems of cocaine codependence as men and have been as effectively treated by methadone.

Gender Differences in Psychiatric Comorbidity

Psychiatric comorbidity is a major problem in both male and female opiate-addicted patients. Thirty percent to 50% have affective disorders, primarily depression; 40%–50% have phobic disorders; and 30%–40% have antisocial personality disorder (Mason et al. 1998). Studies have shown that at the time of entry into methadone maintenance treatment for heroin addiction, women do have a slightly different profile than men with respect to psychiatric comorbidity. Anxiety disorders are more prevalent in women than in men. In contrast, antisocial personality disorder is more prevalent in men than in women. Affective disorders are equally prevalent in men and women. Thus, in addition to treatment of the addiction per se, each of these psychiatric disorders requires management. Alcoholism as a codependence with opiate addiction is less prevalent in women than it is in men. However, cocaine dependency is similarly prevalent in women and men entering methadone maintenance treatment. Our laboratory studies have shown that cocaine, like heroin, profoundly alters stress responsivity, maternal nesting behavior in rodents, and the molecular neurobiology of the endogenous opioid system along with the dopaminergic system, with possible differences in females compared with males (Branch et al. 1992; Kreek 1996c, 1996d, 1996e, 1997; Maggos et al. 1997; Maisonneuve and Kreek 1994; Maisonneuve et al. 1995; Quiñones-Jenab et al. 1997; Spangler et al. 1993a, 1993b, 1996; Tsukada et al. 1996; Unterwald et al. 1992, 1993, 1994a, 1994b, 1995, 1996; Zhou et al. 1996a, 1996b).

Gender Differences in Infectious Disease Comorbidity

In terms of risk factors for HIV-1 infection, sharing of needles and other injection equipment is less common in women than it is in men. However, having sex with other intravenous drug users is more prevalent in women than in men, and selling sex for money or for drugs is much more common in women than in men.

Many other medical diseases complicate addiction treatment, primarily hepatitis B and C as well as HIV-1 infection and AIDS, which are present in 30%–90% of all heroin addicts entering treatment (Cooper et al. 1983; Kreek 1973a, 1973b, 1978; Kreek et al. 1972, 1990; Novick et al. 1985, 1986a, 1986b, 1986c, 1988, 1997). These diseases occur in both men and women. In studies of patients in long-term treatment, it has been found that continuing drug abuse drops precipitously in both male and female patients and that infections with various diseases also decline (Novick et al. 1993).

Benefits of Methadone Maintenance Treatment

Reduction of AIDS Infection Risk

In our early 1983–1984 study, we also found that among those persons who were fortunate enough to have entered an effective methadone maintenance program prior to the HIV-1 epidemic's arrival in New York City in 1978, and who continued in treatment, only 9% were HIV-1 infected—and this at a time when more than 50% of untreated street addicts were HIV-1 infected (Des Jarlais et al. 1984, 1989; Novick et al. 1986a, 1986b). In addition, we found that those at greater risk for HIV-1 infection were men and women who continued to use cocaine (primarily by the parenteral route), both in populations of heroin addicts who were not in and receiving methadone maintenance treatment and in populations of former addicts who were in treatment (Novick et al. 1989). The reduction of cocaine use in codependent former heroin addicts stabilized in methadone maintenance treatment also reduces the risk of HIV-1 infection.

Normalization of Disrupted Physiological Functions

Finally, normalization of the multiple physiological systems and functions that are disrupted by long-term self-administration of the short-acting opiate heroin is achieved during chronic stabilization on steady, moderate- to high-dose methadone maintenance treatment (Cooper et al. 1983; Kreek 1973a, 1973b, 1978, 1991, 1992, 1996a, 1996c, 1996d, 1996e; Kreek et al. 1972, 1976; Rettig and Yarmolinsky 1995). This includes normalization of the important stress-responsive hypothalamic-pituitary-adrenal axis, the survival-based hypothalamic-pituitary-gonadal axis (including, in women, return of normal menses, ovulation, and ability to conceive and deliver normal offspring), and the related neuro-immune system function, along with the normalization of behavior in most patients. Thus, women as well as men benefit profoundly from appropriate pharmacotherapy coupled with counseling and access to medical and psychiatric care (Kreek et al. 1973a, 1973b, 1978, 1991; Novick et al. 1993).

Summary

Both female and male drug abusers suffer from the specific diseases of addiction. Thirty percent to 60% of drug abusers and drug addicts of each of the major abuse classes (heroin and other illicit opiates; cocaine and other illicit stimulants; and alcohol) are women. Women develop special problems during their cycles of addiction as a result of a variety of social and biological factors. Of particular importance, many women have had to work as prostitutes to support their drug addictions. Because women with drug abuse or addiction are exposed—albeit sometimes by different routes—to the same diseases as are men, hepatitis B, hepatitis C, and also HIV-1 infection leading to AIDS are as common in women as they are in men. Neurobiological studies conducted in human patients, as well as ongoing, more extensive studies conducted in appropriate animal models, are beginning to show that although the mechanisms of action of major classes of drugs of abuse (including opiates, cocaine and other stimulants, and alcohol) are similar in males and females, the quantitative degree or magnitude of response to the drug may be different in men and women. Clearly, more laboratory as well as basic clinical research work needs to be done to further elucidate these differences, since they may have profound implications both for the vulnerability to develop an addiction and for the treatment of addiction.

Short-acting opiates, primarily heroin, as one major class of drugs of abuse, have been extensively studied with respect to their negative impact on normal human physiology. Some very important specific alterations occur in women that are related to the suppression of specific components of the hypothalamic-pituitary-gonadal axis by short-acting opioids. Pharmacotherapy with long-acting opioids such as methadone and LAAM has been shown to reverse this disruption of critical reproductive-related biological function. Menstrual cycles, which are usually abnormal in opiate-addicted women, sometimes even to the extent that secondary amenorrhea has developed, become normal during methadone maintenance treatment. Ovulation also returns to normal, allowing normal conception to occur. Many studies have shown that normal pregnancies may ensue in the methadone-maintained former heroin addict who is no longer using any other drug of abuse, and that healthy offspring result.

In addition to these female-specific effects, both males and females experience disruption of another critical survival mechanism—stress responsivity—during cycles of heroin addiction. Again, it has been shown that stress responsivity returns to normal during long-term steady-dose treatment with the long-acting opioid methadone. Although special clinical treatment needs pertain to women, especially those who are mothers and/or heads of households, studies to date have shown that with appropriate adjunctive care, pharmacotherapy for opiate addiction is equally effective in male and female former heroin addicts. Thus, both gender similarities and gender differences exist with regard to the effects of both opiates and cocaine. These similarities and differences have implications not only for treatment but also possibly for the fundamental neurobiology and initial vulnerability underlying the development of addiction.

References

Branch AD, Unterwald EM, Lee SE, et al: Quantitation of preproenkephalin mRNA levels in brain regions from male Fischer rats following chronic cocaine treatment using a recently developed solution hybridization assay. Brain Res Mol Brain Res 14:231–238, 1992

Cooper JR, Altman F, Brown BS, et al. (eds): Research in the Treatment of Narcotic Addiction: State of the Art (DHHS Publ No ADM-83-1281). NIDA Monograph. Washington, DC, U.S. Government Printing Office, 1983

Des Jarlais DC, Marmor M, Cohen H, et al: Antibodies to a retrovirus etiologically associated with acquired immunodeficiency syndrome (AIDS) in populations with increased incidences of the syndrome. MMWR Morb Mortal Wkly Rep 33:377–379, 1984

Des Jarlais DC, Friedman SR, Novick DM, et al: HIV-1 infection among intravenous drug users in Manhattan, New York City, 1977 to 1987. JAMA 261:1008–1012, 1989

Dole VP, Nyswander ME, Kreek MJ: Narcotic blockade. Arch Intern Med 118:304–309, 1966

Finnegan LP, Chappel JN, Kreek MJ, et al: Narcotic addiction in pregnancy, in Drug Use in Pregnancy. Edited by Niebyl JR. Philadelphia, PA, Lea & Febiger, 1982, pp 163–184

Hachey DL, Kreek MJ, Mattson DH: Quantitative analysis of methadone in biological fluids using deuterium-labeled methadone and GLC-chemical-ionization mass spectrometry. J Pharm Sci 66:1579–1582, 1977

Hachey DL, Nakamura K, Kreek MJ, et al: Analytical techniques for using multiple, simultaneous stable isotopic tracers, in Stable Isotopes. Edited by Schmidt HL, Forstel H, Heinzinger K. Amsterdam, Elsevier Scientific, 1982, pp 235–239

Inturrisi CE, Verebey K: A gas-liquid chromatographic method for the quantitative determination of methadone in human plasma and urine. Journal of Chromatography 65:361–369, 1972a

Inturrisi CE, Verebey K: The levels of methadone in the plasma in methadone maintenance. Clin Pharmacol Ther 13:633–637, 1972b

Inturrisi CE, Max MB, Foley KM, et al: The pharmacokinetics of heroin in patients with chronic pain. N Engl J Med 310:1213–1217, 1984

Kaiko RF, Inturrisi CE: A gas-liquid chromatographic method for the quantitative determination of acetylmethadol and its metabolites in human urine. Journal of Chromatography 82:315–321, 1973

Kreek MJ: Medical safety and side effects of methadone in tolerant individuals. JAMA 223:665–668, 1973a

Kreek MJ: Plasma and urine levels of methadone. New York State Journal of Medicine 73:2773–2777, 1973b

Kreek MJ: Medical complications in methadone patients. Ann N Y Acad Sci 311:110–134, 1978

Kreek MJ: Methadone disposition during the perinatal period in humans. Pharmacol Biochem Behav 11 (suppl):1–7, 1979

Kreek MJ: Using methadone effectively: achieving goals by application of laboratory, clinical, and evaluation research and by development of innovative programs, in Improving Drug Abuse Treatment (NIDA Research Monograph Series 106). Edited by Pickens R, Leukefeld C, Schuster CR. Washington, DC, U.S. Government Printing Office, 1991, pp 245–266

Kreek MJ: Rationale for maintenance pharmacotherapy of opiate dependence, in Addictive States. Edited by O'Brien CP, Jaffe JH. New York, Raven, 1992, pp 205–230

Kreek MJ: Long-term pharmacotherapy for opiate (primarily heroin) addiction: opiate agonists, in Pharmacological Aspects of Drug Dependence: Toward an Integrated Neurobehavioral Approach. Edited by Schuster CR, Kuhar MJ. Berlin, Springer-Verlag, 1996a, pp 487–541

Kreek MJ: Long-term pharmacotherapy for opiate (primarily heroin) addiction: opiate antagonists and partial agonists, in Pharmacological Aspects of Drug Dependence: Toward an Integrated Neurobehavioral Approach. Edited by Schuster CR, Kuhar MJ. Berlin, Springer-Verlag, 1996b, pp 563–592

Kreek MJ: Opioid receptors: some perspectives from early studies of their role in normal physiology, stress responsivity, and in specific addictive diseases. Neurochem Res 21 (suppl 11):1469–1488, 1996c

Kreek MJ: Opiates, opioids and addiction. Mol Psychiatry 1:232–254, 1996d

Kreek MJ: Cocaine, dopamine and the endogenous opioid system. J Addict Dis 15 (suppl 4):73–96, 1996e

Kreek MJ: Opiate and cocaine addictions: challenge for pharmacotherapies. Pharmacol Biochem Behav 57:551–569, 1997

Kreek MJ, Dodes L, Kane S, et al: Long-term methadone maintenance therapy: effects on liver function. Ann Intern Med 77:598–602, 1972

Kreek MJ, Gutjahr CL, Garfield JW, et al: Drug interactions with methadone. Ann N Y Acad Sci 281:350–370, 1976

Kreek MJ, Hachey DL, Klein PD: Stereoselective disposition of methadone in man. Life Sci 24:925–932, 1979

Kreek MJ, Des Jarlais DC, Trepo CL, et al: Contrasting prevalence of delta hepatitis markers in parenteral drug abusers with and without AIDS. J Infect Dis 162:538–541, 1990

Maggos CE, Spangler R, Zhou Y, et al: Quantitation of dopamine transporter mRNA in the rat brain: mapping, effects of "binge" cocaine administration and withdrawal. Synapse 26:55–61, 1997

Maisonneuve IM, Kreek MJ: Acute tolerance to the dopamine response induced by a "binge" pattern of cocaine administration in male rats: an in vivo microdialysis study. J Pharmacol Exp Ther 268:916–921, 1994

Maisonneuve IM, Ho A, Kreek MJ: Chronic administration of a cocaine "binge" alters basal extracellular levels in male rats: an in vivo microdialysis study. J Pharmacol Exp Ther 272:652–657, 1995

Mason BJ, Ritvo EC, Morgan RO, et al: A double-blind, placebo-controlled pilot study to evaluate the efficacy and safety of oral nalmefene HCl for alcohol dependence. Alcohol Clin Exp Res 18:1162–1167, 1994

Mason BJ, Kocsis JH, Melia D, et al: Psychiatric comorbidity in methadone maintained patients. J Addict Dis 17:75–89, 1998

Nakamura K, Hachey DL, Kreek MJ, et al: Quantitation of methadone enantiomers in humans using stable isotope-labeled 2H3, 2H5, 2H8 methadone. J Pharm Sci 71:39–43, 1982

National Institute on Drug Abuse: NIDA Capsule: Women and Drug Abuse: A New Era for Research (C-94-02; NCADI #CAP45). Bethesda, MD, National Institute on Drug Abuse, June 1994

Novick DM, Farci P, Karayiannis P, et al: Hepatitis D virus antibody in HBsAg-positive and HBsAg-negative substance abusers with chronic liver disease. J Med Virol 15:351–356, 1985

Novick D, Kreek MJ, Des Jarlais D, et al: Antibody to LAV, the putative agent of AIDS, in parenteral drug abusers and methadone-maintained patients: Abstract of clinical research findings: therapeutic, historical, and ethical aspects, in Problems of Drug Dependence, 1985; Proceedings of the 47th Annual Scientific Meeting, the Committee on Problems of Drug Dependence (NIDA Research Monograph Series 67; DHHS Publ No ADM-86-1448). Edited by Harris LS. Washington, DC, U.S. Government Printing Office, 1986a, pp 318–320

Novick DM, Khan I, Kreek MJ: Acquired immunodeficiency syndrome and infection with hepatitis viruses in individuals abusing drugs by injection. United Nations Bulletin on Narcotics 38:15–25, 1986b

Novick DM, Stenger RJ, Gelb AM, et al: Chronic liver disease in abusers of alcohol and parenteral drugs: a report of 204 consecutive biopsy-proven cases. Alcohol Clin Exp Res 10:500–505, 1986c

Novick DM, Farci P, Croxson ST, et al: Hepatitis D virus and human immunodeficiency virus antibodies in parenteral drug abusers who are hepatitis B surface antigen positive. J Infect Dis 158:795–803, 1988

Novick DM, Trigg HL, Des Jarlais DC, et al: Cocaine injection and ethnicity in parenteral drug users during the early years of the human immunodeficiency virus (HIV) epidemic in New York City. J Med Virol 29:181–185, 1989

Novick DM, Richman BL, Friedman JM, et al: The medical status of methadone maintained patients in treatment for 11–18 years. Drug Alcohol Depend 33:235–245, 1993

Novick D, Reagan K, Croxson TS, et al: Hepatitis C virus serology in parenteral drug users with chronic liver disease. Addiction 92:167–171, 1997

O'Malley SS, Jaffe AJ, Change G, et al: Naltrexone and coping skills therapy for alcohol dependence. Arch Gen Psychiatry 49:881–887, 1992

Pond SM, Kreek MJ, Tong TG, et al: Altered methadone pharmacokinetics in methadone-maintained pregnant women. J Pharmacol Exp Ther 233:1–6, 1985

Quiñones-Jenab V, Batel P, Schlussman SD, et al: Cocaine impairs maternal nest-building in pregnant rats. Pharmacol Biochem Behav 58:1009–1013, 1997

Quiñones-Jenab V, Ho A, Schlussman SD, et al: Estrous cycle differences in cocaine-induced stereotypic and locomotor behaviors in Fischer rats. Behav Brain Res 101:15–20, 1999

Rettig RA, Yarmolinsky A (eds): Federal regulation of methadone treatment. Washington, DC, National Academy of Sciences, National Academy Press, 1995

Substance Abuse and Mental Health Services Administration, Office of Applied Studies: Summary of Findings From the 1998 National Household Survey on Drug Abuse. National Household Survey on Drug Abuse Series: H-10. Rockville, MD, Department of Health and Human Services, SAMHSA, August 1999

Spangler R, Unterwald EM, Branch A, et al: Chronic cocaine administration increases prodynorphin mRNA levels in the caudate putamen of rats, in Problems of Drug Dependence, 1992: Proceedings of the 54th Annual Scientific Meeting, the College on Problems of Drug Dependence. NIDA Research Monograph Series 132; DHHS Publ No ADM-93-3505). Edited by Harris LS. Washington, DC, U.S. Government Printing Office, 1993a, p 142

Spangler R, Unterwald EM, Kreek MJ: "Binge" cocaine administration induces a sustained increase of prodynorphin mRNA in rat caudate-putamen. Brain Res Mol Brain Res 19:323–327, 1993b

Spangler R, Ho A, Zhou Y, et al: Regulation of kappa opioid receptor mRNA in the rat brain by "binge" pattern cocaine administration and correlation with preprodynorphin mRNA. Brain Res Mol Brain Res 38:71–76, 1996

Spangler R, Zhou Y, Maggos CE, et al: Prodynorphin, proenkephalin and kappa opioid receptor mRNA responses to acute "binge" cocaine. Brain Res Mol Brain Res 44:139–142, 1997

Tsukada H, Kreuter J, Maggos CE, et al: Effects of "binge" pattern cocaine administration on dopamine D_1 and D_2 receptors in the rat brain: an in vivo study using positron emission tomography. J Neurosci 16 (suppl 23):7670–7677, 1996

Unterwald EM, Horne-King J, Kreek MJ: Chronic cocaine alters brain mu opioid receptors. Brain Res 584:314–318, 1992

Unterwald EM, Cox BM, Kreek MJ, et al: Chronic repeated cocaine administration alters basal and opioid-regulated adenylyl cyclase activity. Synapse 15:33–38, 1993

Unterwald EM, Ho A, Rubenfeld JM, et al: Time course of the development of behavioral sensitization and dopamine receptor upregulation during "binge" cocaine administration. J Pharmacol Exp Ther 270 (suppl 3):1387–1397, 1994a

Unterwald EM, Rubenfeld JM, Kreek MJ: Repeated cocaine administration upregulates kappa and mu, but not delta, opioid receptors. Neuroreport 5:1613–1616, 1994b

Unterwald EM, Rubenfeld JM, Imai Y, et al: Chronic opioid antagonist administration upregulates mu opioid receptor binding without altering mu opioid receptor mRNA levels. Brain Res Mol Brain Res 33:351–355, 1995

Unterwald EM, Tsukada H, Kakiuchi T, et al: Use of positron emission tomography to measure the effects of nalmefene on D_1 and D_2 dopamine receptors in rat brain. Brain Res 775:183–188, 1997

Volpicelli JR, Alterman AI, Hayashida M, et al: Naltrexone in the treatment of alcohol dependence. Arch Gen Psychiatry 44:876–880, 1992

Volpicelli JR, Watson NT, King AC, et al: Effect of naltrexone on alcohol "high" in alcoholics. Am J Psychiatry 152:613–615, 1995

Yuferov VP, Zhou Y, Spangler R, et al: Acute "binge" cocaine increases mu opioid receptor mRNA levels in areas of the rat mesolimbic dopamine system. Brain Res Bull 48:109–112, 1999

Zhou Y, Spangler R, LaForge KS, et al: Corticotropin-releasing factor and CRF-R1 mRNAs in rat brain and pituitary during "binge" pattern cocaine administration and chronic withdrawal. J Pharmacol Exp Ther 279:351–358, 1996a

Zhou Y, Spangler R, LaForge KS, et al: Modulation of CRF-R1 mRNA in rat anterior pituitary by dexamethasone: correlation with POMC mRNA. Peptides 17:435–441, 1996b

Index

Page numbers printed in **boldface** *type refer to tables or figures.*